A NEW APPROA
DISTRICT NURₛᵢₙ𝗀

A NEW APPROACH TO DISTRICT NURSING

Edited by

Monica E. Baly
BA (Hons), SRN, SCM, HVCert

Lecturer and Examiner for the Diploma in Nursing (London University); formerly Area Officer, Royal College of Nursing

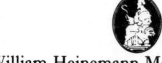

William Heinemann Medical Books Ltd
London

First published 1981

© Monica Baly

ISBN 0 433 01162 9

Printed in Great Britain
by Mackays of Chatham Ltd

Contents

Section IV: Policies for care

Section V: The professional district nurse

Appendices

Contributors

June Clark BA (Hons), MPhil, SRN, HVCert.

Research Fellow, Department of Nursing and Community Health Studies, Polytechnic of the South Bank, London.

Barbara Robottom BA, SRN, RSCN, QN, RNT, CHNTCert.

Principal Professional Officer to the Panel of Assessors for District Nurse Training; formerly Lecturer in Nursing, Department of Nursing, University of Manchester.

Mary Chapple SRN, NDN, HVCert.

Formerly Nurse Adviser to the Society of Primary Health Care Nursing, Royal College of Nursing.

Monica Baly BA (Hons), SRN, SCM, HVCert.

Lecturer and Examiner for the Diploma in Nursing (London University); formerly Area Officer, Royal College of Nursing.

A New Approach to District Nursing is essentially the work of a team; each contributor has learnt from and borrowed from the others. At times material has changed its section regardless of authorship. However, responsibility is primarily as follows:

Chapters 1, 2, 3, 4, 5 and Appendices 1–3	June Clark
Chapters 6, 7, 8, 9, 10 and 11	Barbara Robottom
Chapters 12, 14, 15 and 16	Mary Chapple
Chapters 13, 17, 18, 19, 20, 21 and 22 and Appendices 4–6	Monica Baly

Acknowledgements

As editor of *A New Approach to District Nursing* I would like to acknowlege the many people who gave help and encouragement during the planning and writing of this book. Particular thanks are due to Mr Anthony Carr who chaired the working party responsible for the curriculum the needs of which this book sets out to meet, and whose initial advice and encouragement were invaluable. Other members of the Panel of Assessors, including Miss Margaret Lindars, gave help in the choice of topics and contributors, as did Miss Peggy Nuttall of *Nursing Times*. Further helpful advice came from Miss Clare Brooks, then Senior Tutor at the Institute of Advanced Nursing Education at the Royal College of Nursing, and from Mrs Mary Chapple, at that time Nurse Adviser to the Society for Primary Health Care at the Royal College of Nursing, whom I was pleased to welcome later as a contributor to the book. I was sorry that Miss Elizabeth Raymond, lecturer in community nursing at the Polytechnic of the South Bank, had to withdraw as a contributor, but would like to acknowledge her help in the planning stages.

The Department of Nursing at Manchester University has cooperated to the full in this project, and Barbara Robottom's contribution forms the core of the book, which we have sometimes called the meat in the sandwich around which we have wrapped our bread. Miss Robottom herself would particularly like to thank Mrs Dorothy Jones at the Department of Health and Social Security for her encouragement and interest.

I would personally like to thank the many members of the Society for Primary Health Care at the Royal College of Nursing who had previously sent me case studies to illustrate their professional and ethical dilemmas. These, in spite of organisational changes, have a way of remaining the same, as do the principles that must guide us in dealing with such problems.

M.E.B.

Foreword

The importance of primary health care is increasingly recognised both in developing countries and in highly complex industrial societies. Within the primary health care team in our National Health Service the district nurse makes a contribution of extreme importance. She complements primary medical care with nursing care and it is to her that many individuals and families owe their ability to remain in their own homes rather than receive care in acute hospitals and institutions. For the young and the elderly this facility is particularly important. The range of the work of the district nurse has developed considerably in recent years and the specialised skills and knowledge required for the role have been identified and synthesised in the curriculum drawn up by the Panel of Assessors for District Nurse Training. New and mandatory training schemes will open a new era of professional preparation in district nursing.

The education of professionals draws on many resources. In particular, in a discipline like nursing, the quality and supervision of clinical practice is fundamental, but unless clinical practice is informed by an adequate literature it can devolve into a series of mindless rituals.

This book is a compendium of much of the knowledge needed for practice by District Nurses. It sets district nursing in the context of social policies for care, surveys various approaches and examines the needs of special groups for whom the district nurse is responsible. It stresses the importance of the individual within the group, and the authors are innovative in their use of the histories of seven patients to illustrate the principles outlined in the rest of the book, which serves to give the bones of knowledge flesh and blood.

Many nurses will already be used to the high standards set by Monica Baly in her authorship of *Nursing and Social Change*. She has now gathered together an authorative team to present what should become the standard text for district nurse students, and of use to many others. It should take its place amongst the classics of nursing literature.

McFarlane of Llandaff
August 1981

Preface

The aim of *A New Approach to District Nursing* is to cover the main requirements of the new Curriculum in District Nursing, at the same time being mindful of Miss Nightingale's dictum that 'it is impossible to learn manual skills from a book'. Practical skills and techniques must be learned in a practical situation.

Since problem solving and the nursing process form the core of the curriculum the authors have used this approach to demonstrate the skills, attitudes and knowledge required in meeting the health care needs of patients. By using seven representative patients and their families as examples throughout the book it is hoped that students will relate the nursing process to more than the mere performance of nursing tasks in the home. While it is paramount that the actual nursing care of Mr Adams is planned, implemented and evaluated according to the principles outlined in Section II, it is equally important that the district nurse understands Mr Adams in his sociological setting, and indeed, why there are so many patients like Mr Adams today. At the same time, she must understand his and his family's psychological and social needs and how the complex services contribute to meeting those needs. Mr Adams' housing problem, his entitlement to supplementary benefit and the needs of Mrs Adams are all part of his total care. The authors, all nurses, have become attached to their seven patients, and we hope they will serve to show that district nursing is about people and that the nursing process is not an idle shibboleth.

However, in using the concept of the nursing process the authors were aware of dangers. Like earlier omnibus phrases attempting to describe good nursing, it arouses certain reactions. Some nurses find it pretentious, esoteric and dressed up in unnecessary jargon that has little relation to their daily round and common task in nursing patients. Others declare that this is something that they have always done; therefore, they ask, why elevate it to a theory? Neither group is right. Because a thing is simple it does not mean that it is easy to do. The Sermon on the Mount is simple, but few of

us find it easy to put into practice. The nursing process is total nursing care at its best, but years of task orientation, beating the clock and thinking in terms of practicality rather than in principles have blunted our perceptions about what is 'total nursing' and even what is 'good nursing'.

Because it was important to inculcate new attitudes and encourage a different conceptual approach there has been a tendency to clothe the nursing process in a new language often borrowed from the behavioural sciences; this, it was thought, would emphasise the new approach. While acknowledging that language is dynamic and new concepts justify new words, the result can be counterproductive and the end result can be mystifying rather than enlightening. The authors have tried to sail between the Scylla of over-simplicity and the 'we have always done it' school, and the whirlpool of Charybdis with its arcane language and neologisms that may be misunderstood.

While this book aims to cover the outline of the curriculum it is hoped that students will enlarge their understanding and knowledge by using the suggestions for further reading at the end of each chapter, by regular reading of the nursing journals, and, because they and their patients are citizens, by keeping a vigilant watch on the daily press for matters relating to the health and social services.

M.E.B.
1981

Section I

Background to Care

'Unless the nurse can appreciate the psychological, emotional, spiritual and social needs of her patients and their families, in addition to the physical needs, her assessment of the nursing aspects could be suspect'.

> Panel of Assessors: Report on
> the Education and Training of
> District Nurses.

District nursing is concerned with people in their normal social setting, in their own homes, with their families. The social circumstances are as varied as the individuals themselves, but these circumstances have considerable significance for their health and nursing needs, the way in which they are managed, and the way in which the nurse can respond. The five chapters of Section 1 describe the context in which district nursing is practiced—the physical and social environments in which both nurse and patient live and the organisational setting which provides the framework for the delivery of care.

Chapter 1

Patients are People

Mr Adams

Mr Adams, who is 85 years old, had a cerebrovascular accident two years ago. He now has a right-sided hemiplegia, is incontinent of urine and faeces, his speech is slurred, and he is very confused. He is cared for by his elderly wife, whose mobility is becoming increasingly limited by arthritis.

The couple's only son was killed in France in 1944; a rather faded photo of a handsome young soldier standing between his smiling parents still has pride of place on the mantlepiece. Mr Adams was the youngest of four brothers, all of whom are now dead, and apart from a nephew and niece with whom he lost contact many years ago, he has no other relatives. Mrs Adams has a younger sister, but she lives more than a hundred miles away and so they rarely see each other.

They live in a terraced cottage in a small village. The house has not been modernised, so the only heating is by open fires, supplemented when necessary with a paraffin heater. There is no bathroom, and only an outside toilet.

Mr Adams is cared for in a living room, which, in addition to the large double bed contains a comfortable clutter of rather old-fashioned furniture. Mrs Adams rarely goes further afield than the village post office where she does most of her shopping, especially since the bus service to the nearest town was stopped some months ago.

Mrs Baker

Mrs Baker, who is 48, lives with her three children (girls of 17 and 12, and a boy of 14), her marriage having broken up about six years ago. Her husband has since remarried, and never visits now. The eldest girl, Sarah, is staying at home from work to care for her mother who has carcinoma of the liver and is now in the terminal stages of her illness.

They live in a modern semidetached house on a suburban housing estate. The neighbours are kind, and willing to help, but most of them are at work all day.

Mrs Baker obviously used to take a pride in her house but it is now showing signs of neglect. Sarah does her best, but without much help from her younger brother and sister; Paul spends very little time at home and Angela seems continually immersed in her school work.

Mrs Baker is aware of her prognosis, but she has not shared the knowledge with her children, although she suspects that Sarah guesses the truth. Each morning Mrs Baker dresses herself carefully and comes downstairs. She spends most of the day 'resting' on the settee in the living room. At present her pain is well-controlled and this has helped her to avoid showing the seriousness of her condition to the two younger children and to visitors.

Mrs Cray

Mrs Cray is a 68-year-old widow who lives alone in a flat on the fourth floor of a high-rise block of flats in a big city. She is obese and has varicose ulcers of both legs. She also has mild diabetes which is controlled by diet and drugs. She is not very mobile and is inclined to sit by an electric fire most of the day. She has not been out of the flat for a long time—saying that if the lift broke down (which happens frequently) she could not climb the stairs to get back home.

She has a home help who brings the shopping when she comes on Wednesday mornings to do the housework. A lady came once and offered her meals on wheels, but she refused. Mrs Cray's married daughter lives in one of the new neighbourhoods which have sprung up around the outskirts of the city. She works full-time now that both her children are at secondary school, but she manages to get over to see her mother about once a fortnight.

Mrs Cray's constant companion is a large white cat called Snowie, whom she has had for seven years ever since he was a kitten. Snowie is just as fat as his owner and, like her, he spends most of the day curled up in front of the fire; his sleek white coat is Mrs Cray's pride and joy.

John Davis

John Davis, who is 22 years old, became tetraplegic following an accident on his motorbike two years ago. He is the youngest child of the family; his older sisters are married and living away from home.

Before his accident his main interests were motorbikes and discos and he was engaged to be married but his fiancée now only visits occasionally.

John lives at home with his parents. To enable him to be transferred home from the regional spinal injuries unit where he spent the months following his accident, the family were rehoused into a bungalow which has been converted to accommodate the various equipment he requires. He has a POSSUM apparatus, a pneumatic bed, lifting hoist and many other aids for his care.

He is incontinent of urine and has a condom drainage fitted. Two nurses visit daily in the mornings, his parents managing his care for the rest of the day. John's father works for an insurance company; they have been very understanding about his rather poor work performance since John came home from hospital, but this is, of course, reflected in his commission. John's mother has devoted all her time to his care since giving up her part-time job when John came home.

Mr Evans

Mr Evans has just been discharged home from the local district general hospital following the repair of an inguinal hernia; there is some infection of the wound, so the district nurse has been asked to visit to dress it.

Mr Evans is 38 years old and works as a brick-layer. He was very relieved to get his operation done relatively quickly because he had to have a lot of time off work, and he is anxious to get back to work as soon as possible, before the winter weather starts. Mrs Evans works part-time in a greengrocer's shop now that the youngest of their two children has just started school. The primary school which the children attend and the shop where she works are part of the 'precinct' which is the centre of the big council estate where the Evans family live.

Mr Fisher

Mr Fisher, who is now in his mid-forties, was first diagnosed as having multiple sclerosis about ten years ago. At first he was able to continue his work as an accountant with a finance house in the City by doing most of the work at home instead of commuting daily as he had done before, but he was forced to give up about three years ago; he continues to work from home, however, as an accountant and tax adviser. Mrs Fisher teaches history in the local high school for girls

and has recently been appointed deputy headmistress. The couple
have no children.

The Fishers live in a detached house in a small private cul-de-sac
quite near the station. They chose the house, and indeed the town,
because of its easy access to London, although Mr Fisher came
originally from the North of England and Mrs Fisher from the West
Country.

Alison Green

Alison Green, who is seven years old, has severe cystic fibrosis. She
is the middle of three children; her older sister and baby brother are
not affected by the disease.

The Greens live in a Victorian terraced house in the centre of a
Northern city. Some parts of the city not very far away have been
redeveloped but the Greens' street is not scheduled for development in the immediate future. The waiting list for council housing
is long because people in the redevelopment areas have priority.
Mrs Green has lived in this area all her life; she was born in the next
street where her mother still lives, and her sister, who also has three
children, lives two streets away. Mr Green works for the council, in
the Parks Department. Alison is in and out of the Children's
Hospital most winters, but she has been much better since she
started going to a new special school which opened last year in the
part of the city which is being redeveloped.

District nurses are concerned with patients who have widely
different nursing needs and who are supported by families, or other
carers, who have markedly different abilities and capabilities. Moreover, patients come from the whole social spectrum and live in conditions ranging from the slum to the affluent. All these variations
must be noted by the nurse when she makes her assessment and be
considered when the plan of care is being made. For these reasons
we refer to the histories of these seven patients in all parts of the
book in order to illustrate the complexity of the factors that the
nurse must take into account when carrying out her responsibilities.

Chapter 2

The World We Live In

Compare the seven patients in Chapter 1 with the following account by a district nurse of her 'typical working day', written in 1893.[1]

For instance, a few days ago, starting at 8 a.m., I go first to see the patient who is more dangerously sick than any of the others—a little girl with bronchial pneumonia and whooping-cough. I find her mother has kept the room warm and well-aired, and carefully carried out the directions given about her medicine, stimulant, and nourishment. As her temperature is high, I give her a sponge bath, I then rub her chest with camphorated oil, and put on a cotton jacket I had made for her.

Then I go to see a little boy just recovering from pneumonia, who is weak and very stiff. I give him a good rubbing, and show his mother how to make a custard and beef-tea for him.

Then to see our oldest case, who says she is a hundred. She has had a grippe, has been quite sick, but is now improving. She is not in pain so I wash her face and hands, rub her back with alcohol, make an eggnog, and leave her calling down numberless blessings on me.

The next case is a two-year-old girl who has bronchitis. I have been at this house before, and am glad to find the sick child in bed with a hot flannel on her chest. I give her medicine and milk, which she refused to take from her grandmother.

I notice the four-weeks-old baby is being fed from a cup of tea, as there is no milk in the house. I promise to ask the doctor for a diet order, and show the grandmother how to prepare the baby's food properly.

I next see a woman who has erysipelas. I show her daughter how to make and apply the wash ordered by the doctor, and how to make some beef-tea.

Then I go to the dispensary to get some supplies, and to the loan closet to get some sheets and pillow-cases for a needy patient. I meet the physician at 12 o'clock and report the cases I have seen

this morning and the preceding afternoon; ask for the diet order, get the new orders, and go with the doctor to see a man who has an abscess which needs to be lanced. When this is done I wash the arm, make a poultice, and put on a sling.

After my luncheon I begin the afternoon round by going to see a woman who has a bruised and crushed ankle. This patient ought to be in hospital, but does not want to leave her young baby and five children. I dress the wound, put on a splint, and caution her to use it as little as possible.

Then to see two chronic cases—one a woman with an ulcer on her leg. I show her how to dress this. As she cannot leave her room and is fond of reading, I lend her some of the books given by one of the managers for this purpose. The other patient is a young girl with phthisis, whose mother is glad of any suggestions for Maggie's pleasure or comfort.

The next call is to a family where the seven children have a painful skin disease. I showed their mother how to wash them and to apply the ordered ointment. Any amount of old linen is needed here. One of the children had brought home a stray dog that was afterward found to be covered with sores. The children had all played with the dog, and this was the result—truly a case of mistaken kindness.

The next house I visit is one of the most dismal in the district. Sounds of quarrelling come from every room. The halls and stairs are dark and dirty. The patient's room is up three flights, and contains only a stove, table and old sofa-bed. He is a boy with acute rheumatism. They have not yet sent for the medicine which the doctor ordered the day before. I get the mother to go for this while I do up the patient's knees in cotton-wool and bandage. This boy's sister was also a patient; her neck and face were burned. As I dressed this for her she explained that in a friendly scuffle she fell across the stove. She neglected doing anything for it until afraid that her neck was growing crooked. I have twice since found this young woman so intoxicated that she could not be roused sufficiently to have her neck dressed; so I fear this is one of the few hopeless cases.

The next visit is to a German woman, who is in bed, with her face and head, particularly about her eyes, badly burned. She had been heating a can of milk with the stopper in, and it exploded in her face. One of her neighbours told her to put ink on it. She did so, and the result was startling, to say the least. It takes

much time and patience to get this properly dressed, as the woman is weak and nervous and understands very little English. She has five small children, and her husband is doing the best he can for her. I stay and show him how to make some gruel for the patient and to prepare the milk for the baby.

Then I go to the little girl I saw first in the morning, take her temperature and pulse, and make her comfortable for the night.

The last visit is to a woman who has gastritis. She cannot retain nourishment, and has much pain. A neighbour who had been a patient some time before came in, made the bed, put the room in order, and offered to make a poultice. She did this very nicely while I peptonized some milk which the patient was able to take.

Almost every day I find some former patient carrying out many of the simple directions that have been given during some former sickness. While this may be taken as a fair day's work, there are many cases requiring hours of care, as, for example, where a child is very sick and the mother is also sick, or in emergencies—as haemorrhages, confinements, or operations.

How, and for what reasons, does this nurse's account differ from district nursing today?

The first difference to be observed is in the age structure of the nurse's clientele: of the thirteen patients described, four are small children and only one patient is described as elderly. One family has six children, a second has seven children and a third five children. The clientele of today's district nurse would include relatively few children, and a much higher proportion of elderly people, and most of the families she meets will contain only one or two children. These differences illustrate the effect of demographic changes on the work of today's district nurse.

A second difference is in the kind of illnesses from which her patients are suffering. The terms 'the grippe' and 'phthisis' do not even appear in a modern dictionary although the conditions themselves still exist under the modern diagnostic labels of influenza and tuberculosis. In 1855 one in six of all deaths was caused by tuberculosis. Today, diseases such as tuberculosis, erysipelas, acute rheumatism, skin infections and even pneumonia would only rarely figure in a district nurse's caseload.

A third difference is shown by what the nurse does for her patients. Today's district nurse is unlikely to spend much time rubbing children's chests with camphorated oil or patients' backs

with alcohol, applying poultices, or making gruel and beef-tea. The fact that she does not illustrates the tremendous recent advances in scientific and medical knowledge, especially in the development of new drugs and in modern technology. Yet this difference is perhaps rather superficial—a difference in the technique rather than in the underlying task—because the basic activities described such as monitoring the patient's condition, attending to the patient's toilet needs, dressing wounds, teaching relatives how to care for the sick member of the family, teaching the principles of sound nutrition and healthy living, mobilising resources, these are aspects of the 'unique function' of the nurse[2] wherever and whenever nursing is practised.

Demographic changes

The size and structure of a population over a period of time is determined by the relationships between the number of births and the number of deaths. A population's size will increase rapidly if the birth rate is constant or increasing while the death rate is falling, as in the underdeveloped countries at present; and less rapidly if the death rate falls while the birth rate is constant or falling less than the death rate as in Britain and other developed countries during the past century.

The growth of the population of Britain can be described in four stages:

Stage 1 (up to about 1750), characterised by high birth rates and high death rates; the population increased very slowly and by 1750 had reached approximately 8 million.

Stage 2 (1750–1880), characterised by a high birth rate and a fall in the death rate from about 30–40 per thousand in the mid-eighteenth century to about 20 per thousand by 1850; the result was a rapid increase in population to 38 million by the end of the nineteenth century.

Stage 3 (1880–1950), characterised by falling birth rates and even more rapidly falling death rates, the population had reached 50 million by 1951.

Stage 4 (1951 to present day), characterised by a low birth rate and a low death rate; the population is still increasing but very slowly with slight decreases in some years; it had reached 55 million by 1971 and is expected to reach about 58 million by the end of the century.

The birth rate (the number of babies born per year per 1000 of the population) is determined not only by the number of babies which each woman has, which is in turn affected by a variety of factors, but also by the number of woman of childbearing age in the population. In Britain the birth rate has fallen significantly during the past century, mainly because of the reduction in family size. Two thirds of the women who married about the year 1860 gave birth to six or more children; women who married a century later rarely gave birth to more than four, and the average number of children per family was less than 2·5. Many factors have contributed to this change—among them the advent of reliable contraception and changes in the role and status of women—but the net result is that families are much smaller then they used to be.

The death rate has fallen even more dramatically: from 22·7 per 1000 in 1851 to 11·7 in 1978, mainly as a result of the different pattern of health and disease which is discussed below. The crude death rate figures, however, do not by themselves show the aspect of the change which is even more significant—the change in the age distribution of deaths. A century ago about 30 per cent of the population died before reaching adulthood, and women who survived until maturity faced a high risk of death in childbirth. Now more than 90 per cent of the population can expect to see their 50th birthday and about two thirds their 70th. The significant change is thus not the reduction in the death rate as such, but the increase in life expectancy, from 41 years in 1841, to 69 years for men and 75 years for women at present.

This complex interaction between birth rates, death rates, causes of death, and life expectancy determines the age structure of the population which can be shown in the form of a 'population pyramid'. Figure 2.1 shows how the shape of Britain's population pyramid changed between 1901 and 1978. The most obvious and significant change is the number and proportion of elderly people in the population. Since 1961 the total population has increased by about seven per cent but the over sixty-five population has increased by over 25 per cent and the trend is continuing. There are now, in 1980, more than eight million people aged 65 years or over in the United Kingdom, and they constitute nearly fifteen per cent of the total population.

Figure 2.1 also shows an even more significant change in the age structure *within* the elderly population—the increase in the number and the proportion of the over 75s and the over 85s.

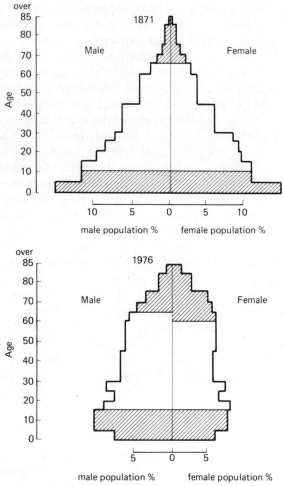

Fig. 2.1. Population profiles, 1871 and 1976 (shaded areas indicate non-workers.

The significance of these changes is not simply the weight of numbers. The elderly, and especially the very elderly, are also the greatest users of health services. More than half of all hospital beds are occupied by patients over the age of 65 years, and more than 80 per cent of district nurses' visits in 1975 were to patients aged over 65 years, 55 per cent being to patients over 75 years.

Other demographic factors increase the difficulties. Smaller families mean fewer children to care for elderly parents—the burden of care falling entirely on the one or two instead of being shared among perhaps six or eight. As life expectancy increases, the sons and daughters caring for their elderly parents are often themselves elderly. Moreover the effects of these demographic changes are exacerbated by social changes. For example, working wives have less time to devote to ageing parents than wives who stay at home; greater mobility means that children have often moved away from their parents' neighbourhood; smaller houses on modern estates do not provide room for accommodating elderly relatives. The 1971 census suggested that more than a quarter of the over 65s and more than a third of the over 75s live alone.

Changing patterns of health and disease

The dramatic decline in mortality is due to changing patterns in health and disease, and in particular to the decline in infectious disease. McKeown[3] has suggested that 86 per cent of the total reduction of the death rate from the beginning of the eighteenth century to the present day is attributable to the decline of the infectious diseases. In 1850 over one third of all deaths recorded were attributable to eight infectious diseases—tuberculosis (which alone accounted for one sixth of the total mortality), typhus, scarlet fever, cholera, smallpox, whooping-cough, measles, and diptheria. In 1978 tuberculosis accounted for $0 \cdot 1$ per cent of all deaths and other infectious diseases for a further $0 \cdot 2$ per cent. In that year one half of all deaths were attributed to circulatory disease (of these half were attributed to ischaemic heart disease and a quarter to cerebrovascular disease), and one fifth to cancer.

Why has this change occurred, and what is the effect of the change on the pattern of present day health care?

Contrary to popular belief the change was not due to the rapid advance in medical knowledge, nor even to the discovery of immunisation, nor to the advent of the National Health Service although all of these things have played some part. As McKeown has shown the decline in the death rate and the change in the pattern of mortality was due primarily to improvements in nutrition, hygiene and sanitation, and in general standards of living. An understanding of this change offers many clues to coping with today's health

problems, and for this reason three examples are considered in more detail:

tuberculosis
cholera
maternal mortality

Tuberculosis

Three hundred years ago John Bunyan described tuberculosis as 'this captain of the men of death', and as already mentioned, in 1850 this disease accounted for one sixth of all deaths. Figure 2.2 shows the decline in the mortality rate from tuberculosis between 1850

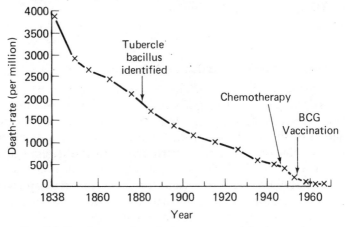

FIG. 2.2. Respiratory tuberculosis: mean annual death-rates (standardised to 1901 population): England and Wales. (From McKeown, T. (1979), *The Role of Medicine:* Blackwell Scientific.)

and the present day. Events which might have been thought to be significant in the decline are shown, but it is clear that these factors alone cannot explain the change although they may have contributed to it. One clue is given by the fact that even before 1900, tuberculosis was far more prevalent in the towns and cities than in rural districts. Another clue is the short-term increase in mortality during both world wars. Yet another is the fact that in Britain today tuberculosis is most common among recent immigrants from developing countries. McKeown has analysed the decline in tuberculosis in detail and has shown convincingly that the major factors in the 'success story' were the improvements in the conditions

which allowed tuberculosis to flourish, namely low resistance as a result of malnutrition and heavy exposure due to overcrowding.[3]

Cholera

It was the great cholera epidemics of the nineteenth century which, in the words of the historian Trevelyan, 'scared society into the tardy beginnings of sanitary self-defence'. Chadwick's great *Report on the Sanitary Conditions of the Labouring Population of Great Britain*, published in 1842, showed that insanitary conditions, defective drainage and inadequate water supply were invariably associated with infectious disease and high mortality, but the great breakthrough in the defeat of cholera is attributed to a London doctor, John Snow, whose detailed records of patients who contracted the disease revealed one factor common to them all: all had drunk water or eaten food prepared with water from the Broad Street pump. When, on his advice, the handle of the pump was removed the outbreak abated, and Snow rightly concluded that the disease was caused by an organism which contaminated the water, although the cholera vibrio was not actually identified until 1883, some thirty years later. Cholera is now confined largely to the tropics—but it is important to recognise that it occurs in certain countries not because they are 'tropical' but because their water supplies are contaminated.

The story of the conquest of cholera illustrates three principles which are as relevant today as they were a century ago in the prevention of disease: firstly, the value of epidemiology in identifying causes and pointing to possible solutions, secondly, the importance of environmental control and thirdly, the fact that preventive action can be effective even in the absence of complete knowledge.

Maternal mortality

At the beginning of this century and before, childbirth was recognised and feared as a life-threatening as well as a life-giving process; upwards of 2500 mothers died in childbirth each year. The novels of the nineteenth century, notably those of Dickens, are rich in accounts of death in childbirth. In 1978 there were only 68 maternal deaths, a reduction of 97 per cent.

The decline in the maternal mortality rate, shown in Table 2.1, shows quite a different pattern from that of tuberculosis and cholera. It can be seen that the decline began much later, during the 1930s.

TABLE 2.1

The decline in the maternal mortality rate 1900–1978

Year	Maternal deaths per thousand live births (United Kingdom)
1900–1902	4·71
1910–1912	3·95
1920–1922	4·37
1930–1932	4·54
1940–1942	3·29
1950–1952	0·88
1960–1962	0·36
1970–1972	0·17
1978	0·08

Source: CSO Annual Abstract of Statistics 1980. London: HMSO

A Departmental Committee to consider maternal mortality which was set up by the Ministry of Health in 1927, suggested that 48 per cent of maternal deaths were avoidable, and recommended investment in antenatal care and provision of more maternity homes and hospital beds. The work of the original committee continues in the Reports on Confidential Enquiries into Maternal Deaths, which were instituted in 1950.

Analysis of the causes of maternal mortality gives some clues to the reasons for the different patterns and provides some lessons which are different from those of the two previous examples. The

TABLE 2.2

Principal causes of maternal mortality 1950–1978

Cause	Number of deaths			
	1950	1960	1970	1978
Abortion	103	62	32	5
Puerperal sepsis	26	8	9	1
Thrombosis and embolism	62	27	10	11
Haemorrhage	82	44	12	4
Toxaemia	185	63	24	23
All other causes	162	106	59	24
ALL CAUSES	620	310	146	68

Source: OPCS. Birth statistics 1978. London: HMSO

principal causes since 1950 are shown in Table 2.2, and they highlight the importance of the contributions made by the control of infection. The prevention of infection was achieved through understanding of the principles of asepsis, and cure through chemotherapy and antibiotics; by the provision of health services, in particular the development of antenatal services during the 1930s and birth control and abortion services in the late 1960s; by developments in medical technology such as anaesthesia and blood transfusions; and by other social provisions such as protective employment legislation and financial benefits, as well as by the general improvement in living standards, especially nutrition. Moreover, it shows more clearly than in any other field (except perhaps for the example of cholera) the importance of a political commitment to take the action necessary to tackle a recognised problem.

Mortality today

The victims of infectious disease were young; today 72 per cent of all deaths occur after the age of 65 years. The change is reflected in the major causes of death: more than half of all deaths nowadays are due to circulatory disease—heart disease and stroke—and a further fifth to cancer. The leading causes of death at different ages are shown in Fig 2.3. Apart from old age, the most vulnerable period is the first week of life, when the main causes are prematurity and congenital malformation. During childhood and early adulthood accidents stand out as the leading cause. During the middle years the pattern is very different for men compared with women: for men the greatest killer by far is ischaemic heart disease, although cancer, especially lung cancer, is also important. For women the cancers are the major cause of death with breast cancer the most important type.

The present pattern of mortality offers new challenges. There is probably still some scope for advances in curative medicine, the investment in the search for a cure for cancer is massive and there is considerable scope for preventive action, e.g. accidents, coronary heart disease, but the greatest challenge is that 'the wheel has gone full circle; what can be prevented has been prevented, what can be cured is largely cured, what is left is care'.[4]

The Prevalence of morbidity

The measurement of ill-health is a far more complex task than the

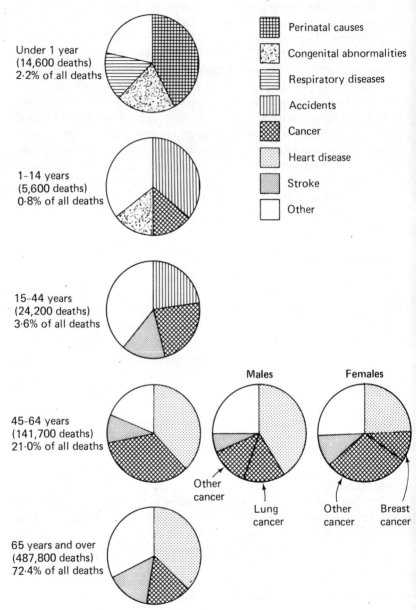

FIG. 2.3. Deaths in age groups indicating the main causes: United Kingdom, 1972. (From *Prevention and Health: Everbody's Business:* HMSO).

measurement of death. There is no clear line between health and illness as there is between life and death, and the definition of illness, which will be discussed in more detail in Chapter 3, is a subjective assessment. In particular, and because these difficulties are increased by changes in diagnostic labels as medical knowledge increases, for example the grippe and phthisis of 1893, it is difficult to trace changes over a long period of time. Several different kinds of yardstick for the measurement of ill-health are currently in use and techniques are still being refined and developed.

The number of people admitted to hospital rises each year, but this may be a truer reflection of demand and of people's expectations about health care than of the prevalence of sickness. More than half of all hospital beds are in psychiatric hospitals, and in general hospitals more than half of all beds are occupied by people over the age of 65 years so the stereotype of the hospital as a place of curative technology is not particularly accurate. Excluding psychiatric and maternity patients, diseases of the digestive and respiratory systems account for a quarter of all admissions, while in terms of the length of time spent in hospital, diseases of the heart and circulation including strokes take first place.

The number of new claims for sickness and invalidity benefits for the year 1978 was 11·2 million; that is, in any given month about one million workers are absent from work by reason of sickness. Sickness accounts for more than 10 times as many lost working days as strikes. The incidence and prevalence of ill-health among the non-working population is difficult to estimate, but in the General Household Survey 1977, 52 per cent of men and 57 per cent of women reported short term health problems, and 56 per cent of men and 70 per cent of women reported chronic health problems; 10 per cent of men and 13 per cent of women had consulted a GP in the two weeks prior to the interview. The discrepancy between the proportions indicates something of the subjectivity of the definition of 'being ill' and also the extent of unreported (and therefore untreated) illness.

Of particular interest to the district nurse, however, who receives her patients by referral from the general practitioner, is the distribution of sickness patterns in a general practice population. A national survey of GP consultation patterns showed that in 1970–71, about a quarter of the population saw their GP about a respiratory complaint, a further 11 per cent for a disease of the nervous system, and the same proportions for skin diseases and mental disorders.

When all the statistics are put together it can be seen that the spectrum of today's health problems contains three main elements:

1   The diseases and disabilities of old age
2   Diseases caused by individual behaviour
3   Hazards relating to our changing environment

Diseases and disabilities of old age

An increasing number of old people inevitably means more cases of disability and chronic degenerative disease. The common chronic degenerative diseases include arteriosclerosis, cerebrovascular disease, cardiovascular disease, multiple sclerosis, osteo-arthritis, rheumatoid arthritis, Parkinson's disease, and chronic chest disease. Defects of sight, hearing and disability increase with advancing years. Troubles rarely come singly: multiple pathology is one of the characteristics of disease in the elderly. Health problems, both physical and mental, are exacerbated by social factors such as social isolation resulting from problems such as bereavement, deafness and immobility, poor nutrition, unsuitable housing conditions and inadequate income. The complexity of the disease and disability in the elderly is well illustrated by our descriptions of Mr Adams and Mrs Cray and this subject is further discussed in Chapter 15.

Diseases caused by individual behaviour

The review of present day mortality and morbity showed that the most common causes of premature death were heart disease, cancer, especially lung cancer, and accidents, and the most common reasons for consulting a doctor were respiratory diseases, nervous disorders, and mental disorders. All these diseases are directly affected, and in some cases actually caused, by aspects of our behaviour—in particular our eating and drinking habits, smoking, sexual behaviour, and our use of leisure. As a nation we eat too much food and food of the wrong kind, drink too much alcohol, smoke too many cigarettes, are sexually promiscuous, and take too little physical exercise.

Diet

The malnutrition associated with poverty and the diseases which flourished as a result (e.g. tuberculosis, rickets) have been replaced by a malnutrition associated with affluence in which general overeating leads to obesity which increases the risk of diabetes and heart

disease and exacerbates other conditions such as respiratory disease and arthritis, and specific dietary habits lead to problems such as dental caries (sugar), coronary heart disease (saturated fats and sugar), bowel cancer and diverticular disease (inadequate roughage) and allergy (food additives). Men who are more than 25 per cent heavier than average for their age and height have a death rate twice as high as those within 5 per cent of the average.

Alcohol

Excessive drinking is the direct cause of disorders such as cirrhosis of the liver and alcoholism, and the indirect cause of a large proportion of road traffic and other accidents. Alcoholism causes serious social problems not only for the victim but also for his family. This problem is discussed in Chapter 13.

Smoking

Smoking is known to be associated with lung cancer, chronic bronchitis, coronary heart disease and increased perinatal mortality. Yet, in 1976, 46 per cent of adult men and 38 per cent of adult women smoked cigarettes. The most dramatic decline in smoking in recent years has, significantly, occurred among doctors, whose death rate has declined correspondingly. The increase in the number of women who smoke is now beginning to be reflected in a reduction of the gap between the sexes in mortality rates.

Sexual behaviour

One change in sexual behaviour—namely the widespread use of contraception—has led to health benefits in the reduction of maternal mortality. However, the increase in sexual activity outside marriage has also contributed to the dramatic increase of more than three-fold between 1959 and 1974 in venereal disease, which is now the most common of all the infectious diseases. The number of sexual partners and the age at which sexual activity was commenced have also been shown to be associated with cervical cancer.

Other behavioural health problems

Reduction in the length of the working week and the increased availability of domestic aids such as washing machines has increased the amount of leisure time available for most people, but not much leisure time is spent on health-inducing activities. The 1977 General Household Survey found that in the four weeks

before interview 97 per cent of the people interviewed had watched television and 63 per cent had been out to a pub or restaurant, but only 42 per cent had done some gardening and only 39 per cent had taken part in an active outdoor sport; moreover, the average person spent 16 hours a week in the summer watching television and 20 hours a week in the winter. More people than ever before work in sedentary jobs and travel by car instead of walking. The result is inadequate physical activity which exacerbates the problems of obesity but in addition is directly associated with an increased risk of coronary heart disease.

Other leisure pursuits carry their own specific hazards. The hazards of hang-gliding may be obvious, but less obvious are the hearing loss and migraines associated with discos, the paraplegia and head injuries associated with motorbikes, and the violence of football terraces.

These patterns of illness are well represented among our seven patients. The health problems of Mrs Adams and Mrs Cray are typical of those of the elderly; Mr Fisher, although comparatively young at present, is the victim of a chronic disease for which there is no known cure and no means of prevention; Mrs Baker will die prematurely from one form of the disease which is the commonest cause of premature death among women; and John Davis is a casualty of his life style.

The physical environment

The importance of environmental factors in the causation of disease has been clearly demonstrated by epidemiological studies in the tradition of pioneers such as Chadwick and Rowntree, but environmental factors are also important in the treatment and care of patients.

The importance of environmental factors is clearly exemplified by chronic bronchitis. The death rate from this disease differs widely in different parts of the country and increases with each step down the social class scale. Other factors which have been shown to be significant include climate, levels of air pollution, occupation and smoking habits. Measures such as smokeless zones, the protection of workers from dust, and a reduction in cigarette smoking, would considerably reduce the prevalence of the disease. For a patient suffering from chronic bronchitis the extent of his recovery and his chances of becoming ill again depend less on the effective-

ness of treatment by antibiotics and bronchodilators than on whether or not he gives up smoking, goes home to a damp house in an inner city area, or returns to work in the same dusty conditions as before.

The following environmental factors have a particularly significant influence upon health:

Nutrition
Environmental hygiene
Atmospheric pollution
Occupational environment
Housing conditions

Consider the effect of these environmental influences on the health problems of the seven families in Chapter 1.

Adequate *nutrition* is little mentioned; there is no evidence that any of the patients are malnourished in the sense of not having enough to eat. However, the effect of misguided eating habits on Mrs Cray's condition can be seen, as well as how much worse the situation might be without the home help to buy the food. Good nutrition is clearly important to Alison Green; her state of health at any time depends greatly on her ability to resist chest infections which in turn depends partly on her nutritional state, and yet a good nutritional state is more difficult to her to achieve than for other children because of the dietary limitations imposed by her cystic fibrosis. Because of the system of protective legislation established over the last century in recognition of the fact that contaminated food is a source of disease, all the families can reasonably assume that their milk will be free from tubercle and other organisms and that their meat will be free from parasites and will have been inspected at the port of entry if it is imported from abroad. One can expect that food will be unadulterated by harmful additives (except for those additives which are specified and controlled), and will be prepared and sold on premises whose standards of hygiene are required to meet a certain standard, and that the nutritional content of staple foods such as bread, margarine and flour meets certain minimum requirements.

Environmental services. These are not mentioned in any of the pen portraits. The reason is not that they are unimportant, but that facilities such as sewage and refuse disposal and a pure water supply are taken for granted in Britain today. One has to read the history of

the nineteenth century to appreciate the difference that these facilities have made to health; the story of the Green family, for example, would have been very different if they had lived in the same street a century ago.

Atmospheric pollution. This is not specifically mentioned, and like the first two factors is subject to legislative controls, but one can guess at the effects on Mrs Cray and Alison Green if this were not so, since both live in city areas where the air is inevitably more polluted than the rural area where Mr and Mrs Adams live, and Alison already has a serious respiratory problem while Mrs Cray could also be considered to be at risk.

Occupation. None of the patients is suffering from an illness which can be directly attributed to their occupation. Prescribed industrial diseases and industrial accidents account for over a tenth of working days lost through sickness. However, it is likely that Mr Evans' occupation has contributed to his health problem and the effect of employment on the management of patient care can be seen in the cases of Mr Evans and Mr Fisher.

Housing. Probably the most influential environmental factor from the district nurse's point of view is housing conditions, and the effects of housing, particularly on the way in which the district nurse can provide care, is seen in the stories of several of our families. The Adams' housing conditions—a small unmodernised cottage with no central heating, no bathroom, and only an outside toilet—lie at one extreme of the continuum. The bungalow which has been specially converted for John Davis lies at the other. Housing conditions affect a patient's susceptibility to certain illnesses and to accidents, and the course of his illness, as well as being an important factor to be considered in the management of illness.

The Green family are lucky in that at least they occupy the whole house, but in the area where they live many larger houses are likely to be occupied by several families. Several families may have to share a single lavatory, water may have to be carried by families living at the top of the house from a tap on the floor below, and cooking facilities may consist of a single gas ring on a small landing. It is not difficult to imagine the risks to health which life in such conditions involves. Overcrowding leads to the rapid spread of airborne infections such as tuberculosis. Damp conditions, caused

by defective roofs or gutters, or the lack of a damp course, lead to exacerbation of rheumatic and respiratory disorders. Poor sanitation and inadequate facilities for food preparation lead to gastroenteritis. There is no space for the children to play, and the inadequate cooking and heating arrangements predispose to accidents, especially burns and scalds. Poor lighting and steep stairs cause falls, especially to old people. Altogether the stress produced by trying to cope with life in these surroundings causes a great deal of mental ill-health.

The implications of housing conditions for the management of care are considerable. For example, a patient suffering from a chronic cardiac condition must avoid stairs. In a modern house it may be possible to turn a downstairs room into a bedroom but the slum dweller may not only have to climb stairs, but have to carry water up and down them as well. Similarly the management of a colostomy may be extremely difficult if the lavatory is at the bottom of the garden and there is no bathroom. Moreover, so far only the physical aspects of housing conditions have been considered. The social aspects, which include location, the type of ownership, the type of neighbourhood are also important.

New environmental hazards

In many respects, our environment today is healthier than it has ever been. We enjoy pure water, clean food, clean air, safe sanitation, drainage and refuse disposal services, and a relatively safe working environment. However, as one environmental hazard is conquered another emerges, and each innovation brings unintended disadvantages as well as its intended benefits. The use of the motor car produces an annual toll of 8000 deaths and almost 100 000 serious injuries; new chemicals are constantly being developed for use in industry and the home; chemical and radiational pollution of the atmosphere is increasingly causing concern. Knowledge is increasing about the effects, particularly on mental health, of less tangible environmental factors such as noise.

Environmental control and personal freedom

Discussion of environmental factors, particularly in relation to the prevention of illness, raises the dilemma of environmental control versus individual freedom. It is a fact that most of the improvements in today's environment compared with that of the last century, and the improvement in health which this has produced, are

due to environmental controls imposed by legislation. Some of today's environmental hazards could be controlled in the same way. Legislation could be used to enforce the wearing of seat belts in cars (it has been estimated that the universal use of seat belts could halve the number of deaths and serious injuries to front-seat occupants of cars), to add fluoride to all drinking water, which has been conclusively shown to reduce the prevalence of dental caries, and to reduce the availability of alcohol and cigarettes. Opponents of such measures argue that they are an unwarrantable intrusion on personal freedom, exactly as did the very many and powerful opponents of the environmental legislation of the last century. The debate is well summarised in the Report of the Royal Commission on the NHS (1979).[5] Meanwhile the dilemma confirms the overwhelming need for health education, which is an integral part of the role of the district nurse in the 1980s as it was in the 1890s.

The social environment

The social environment is as important to patterns of illness and to the management of care as is the physical environment, and the changes which have taken place during the last century have been just as dramatic and their effects no less profound. Demographic changes have already been discussed, but other significant social changes include changes in family structure and patterns of family life, changes in the role of women, in education, in work and in patterns of income and spending. All these factors are closely inter-related; for example, the reduction in family size is both a cause and a result in changes in the role of women and the pattern of women's work outside the home.

Perhaps the most striking changes are those in family structure and patterns of family life, particularly since the 1930s. The family is discussed in more detail in Chapter 4, but must be considered here also as an aspect of social change. Some of the differences are shown in Fig. 2.4. Compared with 1900, more people marry and they marry younger; there is a corresponding decrease in the number and proportion of single women; women have, on average, fewer children, and their childbearing period is completed earlier than previously, releasing them for paid work outside the home; divorce is five times more common than in 1951 and there is a corresponding increase in the number of one-parent families (11 per cent of all families with dependent children in 1976).

To social statisticians the terms 'families' and 'households' mean

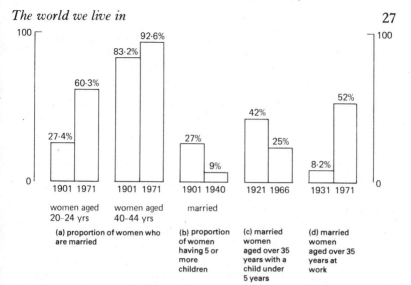

Fɪɢ. 2.4. Changes in family life, 1900–1980.

different things; households are groups of people who live and eat together, while families consist of a married couple with or without children, or a lone parent with children. A household may consist of a single family, or more than one family living together, or occupants who are unrelated. The change in the number and proportion of the different types of households is another indicator of change in family life. The increased number of households reflects a fall in household size, which is due not only to a reduction in family size but a reduction in the number of households containing two or more families and to an increase in the number of elderly people living alone.

Changes in the pattern of family life have been exacerbated by changes in housing patterns and town planning. In city areas the old back-to-back slums have been cleared and replaced by tower blocks of flats; in rural areas the lack of work opportunities for young people and problems of public transport have forced young people to move nearer to towns; the modern semi-detached on a suburban estate is too small to house elderly grandparents and unsuitable for elderly people living alone.

Some of the implications of these changes in the social environment can be seen in the stories of our seven patients but they are no doubt particularly problematic for Mr Adams, Mrs Baker, Mrs

Cray and Mrs Fisher. Who will care for Mr and Mrs Adams as they become older and more frail? Who will care for Mrs Baker's children when their mother is dead? How will Mrs Cray's daughter cope with the conflicting needs of her mother and her children? How will Mrs Fisher resolve the conflict between a promising career and an increasingly disabled husband? and how will Mr Fisher avoid adding the problems of social isolation to the problems of his physical disability? All these questions must be asked by the district nurse—and answered—in assessing each patient's needs and planning and implementing her programme of care.

The effect of technology

The kind of nursing action which was open to our district nurse in 1893 seem extremely limited when compared with the resources which would be available to her today. Such resources include not only increased medical knowledge, but powerful drugs, sophisticated diagnostic techniques, and equipment such as ripple beds and electric wheelchairs, pre-sterilized dressings, disposable syringes and needles. District nurses no longer depend on 'old linen' or dressings sterilized in a biscuit tin in the family's oven. While such modern devices make district nursing much easier in some ways, in others they make it more difficult; the modern district nurse needs greater knowledge and more varied skills than ever before if she is to get the best from the resources available.

One aspect of technological development which has revolutionised the lives of all of us is the development of communication media, especially the telephone and television. Television brings the remote and esoteric into the family living room, increasing people's knowledge and influencing their expectations about health care as about other things; its potential as a medium for health education has scarcely begun to be exploited. Computers and the microchip have already revolutionised the storage, manipulation, and retrieval of information in industry and commerce, and their implications for health care are tremendous.

Technological advance also brings problems in the pace of life and the rate of change which make considerable demands on human adaptability, and produces stresses which may lead to individual and social breakdown.

Social conditions and the role of the nurse

A constant problem for all those who work in the health and social

services is the dilemma produced by knowing that social conditions are affecting a patient's health or recovery from illness and being unable to change those conditions. It is easy to advise a patient suffering from bronchitis that he must change his job and move out of the damp inner-city basement where he is living. In practice, however, it may be quite impossible for him to follow this advice. It is important in planning an individual patient's care to make a realistic assessment of his social circumstances including the possibilities for change, and to plan his care accordingly. It is equally important to recognise the nurse's role as the patient's advocate in attempting to improve his situation. Caring for a patient must include measures to improve in whatever way is possible, the social conditions which are affecting his health, and also the support which may be necessary to help him maintain his health at the optimum level in whatever conditions he finds himself.

References

1. Somerville C. E. M. (1893). District Nursing. In: Hampton I.A. *et al.* (1949). *Nursing of the Sick 1893: papers and discussions from the International Congress of Charities Correction and Philanthropy, Chicago 1893.* New York: McGraw Hill.
2. Henderson V. (1960). *Basic Principles of Nursing Care.* Geneva: International Council of Nurses.
3. McKeown T. (1979). *The Role of Medicine.* Oxford: Blackwell.
4. Baly M. (1973). *Nursing and Social Change.* 1st ed. London: William Heinemann Medical Books.
5. *Report of the Royal Commission on the National Health Service* (1979). Cmnd. 7615. London: HMSO.

Further Reading

Baly M. (1980). *Nursing and Social Change.* 2nd ed. London: William Heinemann Medical Books.
Central Statistical Office (1980). *Facts in Focus.* 5th ed. Harmondsworth: Penguin Books.
Central Statistical Office (1980). *Social Trends.* London: HMSO.
Department of Health and Social Security (1976). *Prevention and Health: Everybody's Business.* London: HMSO.
Halsey A. H., ed. (1972). *Trends in British Society Since 1900.* London: Macmillan Press.
McKeown T. (1979). *The Role of Medicine.* Oxford: Blackwell
McKeown R., Lowe C. R. (1974). *An Introduction to Social Medicine.* 2nd ed. Oxford: Blackwell.
Watkin B. (1975). *Documents on Health and Social Services 1834 to the Present Day.* London: Methuen.

Chapter 3
People as Individuals

The idea that each patient is a unique individual is basic to the philosophy of nursing care. But what do we mean by the term 'unique individual'? Clearly human beings have many shared characteristics and one can detect and describe patterns of bodily function and of behaviour which are common to all mankind. Moreover in accepting Alexander Pope's belief that 'the proper study of mankind is man', one must recognise that man can be studied from a number of perspectives; the disciplines of chemistry, anatomy, physiology, psychology, anthropology, and sociology all make a contribution to our understanding of man both as a species and as a unique individual. It is important that nurses recognise and use the contribution which the theories, concepts and discoveries of other disciplines can make to their own unique function of giving nursing care.

This chapter and the following one draw heavily upon the resources of psychology and sociology. They should not, however, be regarded as a 'potted textbook' of those disciplines, nor is the line between the two disciplines distinct, although this chapter draws more heavily on psychology and the following chapter on sociology.

The uniqueness of the human individual

The complexity of the human individual arises not so much from the number and complexity of the elements from which he is made, as from the infinite variety of ways in which they inter-relate. Of particular importance is the inter-relationship between heredity and environment. Heredity includes all the characteristics with which a person is endowed from the moment of conception as a result of the particular combination of genes carried by the chromosomes contained within the nucleus of each body cell. It is important to recognise that genetic factors determine not only physical characteristics such as sex or eye colour, but also some mental characteristics such as temperament. Except in the case of uni-ovular twins, each individual's genetic endowment is unique. The

term 'environment' includes all the external physical, mental and social experiences which happen to an individual from the moment of conception onwards. In practice each individual's environment is also unique. Studies of twins which have attempted to estimate the relative influence of heredity and environmental factors on many different characteristics have confirmed the complexity and the uniqueness of the human individual. Uni-ovular twins differ from each other because of the differences in their environments, while even if a completly uniform environment could be provided people would experience it differently.

Moreover, a human being is more than simply the sum of certain genetic and environmentally determined elements. As the biologist H. J. Muller has remarked:

> Although parts and processes may be isolated for analytical purposes, they cannot be understood without reference to the dynamic unified whole that is more than their sum. To say for example that man is made up of certain elements is a satisfactory description only for those who intend to use him as fertiliser.[1]

Individual personality

One aspect of the uniqueness of the individual is the phenomenon which we call 'personality'. Personality is the complex of psychological and emotional attributes, of feelings, attitudes, thought patterns, emotions and drives, that characterises a person. Like other attributes, personality is the product of hereditary and environmental factors. Different schools of psychological thought lay different emphasis on the various factors which contribute to personality and offer different explanations of how personality develops and why a particular person's personality is the way it is.

Personality is an important, although not the only, determinant of behaviour. Some people are more consistent in their reactions and behaviour than others because personality is more organised in some people than in others. We apply the terms 'stable' and 'unstable' to the personality as an explanation of the consistency or inconsistency of a person's behaviour, and by using the terms 'mature' and 'immature' we also imply that the acquistion of personality is a developmental process; experience is an important aspect of environment, and childhood experience in particular is an important determinant of adult personality.

Personality is usually described in one of three ways—by attri-

butes referred to as personality traits, by temperament, or by personality type. *Personality traits* are attributes such as patience, tolerance, assertiveness etc., which indicate a tendency to behave in a consistent manner in particular situations; psychologists such as Eysenck and Cattell have devised techniques for testing the strength of various personality traits and have tried to relate them to specific behaviours. *Temperament* refers to a person's emotional state, and in particular to the way in which emotions are expressed over a long period of time, e.g. placidness, irritability. *Mood* describes the emotion prevailing for a short period.

Psychologists such as Kretchmer and Sheldon have associated different temperaments with different body types, and even at an everyday level reference is often made to the 'fat and happy' type of person. The link between temperament and physical factors, especially endocrine factors, has important implications for the nursing care of individual patients. Temperament tends to change with age and may be seriously distorted by endocrine imbalance whether associated with age (e.g. the menopause) or therapy (e.g. steroids). Classifications based on temperament overlap with those based on *personality type*, the most common of which is Jung's distinction between *introverts* and *extroverts*. *Introverts* are defined as people who 'turn inwards' in their behaviour, i.e. are quiet, shy, and reserved with other people, while *extroverts* 'turn outwards' and use their relationship to other people as the main guide to their behaviour.

It is important to recognise, however, that personality is by definition unique to the individual, and no individual exactly conforms to an ideal type.

Individual experience

One definition of psychology is 'the scientific study of behaviour and experience.'[2] Some psychologists believe that behaviour alone is a legitimate subject for study, because only behaviour can be objectively observed; the behaviourist school of psychology, originated by the psychologist Watson, is based on this view. The conception of experience is, however, at least as relevant to the practice of nursing because it explains and justifies the need to adapt nursing care to the individual patient.

When a nurse sticks an injection needle into a patient's buttock, this stimulus produces a behavioural response such as crying (if the patient is a baby) or a grimace (if the patient is a more controlled

adult), which can be observed. The nurse will probably assume that the patient is experiencing pain, inferring this both from the observed behavioural response and from expectations based upon her own experience of receiving injections, but she cannot feel his pain in exactly the way that he feels it, however close her relationship or however great her empathy. This view forms the basis of the work of psychologists and psychiatrists such as R. D. Laing, philosophers such as Husserl and Sartre, and of the sociological approach known as phenomenology. It is particularly important for the nurse because it shows the danger of responding to patients on the basis of what the nurse thinks the patient 'ought' to feel rather than on what he does feel. The nurse must recognise and take account of the limitations imposed by the fact that her only entry to a patient's experience, which is unique and peculiar to him, is by what the patient tells her either verbally or by other behaviour; for example, if a patient says he is in pain, there is no justification for the nurse to say that he is not. When taking into account environmental factors, such as those described in the previous chapter, it is important to recognise that every individual's environment is different and unique because he experiences it differently from other people. Similarly, his experience of his illness and the way in which he responds to it is individual and unique, and his behaviour will vary accordingly.

Individual behaviour

Why do people behave in the way they do? What are the determinants of human behaviour?

Behaviour can be defined as the activity of an organism in response to the situation in which it finds itself. At its simplest level, for example at the level of the amoeba, behaviour is merely the response to a stimulus; the particular response produced by a particular stimulus occurs automatically and is always the same. In more complex organisms, including man, this type of behaviour persists in the form of *reflex behaviour* whose main function is to ensure physical survival, for example protective responses such as blinking or coughing and the maintenance of essential processes such as heart beat and digestion. In complex animals, however, most behaviour is controlled through a *central nervous system*, in which sensory nerves carry information from the receptors to the brain, where the information is sorted, interpreted and translated into instructions which are transmitted by motor nerves to approp-

riate effectors. The processes which take place within the brain are extremely complex and little understood, but it is these activities, or *mental processes*, which direct human behaviour and which are the subject of study of the discipline called psychology.

It would be impossible in this book to describe, even briefly, all the mental processes involved in individual behaviour; this section merely outlines some of the main concepts and factors which the study of psychology has shown to affect human behaviour, and which are particularly relevant to the task of the district nurse; readers are strongly advised to pursue the suggestions for further reading.

Factors which have been the subject of intensive investigation and which have been found to be particularly important include:

Perception
Motivation
Attitudes and values
Memory
Learning

Perception is the interpretation in the brain of the sensory stimuli received by the sense organs. It is a learnt activity which involves remembering previous stimuli, comparing the new stimulus with them, and recognising it as similar or different. Since the amount of information bombarding the sense organs at any one time is greater than the mind can cope with, material is selected through the mechanism of *attention*. No two individuals will make exactly the same selection, and because people's previous knowledge, expectations, and standards of comparison differ, no two people will perceive the same thing or event in exactly the same way; perception, like experience is unique.

Because the process is so complicated and affected by so many factors, misinterpretation of the information received is common, and this is important because it may lead to inappropriate behaviour. Misinterpretation may result from inadequacies in the information gathered by the sense organs, deficiencies in attention, the 'wrong kind' of previous knowledge, or conflict between the new perception and previous perceptions or expectations.

Motivation can refer either to the goal of an action or to the energising force which initiates action, and it is variously analysed in terms of drives, antecedents, or purpose. A *drive* is a state of arousal to remedy a felt need, e.g. hunger drive, sex drive; needs may be physiological, psychological, or social. Explanations based

on *antecedents* try to link cause and effect; for example a child's response to admission to hospital may be determined by his previous experience of separation from his mother. The third approach to motivation sees behaviour as *goal-oriented*; for example a child may respond to the birth of a baby brother by reverting to babyish behaviour in order to obtain more of his mother's attention. It is important to realise that motivation is often unconscious; few people can recognise their own motivation when asked to account for their behaviour although they may recognise that their behaviour was not rational.

An *attitude* is a persistent predisposition to think, feel and act in a certain way, favourably or unfavourably, in relation to something. *Values* are collections of inter-related attitudes. Attitudes and values certainly influence behaviour, but the exact relationship between them is much debated. Attitudes are learned, mainly during the process of socialisation (Chapter 4), and those which are acquired early are usually strongly held and very resistent to change. Attitude change is one of the most important and one of the most difficult tasks of education.

Memory is the mental process concerned with the storage and recall of information; it is therefore an important component of the processes of perception and learning. The process of remembering events just perceived is referred to as short-term memory; the storage capacity of short-term memory is small, so any overflow of information is either forgotten or transferred to the long-term memory. Retrieving information from the long-term memory is often difficult and incomplete and considerable attention has been applied to investigating what factors improve the ability to recall. The inability to recall unpleasant or worrying events acts as a protective mechanism; material which is hidden in the memory in this way is said to be *repressed*. The activity of remembering depends on a healthy and intact brain; brain damage, whether caused by disorders such as epilepsy or by the process of ageing, produces memory impairment.

Learning is the acquistion of a new and better adapted pattern of behaviour; it is the process by which changes are brought about in an individual's response to the environment. Learning is an important topic in psychology which has wide application for nursing and is discussed in more detail in Chapter 9. Not all learning is conscious and this has important implications for behaviour. Experimental work has led to a number of theories to explain

learning, but basically two broad types can be distinguished: stimulus-response learning or conditioning, and cognitive learning or learning by insight. Conditioning was first described by Pavlov who conditioned a dog to salivate in response to a bell by ringing the bell every time the dog was given food until the dog would salivate in response to the bell alone. Pavlov's discoveries were developed by Watson and later by Skinner who showed that a response to a stimulus could be strengthened by consistently following it with a reward (a *reinforcer*); this process of 'operant' conditioning forms the basis of the behaviour therapy used in psychiatric nursing to help patients overcome phobias or unacceptable behaviour (however defined), but the concept of *reinforcement* has much wider application.

Insight or cognitive learning involves solving problems by thinking about the relationships between different ideas and actions and relating general principles to specific problems. An important aspect of learning is the learning of skills, and Argyle has shown that the process of learning a motor skill such as riding a bicycle applies equally to the learning of social skills.

Anxiety and stress

Stress is an important concept in nursing for two reasons: firstly because it has been shown to be an important causative factor in illness and secondly because illness itself is a stress-producing event. At a common-sense level most people would define stress as a 'feeling' which is provoked by any situation which is 'too much to cope with'. On a more sophisticated level stress can be analysed from the physiological and from the psychological perspective. From the physiological perspective stress is a physiological adaptation, manifested by physiological events such as increased heart rate, to physiological threat; from the psychological perspective—which must be included because even physiological stressors depend on the individual's perception of the threat—stress is consciously experienced through the emotions of fear or anxiety as well as through the assessment of the situation made by the rational or cognitive aspect of the mind. We do not know why some people are able to tolerate stress better than others, but we do know that when stress exceeds the level which an individual is able to tolerate—whatever that level may be for the particular individual—it becomes manifest in his behaviour, sometimes to the extent of mental or psychosomatic illness.

Stress mobilises mechanisms which help an individual to cope, and part of the task of the nurse is to enhance these coping mechanisms, for example by listening empathetically and by counselling, as well as to try to reduce the stress wherever possible by removing the cause. Some coping mechanisms, however, operate below the level of consciousness; the form which these *mental defence mechanisms* take depends on the particular individual and the particular circumstances. James[3] has distinguished six types:

1　Mechanisms involving substitution—
　　e.g. *compensation*: when energy is redirected from the problem area into a different and less threatening channel; *sublimation*: when energy is redirected towards a similar but more attainable goal.

2　Mechanisms for improving the chances of coping with the problematic environment—
　　e.g. *regression*: returning to earlier patterns of behaviour which were previously successful; *identification*: adopting the attitudes and behaviour of other people who seem to cope more successfully.

3　Mechanisms for converting mental anxieties into physical terms which are thought to be more acceptable—
　　e.g. *psychosomatic illness*: where an individual develops a physical illness such as asthma or gastric ulcer; *conversion hysteria*: where an individual develops a physical incapacity which enables him to withdraw without loss of face.

4　Mechanisms for ignoring the existence of the problem—
　　e.g. *repression*: when the unpleasant experience is stored away so far into unconsciousness that it cannot be recalled; *rationalisation*: when information about the problem is re-interpreted so that it is made tolerable.

5　Mechanisms for redirecting the conflict—
　　e.g. *projection*: when the blame for one's own unsatisfactory responses is transferred to other people.

6　Mechanisms for avoiding the problem by retreating from it—
　　e.g. *withdrawal*: when the person withdraws from normal social interaction 'into his own shell'; *hyperactivity*: when the person busies himself with so many other activities that he has no time to think about the real problem.

These mental defence mechanisms are used by everyone to some extent, and they are a valuable means of relieving anxiety and

coping with stress, but when pursued to extremes can interfere with normal behaviour even to the extent of mental illness.

Psychological concepts and nursing

All these concepts and theories, which are the specific concern of psychologists and which have been demonstrated and tested in mainly 'artificial', i.e. experimental, settings, are nevertheless directly relevant to the district nurse's everyday task of caring for patients. An understanding of the patient's personality, mental processes and behaviour, and of her own, is fundamental to the nurse's ability to assess and to meet an individual patient's needs. Effective teaching, which is an important part of her role, requires an understanding of how people learn, including the processes of perception, memory and motivation. Effective communication, which is a prerequisite for the use of all other nursing skills, is itself a learnt skill which also incorporates these processes. For this reason, many of the concepts introduced in this chapter reappear in later chapters as practical factors in patient care.

The individual definition of illness

Illness is not merely a physiological phenomenon. People differ in their experience of particular symptoms, in their readiness to accept a particular symptom as a symptom of illness, and in what they decide to do about it. Nor is *illness* the same thing as *disease*; it is possible to feel ill when no disease exists. *Disease* is a medical concept based on the presence of certain observable pathological abnormalities of body function which are indicated by a set of signs or symptoms. *Illness* on the other hand is a subjective experience indicated by the person's feelings of pain or discomfort. The difference was well described by an American lady (note that Americans use the word 'sick' where English people use the word 'ill') as follows:

> I wish I knew what you mean by being sick. Sometimes I felt so bad I could curl up and die but I had to go on because of the kids who have to be taken care of, and besides we didn't have the money to spend for the doctor. How could I be sick? Some people can be sick anytime with everything, but most of us can't be sick, even when we need to be.[4]

Because the 'disease theory' approach to illness, which is the basis of most medical training and practice, is outside the experi-

ence of most patients, it is perhaps not surprising that doctors, nurses and patients may have different perceptions, as shown in Fig. 3.1. Illness is defined by individuals in terms of their own experience, feelings and values and the nurse must recognise that just as she is entitled to her own experience, feelings and values, so that patient is entitled to his.

The term *illness behaviour* is used to describe 'the way in which symptoms may be differentially perceived, evaluated, and acted (or not acted) upon by different kinds of persons'[5], and both the

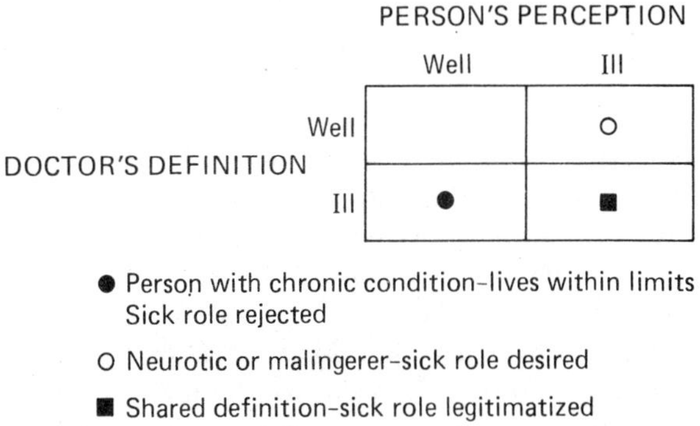

PERSON'S PERCEPTION

		Well	Ill
	Well		O
DOCTOR'S DEFINITION			
	Ill	●	■

● Person with chronic condition–lives within limits
Sick role rejected

O Neurotic or malingerer–sick role desired

■ Shared definition–sick role legitimatized

FIG. 3.1. Perceptions of illness (From Chapman, C. *Sociology for Nurses:* Bailliere Tindall).

concept and the way it is manifested in people's behaviour has been extensively studied by medical sociologists such as Robinson, Mechanic and others.

Individual responses to illness

Balint has pointed out that 'With the starting of an illness a number of secondary processes are also set in motion. One may say that illness creates a new life-situation to which the patient must adapt himself'.[6]

The individual's response depends on his definition of illness, his experience of it, and what it means to him; it will also be coloured by his personality. Illness is a psychological as well as a physiological stressor and therefore provokes various coping mechanisms including all the *mental defence mechanisms* previously described. One of the mechanisms most commonly adopted by people who are ill is regression—that is they revert to previous patterns of behaviour,

especially to those of childhood. They may be unreasonably demanding, seeking constant attention from those around them rather like a toddler constantly demands the attention of its mother, and they may become more dependent on other people, physically and emotionally, than their physical condition warrants. Some people will repress and deny the seriousness of their situation because they cannot consciously face it; this mechanism must always be considered in dealing with patients for whom the prognosis is poor or who are dying (Chapter 16).

Emotional responses are very varied. Almost everybody who becomes ill experiences anxiety not only because of fears about the illness itself but also about consequential events such as having an operation or being admitted to hospital. Relieving anxiety is an important nursing function about which much has been written which is considered in more detail in later chapters. The question 'Why did this happen to me?' often provokes anger, which may be expressed directly in angry behaviour or channelled inwards as guilt or towards other people in the mental mechanism of projection. Some patients feel guilty because they look upon the illness as a punishment for something they have done or not done; this is especially common among children. Guilty feelings are also experienced by anxious relatives and are sometimes the reason for trying to take on too much responsibility for their loved one's care. For some people the worst part of illness is the damage which it does to their self-esteem. It is difficult for a person to think well of himself when he is helpless, robbed of his privacy and his independence, yet self-esteem is a basic human need (Chapter 7).

Some illnesses and treatments cause disturbances in the *body image* which an individual develops in early childhood and which includes not only his awareness and perception of his physical shape but also the values and emotional attitudes which he attaches to it. The way in which people respond to and come to terms with disfigurement depends on many factors, including their age, the speed at which the change occurred and how visible the disfigurement is.

Social responses to illness

Although an individual's experience of his illness is unique, his behaviour also takes account of other people's views about it, and their behaviour towards the sick person depends on their views about illness and their expectations about how sick people behave.

This pattern of expectations and the behaviour which occurs in response to it is an application of the concept of *role* which is discussed in more detail in the next chapter. The pattern of expected behaviour associated with being ill, which is called 'the sick role',[7] has four aspects:

1 The sick person is exempted from his normal social responsibilities. This is accepted as the 'right' of the sick person, but only when it has been 'recognised' or *legitimised* by others, i.e. when *other people* define the sick person as sick.

2 The sick person cannot be expected to make himself well by an act of decision or will. It is recognised that he 'cannot help' his illness. This also depends on *other people's* definition of the sick person's sickness.

These two 'rights' carry associated responsibilities:

3 The sick person should want to get well, and as speedily as possible. Everybody assumes that illness is temporary, and 'makes allowances' for it on that basis.

4 The sick person should seek expert (medical) help and should co-operate with it in order to get well.

While these expectations do govern the behaviour of people who are ill to a considerable extent, and a good deal of our health care system assumes that this behaviour will occur, there are many cases which do not 'fit' the pattern. For example, some conditions require the person to be exempted from normal responsibilities, but there is no possibility that he will 'get well': should one treat as 'sick' a patient who is paralysed after an accident, like John Davis? Similarly some people who have been defined—rightly or wrongly—by other people as 'sick' refuse to behave in the way expected. These discrepancies in behaviour cause problems for the patient, his family, and the nurse, but they confirm the uniqueness of the individual and of his experience.

Another way in which other people's perceptions of the illness affect both their behaviour and that of the sick person is based on the concept of 'stigma'. The word stigma means mark or blemish, but is used as a technical term in sociology to mean any characteristic which marks out an individual as being inferior in some way; in other words it is an expression of people's moral judgements, and is closely related to the idea that illness is a punishment and the

sufferer is 'to blame'. Some illnesses—especially mental illness, mental handicap, epilepsy, and venereal disease—carry a stigma which results in the sufferer being treated by other people as an 'outcast'. This has serious effects not only on the individual patient but also on his family, for frequently the stigma is attached to the whole family.

Individual development

An individual's behaviour and personality are moulded by his life's experiences and must therefore be considered in relation to his age and stage of development. Although the term 'life cycle' conjures up an image of a smoothly rounded circle, the process of individual development is more like a series of steps as shown in Fig. 3.2. The horizontal lines in the diagram represent the relatively stable stages of childhood, adulthood, and old age. The diagonal lines represent the jump from one relatively stable stage to the next; the stages of infancy, adolescence, and middle age are 'critical periods' in development, periods of imbalance before stability returns. During these 'critical periods' the individual is especially vulnerable to stressors in the external environment which are indicated by arrows on the diagram; physical and mental changes coincide with changes in roles and responsibilities, some of which are listed alongside each diagonal line or 'critical period'. The term 'critical period' is also used in another sense, to imply that for each step forward or upward there is a 'right' time; the step cannot be taken before the individual is 'ready' and although some indication of the typical chronological ages at which these changes occur is given in the diagram, the age at which each step forward occurs varies from person to person. Like physical development, psychosocial development follows a characteristic sequence which is the same for everyone although the rate of development, and therefore the timing of a particular step, varies. Like physical and intellectual development, psychosocial development may be arrested—an individual may be unable to achieve the leap from one level to the next.

Different psychologists use different theories of development and concentrate on different stages or aspects of behaviour or personality. However, all agree on two basic principles: firstly, that what happens at one stage of development affects what happens at later stages, and secondly that the earliest stages, especially early childhood, are especially important.

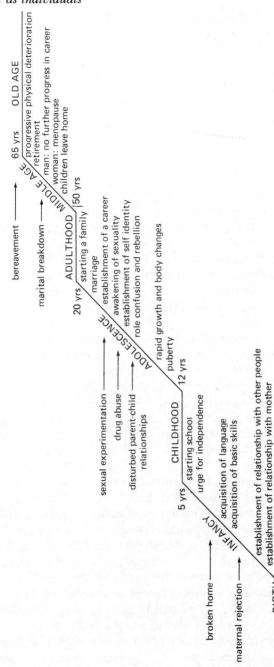

Fig. 3.2. Steps in psycho-social development.

The exact number of stages identified varies but they can be broadly grouped into six:

Infancy
Childhood
Adolescence
Adulthood
Middle age
Old age

Infancy

There are many ways of approaching the study of infant development. For example, paediatricians such as Sheridan and Illingworth have concentrated on establishing norms of physical development; Freud and his followers have concentrated on emotional development; Piaget on intellectual development; Erikson on psychosocial adjustment to developmental 'tasks'. Clearly physical, mental and social development are closely inter-related, but the ages at which children reach particular developmental milestones varies considerably.

From many points of view the first year of life is the most important. During this time the baby develops from the helpless, completely dependent newborn whose range of behaviour is very limited, to the one-year-old who has achieved considerable, although not complete, control over his body movements; has learnt that he exists as an independent being which is separate from the rest of the world; has learnt to use his sense organs as a means of collecting information about the world; and has established social relationships with other people, including a special social relationship with his mother or mother-substitute, and a sophisticated means of communicating with them.

During the second year his ability to walk enables him to explore a far larger segment of the world around him, but his confidence to do so depends very much on the security of a safe and constant base to which he can return at will; the absence of this base, usually his mother, causes considerable distress, and the consequences of long-term absence or complete loss of this base-person may be far reaching. Around the age of two he is beginning to discover the extent of his independence and to use the power which this gives him, in manipulative or negativistic behaviour; he is beginning to use language as the main means of communicating his needs and

feelings to other people. By the age of four or five he is relatively independent in terms of basic self-care skills, completely mobile, manually dextrous, fluent in language, and able to establish and maintain social relationships with relative strangers. By the age of five the foundations of his personality, self-concept, and basic patterns of behaviour are well and truly laid, and the experiences of this early period will have a profound effect on his future development.

Childhood

The rate of change is much slower during the next stage, between the age of about five years and puberty. Starting school, however, is an important step because it provides opportunities for learning far more than facts and skills; the social learning which takes place during the primary school years includes responses to authority and discipline, the establishment of peer-group relationships especially friendships, and the rights and obligations involved in being a member of a group. Social learning is accompanied by moral learning—not only an awareness of right and wrong but of the ability to choose between them—and rapid intellectual development.

Adolescence

Adolescence is a period of transition from childhood to adulthood. The physical changes associated with the development of sexual maturity are reflected in the coming to terms with one's sexuality and in the awakening of sexual feelings. Endocrine instability causes instability of mood which is reflected in instability of behaviour. Socially the transition is from the dependence of childhood to the independence of adulthood. Erikson[8] describes the adolescent mind as 'essentially a mind of the moratorium . . . between the morality learned by the child and the ethics to be developed by the adult . . . an ideological mind' in search of 'identity'; the achievement of 'identity' represents the achievement of maturity.

Adulthood

Although adulthood is associated with the achievement of 'maturity', maturity is an elusive concept. In terms of physical development it carries the connotation of completion, or even of an optimal stage which is followed by a decline. Emotional maturity, however, implies integration and self-control, the ability to give love as well as

to receive it, and the ability to accept responsibility for other people as well as for oneself. Maturity is expressed in attitudes to work, in social responsibility and in the creation—socially as well as physically—of the new generation. Some adults, however, continue to be motivated in their behaviour by emotions which properly belong to childhood, and to persist in behaviour patterns which were appropriate to an earlier stage of development; an adult who behaves in this way could be described as physically mature but emotionally immature. This kind of immaturity is frequently brought to light when the individual has to face a particular stress such as illness.

Middle age

It has been said that middle age is a modern invention which can be attributed to improved standards of living; life has been stretched out in the middle so that what used to be old age is now middle age. Defining the stage in chronological terms is not easy; 'middle age' is usually considered to cover the years from the middle or late forties to retirement, but chronological age may not be exactly reflected in physiological or psychological age. Point of view alters the definition—while the child or the adolescent may consider the 45-year-old to be quite ancient, the 45-year-old may consider himself young.

In terms of psychosocial development, however, middle age represents a critical developmental period analogous to adolescence in that it is a stage of 'becoming'—shown in Fig. 3.2 as a diagonal line. As in adolescence the physiological changes associated with the climacteric, and especially in women with the menopause, have psychological and social as well as physical effects. In the field of family relationships instability may result from the fact that the children are no longer dependent but have left the parental home to establish their own homes and families. This changes the marital relationship at the same time as the menopause may be causing changes in ideas about sexual activity and changing body image. At work a man must accept that he has 'reached his peak' whether this point is at or short of his aspirations or capabilities; for a woman this period may mark a new career. The death of elderly parents may be the first real experience of bereavement. The early stages of degenerative disorders such as arthritis may be beginning to make their presence felt.

This period offers an important challenge for health education because intervention at this stage can considerably mitigate some of the problems of old age; in particular preparation for retirement can

make the adjustment to retirement, for both men and women, considerably easier.

Old age

Ageing, like adolescence, is a social and psychological as well as physical process and as in adolescence, physical changes affect personality and behaviour. Unlike adolescence, however, the onset of old age is not marked by an identifiable event; the onset is insidious and its definition, like that of illness, is very subjective.

Deterioration of the special senses such as vision and hearing have important mental and social consequences. The organic degeneration of the brain which is termed dementia disrupts the personality and affects intelligence, memory, emotional state, and learning—that is, the ability to adapt to a changing environment. One manifestation of these changes is that personality becomes more rigid; old people tend to be set in their ways. Conservatism and apprehension about change increase, although how far this is due to mental changes and how far to social changes is uncertain. The older people get the more dependent they become on the stabilising effect of their own home and their own possessions; familiar ornaments and old photographs are not only treasured mementoes but an important prop to maintaining identity. Short-term memory becomes poor while long-term memory is retained—even appearing, relative to the short-term memory loss, to improve. Old people like to reminisce, and it is possible that this is a means of 'reworking' previous experiences in such a way as to come to terms with them. Erikson sees 'coming to terms' with oneself as the mark of the successful achievement of the last stage of development:

> Only in him who in some way has taken care of things and people and has adapted himself to the triumphs and disappointments adherent to being—only in him may gradually ripen the fruit of these seven stages. I know no better word for it than ego integrity ... It is the acceptance of one's one and only life cycle as something that had to be and that, by necessity, permitted of no substitution ... The lack of this accrued ego integration is signified by fear of death: the one and only life cycle is not accepted as the ultimate of life.[8]

The elderly person's method of adjustment is sometimes called *disengagement*. Disengagement involves reducing the extent of

social interaction, reducing the number of social roles played, reducing life space and social activity. Emotional disengagement involves a flattening of emotion which may be manifested as a certain 'mellowness' or equanimity of temperament. The prospect of death is no longer terrifying and may be looked forward to peacefully.

Conclusion

Each individual experiences illness differently and copes with it differently; this chapter has described some of the factors which explain individual differences. The nurse must consider all these factors in relation to each patient, but one might apply them to just one of the seven patients as follows:

John Davis is 22 years old, and is tetraplegic as the result of a motorbike accident two years ago. At the time of his accident he was at the threshold of healthy adulthood, recently 'flown' from the family 'nest', launched upon a promising career, about to marry. All his hopes and expectations of a wonderful future—and those of his parents—were shattered. Imagine the immediate psychological effects of the accident. John's immediate reactions might have been masked by the intensive care required for his survival, but his parents' response might have been first numbed shock, then anger, then despair. Does John's father blame himself for allowing John to have a motorbike, and is that why he feels he must contribute to John's care even at the risk of his job? During the months in hospital the realities of his situation will gradually have dawned upon John, but the environment of the hospital, where he could identify with and derive support from other patients in similar situations, may have protected him for a time. Now that he is living at home and his condition is stable is he still 'sick'? Do other people treat him as 'sick', and does he want them to do so? How has he adjusted his body image to take account of his paralysis? How does he cope with the fact that his sexual drives, which are strongest at this age, are unimpaired although the means by which they would normally have been expressed are no longer available? What mental mechanisms does he use to cope with his situation—does he compensate for his physical loss by becoming the local chess champion, or deny reality by escaping into daydreams? Does he regress into childish dependency—and do his mother and sisters reinforce his behaviour, compensating for their own loss by regarding him as still their 'baby'? Does he express his frustration and anger in rages and

verbal abuse of his parents and the nurse? Does an extrovert personality help him to establish new kinds of social relationships or does an introvert personality increase his risk of social isolation? Are there strong personality traits such as persistence and determination which will help him to cope?

Since John Davis is a fictional character, one can only speculate, but the answers to similar questions are an important part of the nurse's assessment of each individual patient in her care.

References

1. Muller H. J. (1943). *Science and Criticism.* New Haven: Yale University Press.
2. Altchul A. (1975). *Psychology for Nurses.* 4th ed. London: Bailliere Tindall.
3. James D. (1970). *Introduction to Psychology.* Harmondsworth: Penguin.
4. Koos E. (1954). *The Health of Regionville.* New York: Columbia University Press.
5. Mechanic D. (1968). *Medical Sociology: a selective view.* New York: Free Press.
6. Balint M. (1964). *The Doctor, his Patient, and the Illness.* London: Pitman Medical.
7. Parsons T. (1951). *The Social System.* London: Routledge and Kegan Paul.
8. Erikson E. (1965). *Childhood and Society.* Harmondsworth: Penguin.

Suggestions for Further Reading

Altchul A. (1975). *Psychology for Nurses.* 4th ed. London: Bailliere Tindall.
Argyle M. (1967). *The Psychology of Interpersonal Behaviour.* Harmondsworth: Penguin.
Berne E. (1968). *Games People Play.* Harmondsworth: Penguin.
Erikson E. (1965). *Childhood and Society.* Harmondsworth: Penguin.
Goffman I. (1968). *Stigma.* Harmondsworth: Penguin.
Laing D. (1966). *The Politics of Experience.* Harmondsworth: Penguin.
Lowe G. P. (1972). *The Growth of Personality from Infancy to Old Age.* Harmondsworth: Penguin.
Peplau H. E. (1952). *Interpersonal Relations in Nursing.* New York: Putnams.
Pettitt E. (1980). Body image. *Nursing.* **1,16**:690–692.
Robinson D. (1971). *The Process of Becoming Ill.* London: Routledge & Kegan Paul.
Robinson D. (1973). *Patients Practitioners & Medical Care.* London: William Heinemann Medical Books.
Rutter M. (1972). *Maternal Deprivation Reassessed.* Harmondsworth: Penguin.
Stafford Clark D. (1967). *What Freud Really Said.* Harmondsworth: Penguin.
Stockwell F. (1972). *The Unpopular Patient.* (RCN Research Series No. 1.) London: Royal College of Nursing.
Tuckett D., ed. (1976). *An Introduction to Medical Sociology.* London: Tavistock.
Wilson M. (1975). *Health is for People.* London: Darton Longman and Todd.
Winnicott D. W. (1964). *The Child the Family and the Outside World.* Harmondsworth: Penguin.
Vernon M. D. (1965). *The Psychology of Perception.* Harmondsworth: Penguin.

Chapter 4

People in Groups

John Donne wrote:

'No man is an island entire of itself. Every man is a piece of the Continent, a part of the main'.

Human beings are social beings; they interact with one another in a social world. An individual's behaviour is determined both by his own mental processes and also by the behaviour of other people in the world around him. He responds to their behaviour as they respond to his in the activity called *social interaction*. Just as psychology provides a way of understanding behaviour in terms of individual mental processes, sociology provides a way of understanding behaviour in terms of its social context. Both perspectives are important to the nurse.

Mr Evans, for example, is unique, but he is also a member of several groups—his family, his work group, his trade union, the group of friends whom he meets at the local pub on Friday nights, the local football club—which influence what he thinks and the way he behaves, and must, therefore, also be taken into account in planning his care. These *primary groups* overlap and interact with one another in larger units such as his neighbourhood and his community, which in turn overlap and interact within the overall group which we term *society*. Each group, for example the Evans family, is a social system which can be viewed in the same way as a physiological system such as the digestive or respiratory systems, that is as a collection of inter-related parts and the relationships between them. We can also talk about the educational system or the political system as social systems within a particular society, or we can use the term 'the social system' to describe society as a whole.

Groups in this sense are more than mere collections of people; the key characteristic of a social group is the fact that its members interact with and behave towards one another in ways which other members of the group encourage and respond to and expect. The way Mr Evans behaves towards his wife and children within the

family group would not be the appropriate way to behave towards his boss and his colleagues at work. Each group has its own *values* and *attitudes* which guide its members' behaviour. The expected patterns or *norms* of behaviour are learned: for example, from the day a child is born he begins to learn the kind of behaviour which is expected of him within his family and his parents will, consciously and unconsciously, teach him by encouraging some behaviours and discouraging others. This process of social learning is called *socialization*. By this means, the pattern of expected behaviour is passed on from generation to generation, gradually changing and developing all the time. The totality of the expected behaviour patterns which a society develops, incorporating attitudes, beliefs, morals, laws and customs, is called its *culture*. Although each individual is unique and endowed with what we call 'free will', his patterns of behaviour depend very greatly on his social and cultural background; he cannot escape entirely from its influence, and some would argue that he is the product of it.

Cultural differences

Because our culture is so much a part of us we tend to take it for granted, assuming that our expectations and patterns of behaviour are normal, inevitable, and 'right' while other patterns are abnormal or 'wrong'. We also tend to assume that our particular patterns of behaviour are common to all mankind, whereas any individual's behaviour patterns come primarily from the group and culture into which he is born, and these are not the same for everyone. It is important for nurses not only to recognise that there are social and cultural differences between people which affect the way in which they behave when they are ill or when someone near to them is ill, but also to respect the differences and to take account of them in planning and giving care.

This is particularly important in a multi-racial society such as exists in Britain today, where nurses and patients will quite commonly be of different cultural backgrounds. About six per cent of the population of the United Kingdom were born overseas; in addition there is an increasing number of second generation immigrants whose parents were born abroad but who were themselves born and brought up in Britain. People migrate from one country to another for a number of reasons. Some have come to Britain as refugees from wars or political pressures in their own countries; examples in this century include German Jews, Hungarians, and

Ugandan Asians. Others are drawn by economic factors such as better job prospects and opportunities for their children. At different times different groups of immigrants have been the focus of interest and concern; for example in the censuses of 1901 and 1911 special efforts were made to assess accurately the large number of foreign born Jews who had emigrated to the UK as a result of the political pressures in their own countries at the end of the nineteenth century.

The new immigrant to a country brings with him the culture—including religion, which in some countries is a major determinant of life-style—and the behaviour patterns of his country of origin. For many present day immigrants to Britain the process of *integration*, which is the process by which an immigrant group modifies its old culture and absorbs the culture of its new home, involves a change from life in a simple rural society to life in a complex urban society. There is an enormous difference between life in a small village in northern India and life in a large industrial city in Britain. People's responses to the change differ; some want to preserve as much as possible of their old culture and to pass it on to future generations, while others, although their own patterns of behaviour are established as the result of their former cultural experiences, are anxious to adopt British ways and are particularly anxious for their children to do so. In both groups the second generation immigrants, for example, the teenage daughters of Asian immigrants, may experience conflict between the old culture and the new. An understanding of these factors is particularly important to the district nurse because it is within the home and family setting that cultural differences are most marked; among the most fundamental differences are those relating to family roles (especially the role of women), child-rearing practices, and food habits.

There are also important culturally-determined differences in sickness behaviour. The subjectivity of the definition of illness was discussed in Chapter 3, and clearly the response to sickness of a western European who believes that the 'cause' of his misfortune is a particular disease will be different from the African who attributes it to witchcraft, and from the Arab who believes it to be simply the will of Allah. Such differences affect the decision to seek help in the first place, who to seek it from, and whose advice to follow; the antibiotic cream and the sterile dressing so carefully applied by the nurse may be quietly removed as soon as she has left the house and

replaced by a home-made herbal concoction prescribed by the community's traditional healer. Cross-cultural research has also demonstrated significant cultural differences in the prevalence of various diseases, responses to mental stress and responses to pain.

Religion is a very important aspect of culture, and religious beliefs and practices also influence sickness behaviour and patient care. Like the more general cultural differences, religious differences affect both patient and nurse; for example, Roman Catholic nurses are not required to participate in abortions, but have to find other solutions when they are caring for a patient who has had an abortion or who is seeking contraceptive advice. In some societies, religious belief is a major determinant of the whole way of life; for example, the Muslim holy book, the Koran, specifically lays down dietary restrictions, codes about the regulation of marriage, family roles, dress, and many kinds of social activity. Religious rites associated with death are very important and the district nurse must make sure that she understands her patient's beliefs and wishes. Religious festivals which may involve fasting, such as the Muslim Ramadan and the Jewish Yom Kippur, have implications for planning patient care. Many religious sects have other beliefs which affect specific aspects of health care, for example the Jehovah's Witnesses' refusal of blood transfusion and the Christian Scientists' rejection of drugs.

Social positions and social roles

The terminology which is used to describe the way in which people behave in groups is the language of the stage: each person is an *actor* who is given a part (a *social position*) and when he acts according to his part he is said to be performing a *role*. An individual occupies many social positions and plays many different roles, even within the same group. Within his family, for example, Mr Evans is a husband, a father, and his mother's son; at the same time he plays other roles in other groups—as an employee and perhaps a shop steward in his work group, as a member of the local football club, and, temporarily at least, as a patient. Just as the groups interact and overlap so do the roles of individual actors within them. Fig. 4.1 shows Mr Evans' social network and some of the roles he plays in relation to other people.

The diagram shows that role relationships are reciprocal—husband and wife, father and child, employer and employee; it is difficult to play the role of husband to someone who does not play

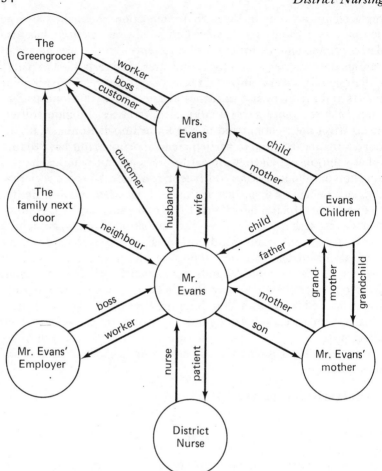

Fig. 4.1. Mr Evans' social network.

the role of wife. Tensions also arise when something prevents a person from playing the role he wants to play or plays it differently from the way other people expect. In the Fisher family, for example, Mr Fisher's physical handicap will interfere with the way he plays the role of husband; one aspect of the normal 'husband-wife' role relationship is reversed in that Mrs Fisher goes out to work leaving her husband at home all day, and is likely to become the main breadwinner. Mrs Fisher, like most people, has multiple roles—as wife, carer and schoolmistress, and these roles may some-

times conflict—for example, if the caring role which she wants to adopt to her husband had prevented her from taking the opportunity for promotion at work.

The concept of social class

In all societies people are differentiated by social as well as by biological criteria into categories which imply that there are not only 'differences' between the groups but also 'inequalities', since the groups can be arranged in some sort of social hierarchy. In ancient Greece and Rome, the basic distinction was between citizen and slave; in India people were differentiated by caste; for Marx the distinction lay in people's relation to the means of production. In an industrialised society occupational status is a convenient and useful indicator of social position, and it began to be used as a criterion by which to 'sort' information about the health of the population from the middle of the last century. In 1911, the Chief Medical Statistical Officer in the General Register Office, T.H.C. Stevenson, developed a comprehensive classification system based on occupation to analyse infant mortality. With relatively minor modifications his scale has survived to be the major classification of social class used today:

Class I	Professional (e.g. accountant, doctor)
Class II	Intermediate (e.g. manager, school teacher, nurse)
Class III (n)	Skilled non-manual (e.g. clerical worker, shop assistant)
Class III (m)	Skilled manual (e.g. bus driver, coal miner, carpenter)
Class IV	Semi-skilled (e.g. agricultural worker, postmen)
Class V	Unskilled (e.g. labourer, dock worker)

This system is used to classify all census data, and in spite of some inherent problems, such as the classification of married women and retired people, it has proved to be an extremely powerful epidemiological tool. One of the reasons why it has proved useful is that it has been shown to differentiate between people on other social characteristics such as education, income, life styles, linguistic codes and even attitudes, values, and norms of behaviour. For this reason, it is a useful way of differentiating between social classes defined in the more general sense as 'segments of the population sharing broadly similar types and levels of resources, with broadly

similar styles of living and some shared perception of their collective condition'.[1]

In interpreting data which has been classified in this way, however, it is important not to impute a *causal* relationship between class and the factor which is being considered: correlation does not necessarily imply causation. While it may be reasonable to infer a causal connection between certain occupations such as coal mining and certain causes of death such as pneumoconiosis on the basis of what is known about the aetiology of the disease, in other cases the relationship is likely to be much more complex; it may even happen that—as has been argued in the case of the epidemiology of schizophrenia—the variable in question is the cause rather than the effect of the social class classification. In social statistics and epidemiology, unlike in some other branches of sociology and political theory, social class is a statistical concept for classifying data, not a means of explaining why or how social differentials exists.[2]

Social class is also *subjectively* defined, usually in the more general terms 'upper class', 'middle class' and 'working class'; this subjective classification is often applied to factors associated with the 'class culture', such as attitudes, values and life-styles. Within this rather less precise classification most people assign themselves either to the 'middle class' which broadly corresponds to the Registrar General's Classes I and II, or to the 'working class' which broadly corresponds to classes III, IV and V; the term 'upper class' is usually applied to the traditional aristocracy.

Some important research studies have analysed the relationship between social class and particular factors, including:

Education[3,4,5]
Child rearing practices[6,7]
Infant feeding practices[8]
Contraceptive practices[9]
Linguistic codes[10]
Family roles[11,12]

A number of studies of more general class-based differences are included in the suggestions for further reading; a summary of the 'working class' and 'middle class' perspectives revealed by one important study[13] is shown in Table 4.1.

TABLE 4.1

Working-class and middle-class perspectives

	Working-Class Perspective	Middle-Class Perspective
General beliefs	The social order is divided into 'us' and 'them': these who do not have authority and those who do The division between 'us' and 'them' is virtually fixed, at least from the point of view of one man's life chances What happens to you depends a lot on luck; otherwise you have to learn to put up with things	The social order is a hierarchy of differentially rewarded positions: a ladder containing many rungs It is possible for individuals to move from one level of the hierarchy to another Those who have ability and initiative can overcome obstacles and create their own opportunities. Where a man ends up depends on what he makes of himself
General values	'We' ought to stick together and get what we can as a group. You may as well enjoy yourself while you can instead of trying to make yourself 'a cut above the rest'	Every man ought to make the most of his own capabilities and be responsible for his own welfare. You cannot expect to get anywhere in the world if you squander your time and money. 'Getting on' means making sacrifices
Attitudes on more specific issues	(on the best job for a son) 'A trade in his hands'. 'A good steady job' (towards people needing social assistance) 'They have been unlucky'. 'They never had a chance'. 'It could happen to any of us' (on Trade Unions) 'Trade Unions are the only means workers have of protecting themselves and of improving their standard of living'	'As good as start as you can give him'. 'A job that leads somewhere' 'Many of them had the same opportunities as others who have managed well enough'. 'They are a burden on those who are trying to help themselves' 'Trade Unions have too much power in the country'. 'The Unions put the interests of a section before the interests of the nation as a whole'

Source: Goldthorpe, J. H. and Lockwood, D. (1970) The changing national class structure. In Butterworth, E. and Weir, D. *The Sociology of Modern Britain.* London: Fontana.

Social class health and health care

Differences in life chances and health patterns between the different social classes begin at birth or even before, and continue throughout life. The baby of an unskilled manual worker (Social Class V) is twice as likely to be still born, twice as likely to die during the first month of life, and five times more likely to die between then and his first birthday than the baby of an accountant or lawyer (Social Class I). The difference persists throughout childhood although it is slightly less for girls than for boys. During adulthood the overall difference is less marked although there are dramatic differences in death from particular causes. Overall the chances of premature death (that is death before retirement) are $2\frac{1}{2}$ times as great in Social Class V as in Social Class I, and the life expectancy for a baby born into Social Class V is five years less than that of a baby born into Social Class I. It has been estimated[1] that if the mortality rates of Class I had applied to Classes IV and V during 1970–72, the lives of 74 000 people aged under 75 years, including 10 000 children and 32 000 men of working age, would not have been lost.

Information about sickness patterns, as was mentioned in Chapter 2, is more difficult to obtain and to assess, but such information as is available reflects the general picture of mortality. Rates of 'long-standing illness' reported in the General Household Surveys are approximately $2–2\frac{1}{2}$ times as high among Social Class V as among Social Class I, and the average number of days lost through illness or accident among unskilled manual workers in 1971–72 was $4\frac{1}{2}$ times as great as the number loss by professional men. There are marked differences in the type of illness experienced by people in different classes; for example, respiratory diseases are much more common in Social Class V while cirrhosis of the liver is more common in Social Class I. Psychiatric illness has recently been shown to be four times as common among working class women compared with middle class women, although it may be less frequently reported or treated.[14]

Differences between the social classes in the availability and use made of health services are also important. Tudor Hart[15] has suggested an 'inverse care law' which states that 'the availability of good medical care tends to vary inversely with the need of the population served'. He argues that in areas with most sickness and death, GPs and hospitals have more work, larger lists, the least

adequate buildings, and less staff and equipment. The removal of such inequalities was one of the stated intentions of the National Health Service; it has never been achieved, although the use of RAWP formulae for the allocation of funds to health authorities is a recent attempt to begin to do so.

Even when the need is evident and the services are available, however, differences persist in the extent to which people use them. The report 'Inequalities in Health'[1] concluded that, although working class adults consulted GPs more and were heavier users of hospital beds than middle class adults, when their increased morbidity was taken into account they made relatively less use of health services, were typically more sick than middle class patients when help was sought, were less likely to seek medical help for their children, and in particular made much less use of the preventive health services. Similar patterns have also been shown in the use of family planning services, dental services, and cervical screening. These differences offer a particular challenge to all those concerned with health education, including district nurses.

Finally, the evidence suggests that there are differences in the quality of care received and in the patient's response to it. For example, studies of the work of general practitioners have shown that working class patients have shorter consultations with their GP. A number of sociological studies have suggested that the social distance between patients and health care professionals—since doctors are defined as belonging to Social Class I and nurses to Social Class II—affects the care given, and that differences in the type of language which they use[10] inhibits doctor–patient communication.

The relationship between health and social class is easy to demonstrate, but extremely difficult to interpret, partly because the concepts 'health' and 'social class' are themselves extremely complex. Sometimes causal factors can be reasonable inferred: for example, some diseases can be directly related to occupation. The ten-fold increase in the risk of death from fire, falls and drowning among boys of Social Class V compared with their peers in Social Class I can be related, at least in part, to environmental factors; the prevalence of respiratory diseases can be related to housing conditions; housing conditions can be related to income levels and both are closely related to social class. Income levels and material resources such as access to a car and a telephone may also explain some of the differences in patterns of usage of health services; education has also been shown to be an important factor. Cultural

behaviour patterns and perspectives such as those which were shown in Table 4.1, and the subjective definitions which were discussed in Chapter 3, are clearly important but are difficult to interpret. What is important from the district nurse's point of view is that she should be aware of the differences and should take account of them in preparing appropriate and realistic care plans for individual patients.

The family

The group which exerts probably the greatest influence on an individual's behaviour is the family, partly because the attitudes and behaviour patterns which are developed in early childhood within the context of a family group become an integral part of an individual's personality and life style, and partly because for most people the family (although in adulthood it may be a different family) is the group with which they have most frequent and prolonged contact.

Fletcher[16] has suggested that the functions of the modern family are as follows:

To regulate sexual behaviour.
To give a legitimate basis for the procreation and rearing of children.
To provide a home for its members.
To serve as the primary agency for socialisation.

To these functions a district nurse would undoubtedly add:

To provide the primary social context for the care of the sick at home.

It is for this reason that district nurses need to understand the sociology of the family, and though some of the most important points are outlined here it is important that this outline should be 'filled out' by reading some of the wealth of specialist literature on the subject; a few of the most useful books are included in the suggestions for further reading. This section concentrates specifically on family responses to illness and the family's role in care.

The family unit

It is common to discuss family structure in terms of two 'ideal-types': the *nuclear* family, consisting of a mother, a father and their children living together, and the *extended* family in which grand-

parents, parents, siblings, aunts, uncles and cousins (or various combinations of these) live together as a single family unit. Other terms used include the *family of origin*, meaning the family into which a person is born; the *family of marriage* meaning the new family which is created by marriage; the *consanguine family*, meaning the family of blood relations; and *kin* or the *kinship network* which is the 'rest of the family' formed by the interlocking network of related nuclear families. The *extended* family is often represented as the 'original' family type, which was economically and socially self-supporting, meeting functions such as obtaining the necessities of life, child-rearing, housekeeping, and caring for sick and other dependent members from within its own resources. The *nuclear* family is represented as the 'modern' family, produced by the consequences of industrialisation in which social and geographical mobility split up extended families and the welfare state took over most of its functions. The extended family type tends to be associated with agricultural communities, immigrant groups, and the working class; the nuclear family type tends to be associated with towns, suburbia and the middle class. Ideal types, however, rarely exist in the real world. There are, and have always been, other kinds of groups in which people live, such as single-parent families, communes of various kinds, unmarried people living alone, and elderly people (often widows and widowers) living alone. The extended family was never as universal as is sometimes suggested, and the modern nuclear family is rarely as isolated.

The social changes described in Chapter 2 have, however, had a significant effect of the structure and life style of the modern family. In general, families are smaller and more socially and geographically mobile; political, legal and economic emancipation of women has profoundly affected traditional male–female, husband–wife, and mother–father–child roles and relationships; social policies in work, housing and welfare services and the development of transport and communications technology have substantially altered social networks between kin.

Many of these factors can be identified in the stories of the seven families. The rural setting has not protected Mr and Mrs Adams from separation from their kin; they, like many other elderly people, do not have children to care for them. The Bakers, as a single parent family, represent one in ten of all families with dependent children. Mrs Cray, her daughter, son-in-law and grandchildren do not live under the same roof, nor do the Greens, but both families

have close contact with their kin which may provide to a lesser or greater degree the same kind of support network as the ideal type extended family was said to provide. Family roles within the Green family and the Davis family probably follow traditional lines; the husband–wife roles of the Fishers were probably different, even before Mr Fisher's illness.

The ideal types of family structures and life-styles may offer a useful framework within which the district nurse can assess a family's social dynamics and coping methods, but it is important to recognise that the complexities of the family system, just as in the individual, make each family and its needs unique.

The family and illness

The family is not only the context within which illness occurs; the family has a direct influence on the illness and its management, and the illness has a direct consequence on the family.

From the district nurse's point of view the ability and willingness of family members to assist in the care of their sick relative is a major factor in the nurse's care plan (Chapter 8). Thus although John Davis' handicap and need for physical care are at least as great as Mr Fisher's, it may be that the district nurse will spend less time with John because a greater part of the burden of care has been accepted, willingly or reluctantly, by John's parents than by Mrs Fisher. The way in which the carers approach their task will also influence the patient's response; for example, will the devotion of John's mother make him more dependent than he needs to be, or make him emotionally as well as physically dependent?

Disturbed family relationships may actually cause illness, especially mental illness. Laing[17] has argued that family pressures are a direct cause of the schizophrenic's withdrawal from reality, and Brown[18] has shown that they are an important cause of relapse and re-admission. Family tensions may cause psychosomatic illnesses as specific as a gastric ulcer or as general as 'tension headaches'. Disturbed parent–child relationships are associated with a wide range of disorders in children including failure to thrive, asthma, vomiting, developmental retardation and accident prone-ness. There is increasing evidence that psychological stress acts as a trigger factor which precipitates or increases susceptibility to diseases such as coronary thrombosis, rheumatoid arthritis, and even infections such as tuberculosis and streptococcal throat infections. The most dramatic example of the effect of family disruption on

physical illness is the increased mortality and morbidity which follows bereavement.[19]

The effect of illness on the family

The effect of illness, particularly long-term illness, on a family is considerable. The practical implications of the 'burden of care' include additional financial expenditure—often at the same time as a reduction in income, having to do too many tasks in the time available—specially if the carer works outside the home and has to manage the home as well as caring for the patient, particular problems such as extra laundry or special food, and the sheer physical fatigue produced by the demands of the day followed by disturbed nights, often for weeks or months without respite. The practical problems are lessened if they are shared among several family members, but it is not uncommon for the burden to be borne almost exclusively by one person—for example, the mother of a handicapped child, a spouse, or the single daughter of elderly parents. Sometimes, the sharing of the common task unites and strengthens a family; often, especially if the demands continue over a long period of time, the stress may become too great, the individuals involved may break down or become ill themselves, and the family as a unit may begin to disintegrate. One might wonder how long Mrs Fisher will be able to cope with the demands of a responsible job, managing the house, and caring for an increasingly disabled husband; quite apart from the demands on her own health, such a situation will impose considerable strain on the marriage.

The practical problems also have social costs. A letter to a woman's journal quoted by Quinn[20] gives some indication of the social cost to the unmarried daughters who even nowadays are often 'expected' to care for their elderly parents:

> I've looked after my mother since she had a heart attack soon after my father's death. She is now 77 and is a wonderful person which makes my duties lighter. But I've no friends or other relatives to turn to for a break, and I feel isolated and lonely. I'm 47 and the only man I ever loved was unwilling to have my mother in our future home, so I lost him. Can you help?

One might consider the social cost to Sarah, Mrs Baker's eldest daughter, in terms of her 'lost adolescence', for Sarah is unlikely to have the time, money, or social contacts to enable her to enjoy many of the activities which her former schoolmates enjoy. Similarly, the

social costs of enabling John Davis to live with his family outside an institution will include the loss of any career aspirations that either of his parents might have had and most of the social activities that they might have enjoyed together. Such costs are borne not only by the adults who have at least some choice, however limited; one might also imagine the price paid by Alison Green's brother and sister as the result of the amount of time and attention which their mother has had to give to Alison. One of the most important, and the least appreciated, costs is the stigma which is still attached to physical and mental handicap, and especially to mental illness.

Illness also disrupts individual roles within the family. Sickness will deprive the patient of some of his normal family roles—for example Mr Evans is temporarily not the main bread-winner of his family—and these roles will have to be taken on by others. This change may not be easy for either the patient or the family to accept. Mr Fisher may not take kindly to the role-reversal implied by the fact that his wife goes out to work every morning while he stays at home and prepares the supper. Mrs Baker will not have found it easy to be father as well as mother to her three children, but the prospect of Sarah trying to be both mother and father to her young brother and sister is even more worrying.

The family's role in care

The miracle is that in spite of these very considerable difficulties, families do care for their sick members and often do so magnificently. The way in which the caring role is played varies according to the family's own resources, and also with the type and stage of the illness. It is important that all health professionals, but especially nurses, recognise that they have no exclusive prerogative to care; care is a partnership between the health professionals, the family, and the individual patient himself.

The community

It is unfortunate that in talking about health services, the word 'community' is sometimes used in antithesis to the word 'hospital'. In one sense the hospital is part of 'the community'; in another sense the hospital is a community in its own right. The word community implies having something in common; the original usage of the word, as the modern usage of the word 'commune',

implies the sharing of goods, interests, and values in a face to face situation. We apply the word community to a number of different kinds of social groups and networks based sometimes on occupation, sometimes on shared interests and purposes, but most commonly on shared locality.

For a geographical area to be called a community, however, implies a certain social as well as geographical cohesion. The degree of cohesion varies. For many people living alone or in nuclear family units in an urban area, the 'local community' means no more than the collection of homes and families around them; in other areas families living within a particular locality are bound together by a strong sense of common identity and share the same cultural background. Families with like characteristics tend to live together in the same neighbourhood. The like characteristics may be race, religion, occupation, income or social class, and the coming together may be either a matter of choice or a lack of any alternative, but the result is a 'consciousness of kind' which gives the neighbourhood a certain social cohesion.

Neighbourhoods, especially in city areas, may change, sometimes quite rapidly, as the result of social policy and planning decisions, for example slum clearance and development programmes. Much of the housing in city centres consists of large houses built by the wealthy during the last century. As they moved outward their large houses, too expensive for a single working class family to afford, were divided into flats and rooms so that one house was occupied by several families; some of the problems which this causes were discussed in Chapter 2. Neighbourhoods may also change because of patterns of immigration. As a new immigrant group settles in a neighbourhood and begins to expand, the former residents move out, and as these immigrants prosper and integrate, they move to better neighbourhoods making room for new and sometimes different groups.

As in the case of families, communities are often analysed in terms of ideal types, and a number of sociological studies have described the ways in which different types of community, and the family and kinship groups within them, function; some are included in the suggestions for further reading. While very few communities in reality conform exactly to the ideal type, the framework which the ideal types provide can help the nurse to appreciate and understand the structure and dynamics of the community within which she works.

Rural communities

A rural community is small in scale with few social groupings so that there is frequent face to face contact among its members; everyone knows everyone else, their activities and their attitudes. Residents have often lived in the village for many years, sometimes for several generations; the extended family is more common, and the kinship and neighbourhood networks provide considerable social support in time of need. Social institutions such as the local church and the local school, and 'village activities' like the annual fête, foster 'togetherness'. Cultural traditions are strong and slow to change, and considerable time may be needed for new residents to become integrated and accepted as 'members' of the community.

Urban communities

Population density in cities and towns produce communities on a larger scale. The population is often more mobile, so that families are separated and the kinship network is less strong. Because a large community can support a large number of social organisations, especially occupational and recreational organisations, social networks may be based on these groupings rather than on kin, and these networks do not usually carry ties of mutual obligation as strong as those between kin. One problem of urban life is that many individuals are isolated from their original family and neighbourhood groups, but do not become members of new groups, and are, therefore, at risk of loneliness and social isolation; Mrs Cray is one such example. On the other hand, large cities may contain smaller communities whose social cohesion, which is often based on the extended family or on occupation, is just as strong as the most tightly-knit rural community; an example of this kind of community is the neighbourhood in which Alison Green's family lives.

Suburban housing estates

In the past the strongest influence on a residential pattern was a man's occupation. He had to live near his place of work. The development of public transport and the growth of car ownership, however, now allow people to work in the city but to live outside. In most of our great cities the population of the central area is decreasing while the population of the 'suburban ring' around the city is increasing.

One of the characteristics of many suburbs, especially where

large new housing estates have been built, is the relative homogeneity of the population in age and income; in some areas the population may consist entirely of young married couples or families with small children. The new estates may be at a considerable distance from people's original homes, and nuclear families are thus separated from their kin at what may be a very vulnerable stage in family development.

In Local Authority estates these difficulties may be exacerbated by the fact that the council tenant does not have the same degree of choice as the home owner. By slum clearance or through housing shortage the council tenant has to live wherever there is a house or flat available for which he is eligible, and near neighbours whom he does not know and did not choose. The social adjustment which this makes necessary may give rise to many problems, especially when the estate is new.

Retirement areas

At the other extreme, but sharing the characteristics of homogeneity of population, are the 'retirement areas' such as the towns of the South Coast to which elderly people like to move on retirement because of the pleasant surroundings and climate. In some areas up to half of the population may be over retirement age. These elderly people are isolated from their kin at an equally vulnerable period, and their problems of social isolation may be exacerbated by bereavement and increasing frailty due to age. However, recently retired people often enjoy good health and have considerable energy which can be committed to the development of a lively and supportive community.

New towns

New towns differ from other neighbourhoods in that they are deliberately created and planned; housing, jobs, recreational facilities and social services are balanced to provide a planned 'social mix'. Some of the housing is available for private ownership and some is owned by the public authorities through the Development Corporation which is responsible for controlling the development and expansion of the area.

Conclusion

The term 'community care' implies a caring community, and assumes that 'the community' is a cohesive entity capable of

thought, decisions and action. The dangers of this assumption should be recognised, for, as has been shown in this chapter, communities are made up of individuals, and as the previous chapter showed, individuals respond differently to the various aspects of their environment.

Sociology is the study of groups, of social interaction and social behaviour. The concepts of sociology enable us to identify and understand in a patient those social experiences which most affect his behaviour, symptoms, perception of illness, and the strategies for coping with it. But it is important always to remember, as was stressed in Chapter 3, that in each individual the particular combination of these factors is unique.

References

1. Black D., Morris J. N., Smith C., Townsend P. (1980). *Inequalities in Health: Report of a Research Working Group.* London: HMSO.
2. Central Statistical Office (1975). Social Commentary: Social Class. In: *Social Trends 1975.* London: HMSO.
3. Douglas J. (1964). *The Home and the School.* London: McGibbon & Kee.
4. Central Advisory Council for Education (1967) (Plowden Report). *Children and their Primary Schools.* London: HMSO.
5. Ministry of Education (1963) (Robbins Report). *Higher Education: A Report of the Committee on Higher Education.* London: HMSO.
6. Newson J., Newson E. (1965). *Patterns of Infant Care in an Urban Community.* Harmondsworth: Penguin.
7. Newson J., Newson E. (1970). *Four Years Old in an Urban Community.* Harmondsworth: Penguin.
8. Martin J. (1978). *Infant Feeding 1975: Attitudes and Practice in England & Wales.* London: HMSO.
9. Bone M. (1975). *Family Planning Services in England and Wales.* London: HMSO.
10. Bernstein B. (1973). *Class, Codes and Control.* London: Routledge and Kegan Paul.
11. Bott E. (1971). *Family and Social Network.* 2nd ed. London: Tavistock.
12. Young M., Willmott P. (1962). *Family and Kinship in East London.* Harmondsworth: Penguin.
13. Goldthorpe J. H., Lockwood D. L., Bechofer F., Platt J. (1969). *The Affluent Worker in the Class Structure.* Cambridge University Press.
14. Brown G., Bhrolchain M., Harris T. (1975). Social class and psychiatric disorder among women in an urban population. *Sociology,* **9**, 2:225–55.
15. Tudor Hart J. (1971). The Inverse Care Law. *Lancet,* **i**:405–412.
16. Fletcher R. (1966). *The Family and Marriage in Britain.* Harmondsworth: Penguin.
17. Laing R. D., Esterton A. (1964). *Sanity, Madness & the Family.* Harmondsworth: Penguin.

18. Brown G. W., Birley J. L. T., Wing J. K. (1972). The influence of family life on the course of schizophrenic illness. *British Journal of Psychiatry*, **121**:241–58.
19. Parkes C. M., Benjamin B., Fitzgerald R. G. (1969). Broken heart: a statistical study of increased mortality among widowers. *British Medical Journal*, 1969, i:740–43.
20. Quinn S. (1981). Promise to care. In: Clark J., ed., *Readings in Community Health*. Edinburgh: Churchill Livingstone. (In Press.)

Suggestions for Further Reading

Anderson M., ed., (1971). *The Sociology of the Family*. Harmondsworth: Penguin.
Banton M. (1965). *Roles*. London: Tavistock.
Bott E. (1971). *Family & Social Network*. 2nd ed. London: Tavistock.
Butterworth E., Weir D. (1970). *The Sociology of Modern Britain*. London: Fontana.
Central Statistical Office. *Social Trends*. London: HMSO (published annually).
Chapman C. (1977). *Sociology for Nurses*. London: Bailliere Tindall.
Cuff E. C., Payne G. C., eds, (1979). *Perspectives in Sociology*. London: Allen & Unwin.
Fletcher R. (1966). *The Family and Marriage in Britain*. Harmondsworth: Penguin.
Frankenberg R. (1966). *Communities in Britain*. Harmondsworth: Penguin.
Henley A. (1979). *Asian Patients in Hospital and at Home*. Tunbridge Wells: Pitman.
Rex J., Moore W. (1967). *Race Community & Conflict*. Oxford: Oxford University Press
Susser M. W., Watson W. (1971). *Sociology in Medicine*. 2nd ed. London: Oxford University Press.
Townsend P. (1963). *The Family Life of Old People*. Harmondsworth: Penguin.
Tuckett D., ed., (1976). *An Introduction to Medical Sociology*. London: Tavistock.
Turkett D., Kaufert J. M. (1978). *Basic Readings in Medical Sociology*. London: Tavistock Publications.
Worsley P. (1970). *Introducing Sociology*. Harmondsworth: Penguin.
Worsley P. (1978). *Modern Sociology*. 2nd ed. Harmondsworth: Penguin. (Especially Part 8: Communities and cities).
Wright-Mills C. (1970). *The Sociological Imagination*. Harmondsworth: Penguin.
Young M., Willmott P. (1962). *Family and Kinship in East London*. Harmondsworth: Penguin.

Chapter 5

The Primary Care Setting

District nursing is not hospital nursing in a different environment. While the basic function of the nurse and many of the skills she uses are the same, the setting has a profound effect on the approach to care.

The role-reversal of community care

The concept of 'role' was discussed in Chapter 4 and the role which the patient plays as a 'sick person' was outlined in Chapter 3. It was suggested that social roles were learnt through the process of socialisation, the most important part of which was childhood experience in the family setting. The roles of patient, nurse, and doctor, however, are learnt mainly in the setting of the hospital, and the setting itself largely determines the way in which the roles are defined and played. The role-styles of the hospital, in which the professionals are all-powerful and the patient is a passive recipient, are, however, inappropriate for the community setting and have to be modified.

In one sense the roles of patient and nurse are actually reversed, for in the hospital setting the nurse is the 'host' and the patient the 'guest' while in the community setting the opposite is true: the patient is in his own territory which the nurse enters by invitation, not by right. This changes the locus of control; while it may be possible in the ward for a nurse to insist on a particular treatment and difficult for a patient to refuse, in the home a much more subtle approach is required. The patient is king of his own castle, and the nurse who fails to win the confidence and co-operation of the patient on her first visit may next time find the door shut in her face. Apart from the equipment she brings with her, all the equipment she uses—drugs and dressings prescribed by the doctor as well as the table on which she lays out a dressing pack, is the patient's personal property, not the nurse's. The nurse would do well to remember this before ruining the french-polished table by a carelessly placed spirit swab.

The isolation of a private home means that the district nurse carries a greater responsibility because there is no-one on the spot to whom she can immediately refer; she has to make her own decisions based on her individual professional judgement. Because she is frequently working single-handed she has to adapt such things as her lifting technique. Specialist services such as physiotherapy may not be available outside hospital and the district nurse may have to extend her role to fill the gaps; she may find herself playing the roles of physiotherapist, dietician, occupational therapist, home help and social worker, all rolled into one.

A third difference in role style arises from the fact that the nurse has continuous responsibility for the nursing care of her patients even though she is not with them all the time. In the community it is often the relatives who provide most of the nursing care between the nurse's visits. The nurse has to learn to share her role and the teaching component becomes relatively much more important.

The settings of district nursing

A considerable proportion of the district nurse's work is carried out in the setting of the patient's own home, but district nurses also work in community hospitals, in clinics of various kinds, in GPs' surgeries and treatment rooms, and in residential homes administered by social services departments. The proportion of first contacts with patients undertaken in the different settings is shown in Table 5.1. In each case the nurse's role changes slightly with the setting.

The most important part of the concept of *the community hospital* is that it is seen as a part of the community services and not an attempt to reproduce in miniature the activities of the specialist services of district general hospitals. Medical advice is provided by general practitioners not hospital consultants, and although most of the nursing staff may be appointed to work only in the community hospital, in many areas district nurses work on a rota basis partly in the hospital and partly outside. Ideally the community hospital provides services for patients needing full-time nursing care —including holiday admissions for those normally nursed at home—but not the specialist services of a District General Hospital. Such hospitals may provide day care services and rehabilitation services, and are linked to the health centre at which the general practitioners, health visitors and district nurses are based.

Clinic-based services of various kinds are provided by health

TABLE 5.1

The settings in which district nurses work

	1973		1979	
Place where first treatment during year took place	number of persons	proportion of all first treatments	number of persons	proportion of all first treatments
Patient's home	1 066 241	51·43	1 317 803	40·6
Health centre	303 082	14·62	986 348	30·4
GP premises	636 552	30·72	866 958	26·7
Maternity and child health centres	21 047	1·01	17 962	0·6
Hospital	13 773	0·7	12 159	0·4
Residential homes	17 044	0·9	29 870	0·9
Elsewhere	15 249	0·8	11 642	0·4
TOTAL	2 072 988	100	3 248 498	100

Source: Annual Reports of the DHSS

authorities either in their own premises or those belonging to general practitioners, and also by general practitioners themselves. The district nurse may find herself depending on her specialist skills and interests and on local facilities, giving immunisations in child health clinics, participating in family planning clinics, and—especially where her work-base includes a treatment room—running her own clinics for special purposes such as the treatment of varicose ulcers.

Most health centres, and an increasing number of general practitioner premises, include a *treatment room,* and sometimes a specialist treatment room nurse is employed to undertake nursing treatments such as dressings, removal of sutures and ear syringing. Sometimes however the 'treatment room service' is provided by the district nurse, and an increasing proportion of her contacts with patients is made in the treatment room rather than in the patient's own home (Table 5.1).

As the average age of residents in old people's home increases, and with it their frailty and need for nursing care, an increasing number of the district nurse's patients are nursed in this setting. In one sense the residential home is the patient's own home, but this setting also provides opportunities for work with groups of peo-

ple—both 'treatment room services' and many forms of rehabilitation and health education.

The district nurse is employed by the health authority and works in close co-operation with the general practitioner in all these settings. The organisational framework, however, varies, and with it some of the nurse's role relationships. Traditionally, district nurses were responsible for providing care for patients living within a defined geographical area. Increasingly since the mid-1960s, however, district nurses have worked as members of a team of doctors, nurses, health visitors and sometimes other specialists, providing services for all the patients who are registered with a particular general practitioner. This system is known as *attachment* to general practice, and the people who work together in this way are collectively described as the *primary health care team*.

Primary medical care

When medical help is sought, the person whom the patient first approaches is normally the general practitioner. Because it is the point of first contact, this part of our system of health care is called *primary medical care*. The general practitioner may request assistance in his diagnosis or treatment in the form of special investigations or the opinion of a colleague, or he may refer the patient to another doctor who is a specialist in the relevant field of illness. The specialist services, based on the hospital, to which the primary care doctors may refer his patient form the 'secondary' part of medical care. When intensive treatment at the secondary level has been completed, the patient returns to the primary level for continuing health supervision and care.

The system of primary medical care which has developed in this country is quite different from the system in other countries; in the USSR, for example, a patient would go to the nearest polyclinic, while in the United States he would decide for himself which specialist he needed and would approach the specialist directly.

General practitioners are not directly employed by health authorities as are other staff in the NHS, but are independent contractors who contract with the local Family Practitioner Committee to provide general medical services to people who register with them. They may also accept private patients in addition to NHS patients. Part of their income is in the form of basic allowances similar to salary, but a considerable proportion is made up of fees for 'items of service'; the money comes out of the central NHS

budget but is channelled through the Family Practitioner Committees and not through the health authorities. This gives the general practitioner considerable independence to decide the way in which services will be provided; for example he may build and equip his own premises and employ his own staff, including nurses, over whom he therefore has direct control.

More than 80 per cent of general practitioners work with other general practitioners in groups of between two and ten, although there are still many single-handed practitioners especially in urban areas. A group practice enables a more comprehensive service to be provided because doctors can deputise for one another for off-duty periods and facilities such as premises, equipment and staff can be shared.

About one sixth of general practitioners work in *health centres* owned by health authorities. One of the responsibilities laid on local health authorities by the NHS Act 1946 was to build health centres at which facilities would be available for general medical (general practitioner), general dental, and pharmaceutical services, and hospital outpatient sessions, together with the (then) local authority health and welfare services. For various reasons health centres were at first slow to develop, but by 1977 there were 824 health centres in operation in the United Kingdom.

The primary health care team

The aims of primary health care have been described as:

1 The promotion of health in its broadest terms, through education, support and the encouragement of self-care.
2 The prevention of ill-health by prophylaxis, early diagnosis, education and advice on the value of early contact with the primary health care services.
3 The care, treatment and rehabilitation of those who are acutely or chronically ill.
4 The referral of patients to specialist services where necessary, and the provision of continuing care following specialist treatment.[1]

The fact that these aims are far too wide to be achieved by any one person or any one discipline has led to the development of the concept of the multidisciplinary primary health care team. A BMA working party on primary health care teams[2] listed the advantages

of team care for both givers and recievers of care as follows:

1 Care given by a group is greater than the sum of individual care.
2 Rare skills are used most appropriately.
3 Peer influence and informal learning within the group raise the standards of care and the corporate status of the team in the community.
4 Team members have increased job satisfaction.
5 Team working encourages co-ordinated health education.
6 Team working lowers the prevalence of disease in the community.
7 The individual gets more efficient and understanding treatment when ill.

It would be difficult to prove some of these contentions, and some people would disagree with some of them, but it is reasonable to assume that a service provided by a team would be at least more comprehensive than a service provided by a single individual or by a single discipline. Lamb[3] has described a primary health care team as a partnership between individuals—each professional discipline having its own specific contribution to make—who were unable to meet present day needs in isolation and who came to realise the benefit that their co-operation could provide.

The members of the primary care team
The most effective composition and size of the nucleus of a team is much debated; the Harvard Davis Report[4] favoured basic units of one doctor supported by nurses and secretarial staff who all relate their work to a defined population, although for practical reasons these units would need to be organised in groups of five or six. In practice the size depends considerably on the number of general practitioners in a group practice and on what health authority staff are available. Nationally the ratio of district nurses to general practitioners is one to 1.7, and the ratio of health visitors is one to 2.4. The BMA[2] has distinguished between the 'nucleus' team composed of doctors, nurses, health visitors, social workers and medical secretaries, and the wider team which includes allied professions such as physiotherapists and pharmacists, the administrative auxiliaries such as receptionists and practice managers, and other services provided by hospitals, local authorities and voluntary agencies. Within the multidisciplinary team is the nursing team,

which consists of the health visitor, the midwife, the district nurse and the treatment room or practice nurse.

The *health visitor* is the team's expert in preventive health care. She* is required to be a state registered nurse, but some health visitors would argue that because of its historical independence and different approach from hospital nursing, health visiting ought to be regarded as a separate profession. She has a statutory responsibility to visit every baby born in her area or registered with the general practice to which she is attached, and to watch over each child's health and development until he reaches school age. But she is also a family visitor[5] who is concerned with the health of the whole family whether there are young children or not, and a considerable proportion of her work may be with elderly people. She visits families in their own homes either on her own initiative or at the request of other members of the team, other health and social agencies, or the family itself, or patients may come to see her at her work base or at the child health clinic. Her job is defined[5] as 'health education and social advice'—that is, to assess the individual or family's health needs, to offer advice or counselling, and to mobilise the resources of other services where necessary. Unlike the district nurse, her clientele is independent of the doctor's referral, and in addition to her work within the practice she is also responsible for work in child health clinics, formal health education in schools and other places, and, in many areas, for school nursing.

The *midwife* is the expert in the care of mothers before, during, and immediately after the birth of their babies, and in the care of the newborn baby. Midwives increasingly work in integrated maternity services which straddle hospital and primary care services, and in this sense could be regarded as part of the 'wider' team rather than the nucleus; but within the primary health care team they play an important role in the provision of antenatal and postnatal care in co-operation with the GP obstetrician.

The *district nurse* is the expert in the care of the sick at home although she also works in other settings (Table 5.1). The SRN district nurse—who is often referred to as the district nursing sister—is responsible, like the ward sister in hospital, for deciding the nursing care which each patient needs and for seeing that it is carried out. She is the leader of a nursing team which includes

---

* Until 1973 only women were allowed to become health visitors; the proportion of men in health visiting is still very small.

SENs and nursing auxiliaries, to whom she delegates work as appropriate; she is accountable for the work delegated to them in addition to her own work.

The SEN district nurse may have her own caseload, but she remains accountable to the SRN for the care given to patients, although this issue is much disputed among district nurses of both grades. Hockey[6] found that although SENs did more basic nursing than SRNs, there was nothing that the SRN did that was not at some time done by an SEN, the level of responsibility fluctuating in response to expediency. Following this report attempts have been made to produce a clearer definition of the role and function of the SEN[10] and since Hockey's report also demonstrated how much of the work of district nurses did not require their professional skills, many more nursing auxiliaries have been employed.

Since 1947 male nurses have been accepted for district nurse training but they comprise only a small proportion of the total district nursing workforce. Depending on the number available within a health authority they may be attached to group practices or work on a geographical basis. Although many have as their main responsibility genito-urinary work with male patients, it is becoming increasingly common for the male nurse to care for female patients; before this is planned, however, it should be agreed with the patient concerned, recognising and respecting different people's prejudices and cultural backgrounds.

Some health authorities provide a 24 hour nursing service in which the evening and night hours are covered by nurses specially recruited for this purpose. The number of staff available is usually small so care in the selection of patients for referral for night care is essential. Where there is no special service the district nursing team will meet patients' needs as far as it is possible to do so by staggering their working hours or by 'on-call' rota systems.

The factors which the district nurse must consider in allocating the work among the various members of her team are discussed in more detail in Chapter 8.

In some very rural areas the work of the health visitor, the midwife and the district nurse may be undertaken by one person, who is often called a 'triple-duty' nurse. Occasionally the duties of district nurse and midwife are combined. The nurse who undertakes combined duties must be appropriately qualified in each speciality.

The *treatment room nurse* may be employed by the health author-

ity and attached to a general practice in the same way as the health visitor or district nurse, or she may be directly employed by the general practitioner under the terms of service[7] which allow him to employ 'ancillary staff' and to be re-imbursed for 70 per cent of their salaries; the directly employed nurse is usually called the *practice nurse.* Reedy[8] has studied the historical development of the private employment of practice nurses, and has compared their work and their occupational characteristics with those of attached district nurses.

In some areas a *social worker* employed by the social services department is attached to general practice in the same way as nurses. There is still a good deal of mutual distrust between doctors and social workers, and social workers have been less ready than nurses to accept the concept of attachment because they see it as a threat to their professional autonomy. However, a number of notable accounts[9] have demonstrated the contribution that social work can make to patient care within the context of the primary health care team.

Without the support of *administrative staff* the professionals in the primary health care team would be unable to function. This group of staff includes receptionists, secretaries, and in some large practices practice managers. Sometimes tensions arise between lay staff and nurses where a member of the lay staff such as the receptionists—who is sometimes an ex-nurse—takes on what the nurses perceive as nursing duties or offers patients advice on matters which the nurses believe to be more appropriate to professionals.

The wider team
The wider team with whom nurse members of the nucleus team must maintain close contact includes:

Other community-based nurses
Specialist nurses
Hospital nurses
Volunteers

Other community-based nurses include school nurses, clinic nurses, and family planning nurses. These services are briefly described in Appendix 2. They also include nurses working in occupational health services which, although they are outside the

administrative framework and finance of the NHS, make an important contribution to community-based health care.

Specialist nurses include, among others, the community psychiatric nurse, the domiciliary family planning nurse, the specialist paediatric nurse, and the stoma therapist. The district nurse works with patients of all age groups who have a wide range of medical and surgical conditions and a variety of nursing problems, and she must recognise that she cannot hope to develop and maintain expertise in all specialist fields. She will therefore need to seek advice from others with up-to-date specialist knowledge, using them as 'consultants' both for advice and referral, similar to the ways in which general practitioners use hospital consultants; the other disciplines represented within the primary care team are a resource which should be used in the same manner.

The Society of Primary Health Care Nursing of the Royal College of Nursing identifies two groups of patient needs which can best be met by specialist intervention: those where a different basic training is required, and those where the problem concerned is relatively rare in general district nursing practice.[11] An example of the former kind of specialist is the community psychiatric nurse who provides support and specialised care for patients with a psychiatric illness; the CPN may provide care to those who have received treatment as in-patients but have now returned home, those who are receiving treatment as day patients or out-patients, and those who can be treated by the general practitioner in the community without hospital referral. An example of the latter kind is the stoma therapist who offers an advisory service to patients with a colostomy, ileostomy or an ileal conduit. This kind of specialist nurse is usually based in the specialist department of the hospital, but although most of her work is carried out in the wards and outpatient department she may also make follow up visits to former patients in their own homes.

The use of specialist nurses in primary health care is an issue which provokes considerable debate. The district nurse needs to be aware of the availability of such services in her locality and should be willing to seek advice or to transfer care where appropriate. Concern is however felt, as noted in the Rcn report, where specialist nurses are used 'to give a type of care which it should be possible for every district nursing team to give, provided that the size of caseload allows the time to give each patient of this type the appropriate level of care.'[11]

Another group of nurses who are hospital based but whose role is different from that of the specialist nurse are *liaison nurses*. These nurses are appointed specifically to promote continuity of care between hospital and community when patients are discharged from hospital. They are often associated with a specialty such as paediatrics but do not provide specialist care as such. Their role is to visit the wards on a regular basis, to collect information concerning the nursing care of patients who are about to leave hospital but who will require continued care or supervision, and to relay this information to the nurse member of the primary care team who will be responsible for providing this care.

Even if such liaison staff are available, however, and particularly where they are not, the nursing members of primary care teams need to maintain close contact with their hospital-based colleagues. The district nurse needs to be able to *give* information to hospital staff about patients for whom she has been caring before their admission to hospital, and also to *receive* information directly from ward staff to enable her to continue care after a patient has been discharged.

This 'wider team' also includes *volunteers*. The contribution of the family and neighbours to care, and the importance of the nurse's willingness to share her role with them has already been stressed. In particular, 'night sitter' and 'good neighbour' services are invaluable in meeting needs which are far beyond the resources of the statutory services.

The concept of a team

A team is more than a collection of individuals; it implies that a number of people are working co-operatively together to achieve a common goal. MacIntosh has defined a team as 'a group of people with diverse but related knowledge and skills who associate for the purpose of directing, co-ordinating and developing the separate parts as well as the sum total of their expertise in order to create new, and maximise existing opportunities for achieving their common goals'[12]. It has been pointed out that the attachment of nursing staff to general practice does not itself constitute the creation of a primary health care team, and that teamwork can be encouraged but it cannot be created by managerial decision.[1] In their study of the work of the nursing team in general practice sponsored by the Council for the Education and Training of Health Visitors, Gilmore *et al.*[13] commented 'there is a widespread assumption amongst

administrators and practitioners that when health visitors and district nurse have been attached to general practitioners, teamwork will automatically evolve. The findings of this study suggest that such a development may not occur without conscious planning based on the promotion of awareness amongst all team members of what is involved in teamwork and of the factors which hinder and accelerate the process'.

The dynamics of teamwork

The effectiveness of multi-disciplinary teams, including the primary health care team, is much debated; it would seem that the characteristics of good teamwork are well known but inadequately applied. Gilmore *et al.* list four requirements:

1   The members of a team share a common purpose which binds them together and guides their actions.
2   Each member of the team has a clear understanding of his own functions, appreciates and understands the contributions of other professions, and recognises common interests.
3   The team works by pooling knowledge, skills, and resources, and all members share responsibility for outcome.
4   The effectiveness of the team is related to its capabilities to carry out its work and its ability to manage itself as an independent group of people.

The Chief Nursing Officer's letter on primary health care nursing[1] adds a very important fifth requirement.

5   A mutually agreed system for communication and referral both within the team and between the team and other agencies.

Common purpose and goals

Teamwork involves the definition of common goals and the development of a plan of action in which each member makes a different but complementary contribution towards the achievement of the team's aims. In a primary health care team this includes general goals related to meeting the needs of the practice population and specific goals related to the care of individual patients. Because the perspectives and values of the various professions differ, there will sometimes be disagreement over the goals to be set at both

levels; for example the doctor may not welcome the extra work-load which the health visitor's case-finding activities create. Conflict is not necessarily destructive, but problems have to be talked through frankly for agreement to be reached, and it is not helpful if team members deal with it, as Gilmore *et al.* found, by simply going their own ways. Each individual professional must set her own goals for patients within her care, but in doing so must take account of and share in the achievement of team goals.

Understanding different roles

Professional roles are learned alongside the appropriate knowledge and skills during the process of professional training, and the process of socialisation which takes place during this time is as influential in respect of professional attitudes and behaviour as are the experiences of childhood in other attitudes and behaviour. Unfortunately, because the different health care professionals have quite separate educational programmes, their understanding of one another's roles may be very limited.[1] Moreover, at the same time as the student professional is learning his own role, he is also developing ideas about the roles of other people around him—as he sees them performed in the setting in which the learning takes place. Medical students and nursing students learn the roles of doctor and nurse in the setting of an acute general hospital where their goals and values will reflect the purpose of the institition—which is curing patients afflicted by serious acute illness; and their relationship with each other is one of 'director' and 'assistant' in the function of curing. Although these role styles are no longer appropriate in the primary care setting, where the illness conditions and the needs of patients are very different, they may persist. Thus the doctor may regard the health visitor's routine surveillance of healthy children as 'a waste of time', the health visitor may regard the district nurse as 'incapable' of social assessment and health education. Gilmore *et al.*[13] and Milne[14] have found that serious misconceptions about one anothers' roles abound among team members.

Unless each member of the team understands and appreciates the roles and functions of the others, there will be gaps, duplications, and inconsistencies in the care available to patients. It is inevitable that roles will overlap, and it is important that they do, but there must be agreement, based on discussion among team members,

about who does what in what circumstances, and there must be sufficient trust to enable a patient to be 'shared' or referred.

Pooling knowledge and skills

Each professional has his own particular area of expertise, but there are many tasks, e.g. supportive counselling and referral to other agencies, which can and should be undertaken by whichever member of the team is in direct contact with the patient. Close liaison is essential to avoid conflicting advice, and each member of the team should be able to use the expertise of the others by using them as consultants.

One mechanism for pooling knowledge and skills, and ensuring at the same time the close liaison which is necessary to avoid duplication and gaps, is the *case conference,* in which the members of the team involved with a particular patient discuss their individual assessments of the patient's needs and the possible strategies for meeting them, and agree a common plan of care.

Team management

If a team is to function as a cohesive unit it must have the ability to manage itself as a unit, including the mechanisms for achieving this; this aspect might be called the team's internal management. The need for common aims and policies, which can be arrived at only by discussion and agreement between members, has already been stressed. A critical question, however, is 'Who leads the team?' The role of leader is closely linked with status, authortiy and power. A difference in status between doctors and nurses is often felt by both and acted upon in a way which inhibits the achievement of true professional partnership and a complementary approach to patient care; for example Gilmore et al.[14] found that in team discussions nurses initiated less, spoke less, and rarely disagreed with the doctors. In the primary health care team the doctor often takes the leadership role on the assumption which is made both by doctors and by nurses that it is 'natural' and 'right' for him to do so. Doctors tend to justify this situation—if they think about it at all—on the basis of their comprehensive responsibility for patients, but the real reason often lies in the role perceptions learnt by both doctors and nurses in the hospital setting. Leadership within any team is a matter for the team itself to decide, and it is important that the issues of leadership, authority, and co-ordination of team action are consciously considered rather than taken for granted.

Although nurses are members of the team and are directly involved in its internal management, they are also, as employees of the health authority, managerially responsible and accountable to a nurse manager who is outside the team. Sometimes this causes tensions within the team, especially where the general practitioner, who is not managerially accountable to anyone because he is an independent contractor, does not understand either the nursing management structure or the differences between nursing and medical services which make it necessary. The tension may be increased, and the role relationships become even more complex, if the team includes both attached nurses who are managerially accountable to a nursing officer, and a directly employed practice nurse who is managerially accountable to the doctor because she is directly employed by him. It is usually in the determination of priorities or the allocation of work that these tensions become visible, not in the area of direct patient care.

Such conflicts can only be resolved by frank discussion. Perhaps the best guideline is given by Henderson in her well known discussion of the role of the nurse.[17] 'No one member of the team should make such heavy demands on another member that any one of them is unable to perform his or her unique function . . . All members of the team should consider the person (patient) served as the central figure and should realise that they are all "assisting" him.'

Communication

The necessity for good communication among team members is implicit in the need to agree common purposes, to understand one another's roles, to pool knowledge, to develop co-ordinated plans of care for individual patients, and to resolve tensions and conflicts. In other words, achievement of all the characteristics of good team-work which have been discussed depends upon good communication. Good communication requires not only a willingness to communicate and a recognition by all the team members of the importance of communication, but also appropriate and easy-to-use channels for communication, and—perhaps most important of all—time. One of the advantages of a health centre or good practice premises is that members of the team are on the same premises and this facilitates informal face-to-face interaction, but it is often assumed—wrongly—that this obviates the need for more formal communication. It is important that there are recognised systems and mechanisms, including time specially set aside for the purpose,

for meetings of the team and of sub-groups within it both for joint discussion of individual patients and for discussions relating to the policies and management of the team as a whole.

An important issue in team communication is the use of records, and in particular the problems of confidentiality which this raises. These problems are discussed in more detail in Chapters 9 and 22. Access to one another's records is important for the planning and implementation of a co-ordinated plan of care for an individual patient, and in some teams all the notes relating to a particular patient are kept together and the whole team records information on the same document.

Conclusion

The extent and methods of inter-disciplinary co-operation in primary health care vary greatly from one part of the country to another. The development of primary health care teams is poor where, for example, the numbers of nursing staff employed are insufficient, where general practitioners do not accept this concept of care, where they work in single-handed practices rather than group practices, where it is impossible to provide adequate accommodation to enable staff of different professions to work from the same premises, where there is considerable overlap of the geographical areas covered by general practitioners, and in inner city areas where there are special health and social problems.

It is important to recognise, however, that teamwork does not necessarily depend on attachment, and equally that attachment does not of itself create teamwork. Whatever the local and practical difficulties, the importance of the concepts of a multi-disciplinary approach to patient care and of co-operative patterns of working is undiminished.

References

1. DHSS (1977). *Nursing in Primary Health Care.* (CNO(77)8). London: HMSO.
2. British Medical Association Board of Education and Science (1974). *Report of the Panel on Primary Health Care Teams.* London: British Medical Association.
3. Lamb A. (1977). *Primary Health Nursing.* London: Bailliere.
4. DHSS and Welsh Office (1971). *The Organisation of Group Practice: A Report of a Sub-committee of the Standing Medical Advisory Committee* (Harvard Davis Report) London: HMSO.
5. Ministry of Health, Department of Health for Scotland, and Ministry of Education (1956). *An Enquiry into Health Visiting* (Jameson Report). London: HMSO.

6. Hockey L. (1972). *Use and Abuse?* London: Queen's Institute for District Nurses.
7. DHSS (1972). *NHS (General medical and pharmaceutical services) Regulations.* Schedule 1 Part 1, 16 (2). London: HMSO.
8. Reedy B. *et al.* (1980). The social and occupational characteristics of attached and employed nurses in general practice and a comparison of the activities and opinions of attached and employed nurses. *Journal of the RCGP;* **30:** 477–489.
9. For example: Forman J., Fairbairn E.M. (1968). *Social Casework in General Practice.* Oxford University Press.
   Goldberg E.M., Neill J. (1972). *Social Work in General Practice.* London: Allen and Unwin.
10. Panel of Assessors for District Nurse Training (1980). *Report of the Education and Training of District Nurses (SEN).* London: DHSS.
11. Royal College of Nursing (1980). *Primary Health Care Nursing: A Team Approach.* (Report of a working party of the Rcn Society of Primary Health Care Nursing.) London: Royal College of Nursing.
12. McIntosh J.B. (1974). Communication in teamwork: a lesson from the district. *Nursing Times* 1970, 85–88.
13. Gilmore M., Bruce N., Hunt M. (1974) *The Work of the Nursing Team in General Practice.* London: Council for the Education and Training of Health Visitors.
14. Milne A. (1979). Students views of the primary health care team. *Nursing Times* (Occasional Papers); **75,** 28: 113–116.
15. Henderson V. (1960). *Basic Principles of Nursing Care.* Geneva: I.C.N.

Further Reading

Bloomfield R., Follis P. (1974). *The Health Team in Action.* London: BBC Publications.
Fry J., ed. (1977). *Trends in General Practice 1977.* London: British Medical Association.
Hicks D. (1976). *Primary Medical Care.* London: HMSO.
Gilmore M., Bruce N. Hunt (1974). *The Work of the Nursing Team in General Practice.* London: Council for the Education and Training of Health Visitors.
Royal College of Nursing (1980). *Primary Health Care Nursing: A Team Approach.* (Report of a Working Party of the Rcn Society of Primary Health Care Nursing.) London: Royal College of Nursing.

Section II

Approaches to Care

Section 1 described the setting in which the district nurse works, and this section will consider approaches to care at home. Florence Nightingale (1859)[1] wrote 'I do not pretend to teach her how, I ask her to teach herself, and for this purpose I venture to give some hints', and following this precedent guidelines and principles are offered, but not details of techniques nor a prescriptive approach.

Chapter 6 looks at the question 'What is district nursing?' and gives a brief outline of the nursing process approach to care. This problem solving approach provides a logical framework for the care of patients and their families and it forms the core of 'The Curriculum in District Nursing for State Registered Nurses and Registered General Nurses'[2] on which all district nurse education and training will be based after September 1981. Many readers will be familiar with the nursing process as used in hospital, and there is therefore no attempt to give a detailed account of the process itself, but rather to present its particular application to district nursing. The application of the nursing process to the care of the seven patients who serve as our examples is included in Chapters 7–11, each chapter dealing with a stage of the process. It is only possible to deal with a few of the problems that may arise with these patients, and it would be a useful learning exercise for readers to identify other problems which could arise in any stage of the sen patients who serve as our examples is included in beginning of this section, Chapters 12–17 devote more attention to some of the special groups of people who require care at home.

Some Health Authorities will have established the nursing process in the district nursing service, others will be in the early stages of its introduction while others will not have begun. The introduction of a new system of nursing care requires a commit-

ment from all concerned, but it is worthwhile taking trouble to gain this commitment because it eventually leads to an improvement in the quality of care. Change is often uncomfortable and initially time has to be spent on discussion, but a critical evaluation of the current nursing practice showing that this is not change for the sake of change. It was no accident that the nursing process was chosen as the framework for the district nursing curriculum: it was adopted because it was felt that this method would increase the standard of care provided by the nursing team.

When change is being inaugurated it is important to look at what is good and worth preserving in the present system and to see if there is a present foundation on which to build a new system. Many district nurses have always used some of the skills required for the nursing process, but some will need to develop certain new skills and attitudes in the provision of care.

References

1. Nightingale F. (1859. Facsimile ed. 1970). *Notes on Nursing.* London: Duckworth.
2. Panel of Assessors for District Nurse Training (1978). *Curriculum in District Nursing for State Registered Nurses and Registered General Nurses.* London: Department of Health and Social Security.

Chapter 6

The Nature of District Nursing

The patient profiles at the beginning of this book give examples of patients and their families requiring the services of a district nurse. Most district nurses will 'recognise' these patients and know that what seems to be the straightforward care required by Mr Evans may turn out to be complicated but in the case of John Davis the district nurse may find she has a minimal role because of the part played by the patient and his parents. Care provided by the district nurse may be relatively simple or involve not only physical needs but a whole range of psychological and social needs as could well be so with Mrs Baker and her family.

Before discussing the methods of care for these and other patients it seems worthwhile to consider first what is district nursing. The well-known definition of nursing by Henderson[1] serves as a good basis for discussion. She states:

> The unique function of the nurse is to assist the individual, sick or well, in the performance of those activities contributing to health or its recovery (or to peaceful death) that he would perform unaided if he had the necessary strength, will or knowledge. And to do this in such a way as to help him gain independence as rapidly as possible.

Two other definitions that complement Henderson's are those given by Orem[2] and Rogers[3]. Orem states that:

> The condition which validates the existence of a requirement for nursing in an adult is the absence of the ability to maintain for himself continuously that amount and quality of *self-care* which is therapeutic in sustaining life and health, in recovering from disease or injury, or in coping with their effects . . . Self-care is an adult's personal continuous contribution to his health and well-being.

Self-care, therefore, is the care that everyone requires each day which includes the care of the person and where appropriate the following of medical directives.

Rogers definition states that:

> Nursing aims to assist people in achieving their maximum health potential. Maintenance and promotion of health, prevention of disease, nursing diagnosis, intervention and rehabilitation encompasses the scope of nursing's goals. Nursing is concerned with people—all people—well and sick, rich and poor, young and old.

There are several factors common to each of these definitions. Firstly, the implication that nursing is *assisting* the patient with those activities he would normally do for himself, which itself implies complementing the person's abilities and compensating for his disabilities. Such assistance may involve:

Acting for or doing for the patient;
Guiding the patient;
Supporting the patient physically, psychologically and socially;
Providing an environment that promotes personal development;
Teaching the patient and the family.

All of these activities involve working *with* the patient, who may be deficient in quantity or quality of self-care; and these deficiencies may be physical, social or psychological. Assisting the patient with the activities he would normally do for himself implies that the care for each person must be planned on an individual basis and in order to do this the nurse must tactfully find out how the patient usually lives.

Shetland[4] describes nursing as a process which is:

> '. . . one of interaction. The nurse enters imaginatively and sensitively into the lives of the people she serves in order to understand their health needs, determine the perception of their needs, reconcile the difference between the two sets of perceptions and institute appropriate nursing measures in interaction with the recipient(s) of her service'

Means of interaction with patients will be discussed subsequently but this definition again shows the importance of working *with* the patient and his family. For example if Mrs Adams believes that it is best for her husband to be left in bed and the district nurse believes

it is preferable for him to be turned regularly and sat out of bed for part of the day there will be conflict until the varying points of view are reconciled. It is obviously not always possible to make all the decisions about care with the patient and/or his family but it is important they are involved in the planning whenever possible. Such involvement is always desirable but is particularly important when the patient is cared for in his own home because most of the care is provided by the patient himself or his family.

Figure 6.1 shows how much a patient and his family were involved in his care following amputation of a limb for diabetic gangrene.[5] Apart from the immediate post-operative period the patient and family 'gave' more care than any other person. This would appear to be a typical picture for the majority of patients cared for at home; the district nurse may visit once, twice or even three times a day and during her visit may give intense nursing care, but this is a small part of the twenty-four hours.

Common to the three definitions of nursing is the fact that the nurse is not only working with the sick but also with the well and that she has a role in the prevention of ill-health and the promotion of health. The district nurse is invariably in a good position to carry out this aspect of her work, with the people directly under her care and also with their families or with members of the wider community. The preventive aspect is stressed by the well known definition of health by the World Health Organisation which states: 'Health is a state of physical, social and mental well-being not merely the absence of disease'.

People's perceptions of health may vary according to their experiences, expectations, age, activities and interests (Chapter 3); for example John, in spite of his disability and with his considerable degree of dependence, may say he feels 'well' once he has adapted to his limitation, whereas Mr Evans may complain of feeling 'poorly' with far less physical disability because he has not adapted to the breakdown in his usual health pattern which limits his normal activities. This comparison emphasises the need for an individual approach to care for each patient.

Individual care and the nursing process

Many would argue that because the district nurse visits one patient at a time her care is individual, but this is not necessarily so, for the care given may be centered on the disease or the task in hand and be merely ritualistic. However, in order to fulfil the criteria outlined

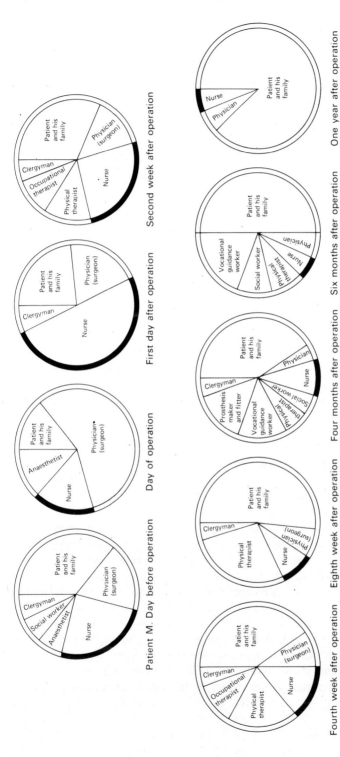

Fig. 6.1. The changing importance of the nurse's role as rehabilitation progresses in the case of a young man having a leg amputated.

above, more is required; it is necessary to discover the patients normal life style, habits and preferences and then identify his problems. The next step is to set the goals of care *in conjunction with* the patient then plan to meet these goals; subsequently carry out the care and finally check that the goals have been achieved. This is the approach known as the nursing process and a brief outline follows.

Jones[6] states that the nursing process is 'an interactive, problem solving, decision making procedure for assessing, identifying, selecting and implementing approaches and evaluating results in relation to the care of the ill or potentially ill person'. It can be seen that this definition provides a logical framework for nursing care and is based on four main stages:

1. Assessment
2. Planning
3. Implementation
4. Evaluation

The assessment stage involves the nurse in gathering, analysing and synthesising pertinent information from all sources, and from this information identifying the problems that are amenable to nursing action. Having identified the problems the nurse can then, in conjunction with the patient, determine the desired goals of care and plan to achieve these. The planning stage is followed by the implementation of the specific measures decided upon, and the final step is the evaluation and determination as to whether the goals have been achieved. The evaluation may result in new information being available, leading to a modification in the initial assessment, and this might change the problems identified and require a restatement of goals and a subsequent change of plan. Thus the nursing process needs to be seen as an ongoing cyclical process rather than one that neatly proceeds from one stage to the next.

This problem solving approach is an orderly and systematic way of providing nursing care. It should not remove any spontaneity from care giving, in fact if a plan for care is carefully made it can save time and allow for the unexpected. The nursing process can be used for patients requiring short-term care, but is of particular value for those patients needing long-term care which tend to predominate in the caseload of the district nurse. If this systematic approach is used universally the quality of information will be

improved and faults in communication when transferring patients to and from hospital will be diminished.

Through the use of the nursing process the district nurse can identify her unique contribution, plan the patient's care and be master of her work. This accords with Henderson's[1] comment: 'This aspect of her work, this part of her function, she initiates and controls; of this she is master'.

The role and function of the district nurse

The role and function of the district nurse can now be clarified. Her *role* is the part she plays in relation to other members of the caring team and her *function* is the job she does, which can be summarised as the provision of skilled nursing care for any person living in the community. The definition of the district nurse as given by the Chief Nursing Officer at the DHSS[7] emphasises the many aspects of her role and function. She states:

> The District Nurse is a SRN who has received post-basic training in order to enable her to give skilled nursing care to all persons living in the community including in residential homes. She is the leader of the district nursing team within the primary health care services. Working with her may be SRNs, SENs and nursing auxiliaries. It is the District Nurse who is professionally accountable for assessing and re-assessing the needs of the patient and family, and for monitoring the quality of care. It is her responsibility to ensure that help, including financial and social, is made available as appropriate. The District Nurse delegates tasks as appropriate to SENs, who can thus have their own caseload, but who remain wholly accountable to the District Nurse for the care that they give to patients. The District Nurse is accountable for the work undertaken by nursing auxiliaries who carry out such tasks as bathing, dressing frail ambulant patients, and helping other members of the team with patient care.

The Scottish Home and Health Department, in a report on the work of the district nurse in 1978[8], listed the following capabilities that were required in addition to professional knowledge and skills:

Making independent professional judgements
Taking decisions on nursing matters
Accepting responsibility and exercising authority

Taking action in an emergency pending medical intervention
Acting independently
Establishing and maintaining good personal relationships
Reflecting objectively and logically
Thinking in abstract and planning ahead.

These two accounts of the work of the district nurse complement one another and both emphasise her responsibilities and her accountability for the care carried out by herself and others in the nursing team and both show the need to develop and maintain good personal relationships and managerial skills.

The district nurse has several roles in the giving of care. She has an independent role where she is responsible for the initiation of nursing care, for example, she makes a nursing decision that Mrs Baker's mouth needs care because it is dry due to an inadequate fluid intake. On the other hand for some work she has a dependent role when she gives medication prescribed by the general practitioner. Above all she has an intermediary role when working in collaboration with other workers, for example, many services and personnel will need to be co-ordinated in the provision of care for John.

The district nurse works with other members of the primary care team and is also often involved with hospital and social service personnel, as well as voluntary workers. Within the team the contribution of any particular member may predominate at any time according to the circumstances; for example, the district nurse is the paramount person in the care of Mrs Cray while her ulcers require intensive treatment but if these heal the social worker may well play a more significant role. In the case of Alison the health visitor may be the person to provide continuous support for the family but in an acute episode the role of the district nurse may become crucial. The independent, dependent and intermediary roles may all be integrated in the care of a single patient. The district nurse may make independent decisions about the positioning of Mr Fisher in his wheelchair to prevent pressure sores from occurring; his weekly injection of cytamen is determined by the general practitioner; and the district nurse liaises with the personnel from the Social Services Department to discuss the provision of aids and adaptations to the home.

It is important that district nurses, as members of a team, work out a personal philosophy for themselves concerning their various

roles, for only when they have done this can they develop a commitment to care. Traditionally in hospital as nurses become more senior they perform the more complex technical tasks; however, the district nurse is in the unique position of having only one patient to care for at a time, and carries out the whole range of care. Much of the work of the district nurse is what is commonly called 'basic nursing care' which in hospital all too frequently is left to junior nurses or auxiliaries; but what can give more satisfaction to the nurse, and benefit to the patient than to be able to give and receive total care from one person. This is quintessential nursing.

References

1. Henderson V. (1960. Revised 1969). *Basic Principles of Nursing Care*. Geneva: International Council of Nurses; pp. 12–13.
2. Orem D. (1971). *Nursing Concepts of Practice*. London: Collier Macmillan; pp. 2 and 6.
3. Rogers M. E. (1970). *An Introduction to the Theoretical Basis of Nursing*. Philadelphia: F A Davis; p. 86.
4. Shetland M. L. (1965). Teaching and Learning in Nursing. *American Journal of Nursing*; **9**: 112.
5. Henderson V. (1966). *The Nature of Nursing*. London: Collier Macmillan.
6. Jones C. (1977). The nursing process—individualised care. *Nursing Mirror* Oct. 13 1977: 13–14.
7. Department of Health and Social Security (1977). *Nursing in Primary Health Care*. CNO (77) **8**: 2.
8. Scottish Home and Health Department. (1978). *District Nursing in Scotland*. (Chairman, Hockey L.) Edinburgh: HMSO; p. 18.

Further Reading

Hunt J. M., Marks-Maran D. J. (1980). *Nursing Care Plans: The Nursing Process at Work*. Aylesbury: H. M. and M. Publishers.
Marriner A. (1978). *The Nursing Process: A Scientific Approach to Nursing Care*. 2nd ed. St Louis: C. V. Mosby.
Mayers M. G. (1978). *A Systematic Approach to the Nursing Care Plan*. 2nd ed. New York: Appleton-Century-Crofts.
McFarlane J. K. (1976). A charter for caring. *Journal of Advanced Nursing;* **1**, 3: 187–196.
Tinkham C. W., Voorhies E. F. (1977). *Community Health Nursing: Evolution and Process*. 2nd ed. New York: Appleton-Century-Crofts.

Chapter 7

Assessment of Need

In order to provide realistic care it is important to get to know the patient, his family, and the community in which he lives. For example, Mr Adam's care will be different from that required by a 56-year-old with the same degree of physical disability cared for by a young, fit wife living in a bungalow with all modern facilities. Differences between patients, with regard to their families, their environments and their lifestyles, affect and determine the care to be given. The district nurse needs to find out about these details in order to plan and give the best possible care, and assessment is the first stage of the nursing process. It begins with the collection of all the information about a patient having implications for nursing action and ends with a statement of the patient's problems. The aim of the assessment stage is to obtain sufficient information on which to plan a programme of care designed to meet the physical, social and emotional needs of the patient.

Information required

In considering what information is required to make the nursing plan it is necessary to look again at the aim of district nursing. If it is agreed that those aims include 'assisting the patient in those activities which he would normally do for himself' it is clearly necessary to know what those activities were. Therefore it follows that the most important information is that which concerns the patient's normal daily routine and behaviour, for only when this is known can a programme acceptable to the patient be drawn up. If Mrs Cray always had her main meal at night it is of little avail trying to get her to have 'Meals on Wheels' in the middle of the day. Although Mr Adams has difficulty in communicating, his wife can tell the nurse about the fluids he normally drinks; if the nurse does not find out this information she may well be advising something like 'plenty of milk', which he abhors.

Apart from the physical and environmental needs of the patient, the assessment should include information about possible

psychological and social needs. John may well need counselling on his enforced lack of sexual activity and if the district nurse has not the will, ability or training herself to deal with this problem then she has a duty to ensure that advice is given by another appropriately qualified person. The emotional and financial needs of patients may very well be interrelated with their physical needs, and it is important that in dealing with the complex problems of the Baker family that all aspects are taken into consideration; concentration on the physical needs at the expense of other factors means failure to give total care.

A complete assessment involves information gathered by the district nurse, which forms the nursing history. In addition the assessment should include information from medical records, referral notification from hospital, information from other health workers and information gathered by observation of the patient, family and environment.

The nursing history

District nurses are in a unique and privileged position to gain information about the patient, his family and his environment. Visiting the patient in his own home enhances a free exchange of information, and the district nurse probably gains more knowledge about the patient and his family than most health workers. But for the information to be of use it needs to be written down and available to others involved in the care of the patient.

The nursing history differs from the medical history in that it is required to form a basis for planning *nursing* care and concentrates on the effect of illness rather than on the illness itself. Nevertheless, the medical history and the nursing history should be complementary to one another. The actual taking of a nursing history enables the district nurse to learn about the patient and his normal lifestyle and is a beginning of the nurse-patient relationship. If this is done well time will ultimately be saved, as the information obtained will be available to others caring for the patient.

To be sure that all aspects of need are considered it is advisable to use a recognised layout which will probably be a printed form or Kardex, the design of which will differ in various Health Authorities. It is important that the design of such a form is developed by the staff using it since it needs to reflect their philosophy for care and local idiosyncrasies.

Henderson[1] lists 14 needs of all people which she feels form the

components of basic nursing care. The nurse may need to assist the patient with these functions or provide conditions that will enable him to:

1   Breathe normally.
2   Eat and drink adequately.
3   Eliminate by all avenues of elimination.
4   Move and maintain desirable posture (walking, sitting, lying and changing from one to the other).
5   Sleep and rest.
6   Select suitable clothing, dress and undress.
7   Maintain body temperature within normal range, adjusting clothing and modifying the environment.
8   Keep the body clean and well groomed and protect the integument.
9   Avoid dangers in the environment and avoid injuring others.
10 Communicate with others in expressing emotions, needs, fears etc.
11 Worship according to his faith.
12 Work at something that provides a sense of accomplishment.
13 Play, or participate in various forms of recreation.
14 Learn, discover or satisfy the curiosity that leads to 'normal' development and health.

If it is agreed that this list covers the needs of each person then it is possible to use these fourteen components as headings on the patient assessment chart, and under each heading there will be a record of how the patient is coping with the activity in question. It is important that all staff understand what each heading includes; for example although integument is primarily the skin it also includes coverings such as the mucus membrane, hair and nails. The terminology in the Henderson list is American but it does have the advantage of covering the range of physical, psychological, spiritual and social needs of all people.

This links with Maslow's[2] hierarchy of needs where he suggests that an individual operates on ascending levels and that once the lower needs have been satisfied they lose their urgency and then the person requires his needs at a higher level to be met (see Fig. 7.1).

When a person is sick it is generally the physiological needs that take precedence, but it is important that all these needs are recognised; for example, with Mr Adams it would be all too easy to concentrate on his problem of immobility and incontinence but it is

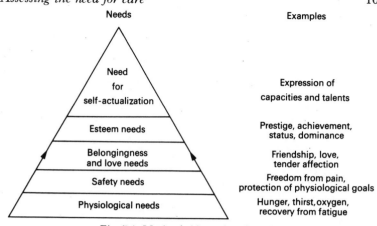

Fig. 7.1. Maslow's hierarchy of needs.

equally important to preserve and respect his dignity as a person of worth. In the case of John, means must be found to achieve a state of self-fulfilment, but to do this other levels in the hierarchy must first be dealt with such as helping him to cope with his incontinence and problems of immobility.

Besides giving information about the patient's physical, social, psychological and spiritual needs the nursing history should also include personal data about the patient and his family, and an assessment of the strengths and weaknesses of the various people giving care. It is also helpful to find out and note what the patient and family understand about the illness and their expectations of care. Wolff and Erikson[3] use 'The Assessment Man' in Fig. 7.2 which serves as a visual reminder of what needs to be considered when making an assessment.

Gathering information

It is essential to get adequate information on which to base care, and therefore the skills needed to acquire this are important. The most important single source of information is the patient and taking his nursing history allows the district nurse to begin to establish a positive nurse-patient relationship, to observe the patient's condition and to obtain information from the patient and where applicable from his family.

If the nursing history is to be used as a basis for planned care it needs to be taken as soon as possible. Apart from recording the condition of the patient and estimating how much information is

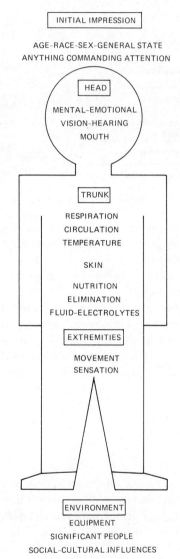

Fig. 7.2. The assessment man. (Based on a figure from *Nursing Outlook* Vol. 25, No. 2 (1980). Copyright: American Journal of Nursing Company).

needed to give optimum care, it is important to note how much information the patient or his family are willing to divulge on their initial contact with the nurse, for the reasons for withholding information may be an unwitting part of the nursing history. John would be unlikely to discuss his sexual problems on the first visit and probably Mrs Adams was so anxious about her husband that she disclosed nothing more than the bare details. On the other hand anxiety and insecurity may make some patients or their relatives over-talkative.

The district nurse may recognise that it is not necessary to take a full history, as when one visit is all that is needed, for instance to remove sutures from a clean wound. However even in such a case the nurse, from her initial impression of the patient, his family, or the environment, may realise that the full history is required. It is important to remember that the nursing history is not static and completed at the first visit but needs constant addition and modification as new information is revealed or the situation changes. As Shetland[4] states: 'the content and context of the interaction are kaleidoscopic rather than static and change constantly as one factor in the total situation changes'

Before the first visit

The district nurse should make sure she has sufficient information to enable her to plan the time of her visit, its approximate length, some knowledge of the patient's condition and the treatment he has received and, of course, the accurate name and address of the patient. The patient will feel more confident if the nurse obviously knows his name and the care he requires, and the district nurse will feel more confident if she knows about the patient. Before visiting a patient for the first time the district nurse may be able to get information from the doctor and the patient's records in the surgery, she may also obtain information from the hospital or from other health and social service personnel. For example, in the case of Mrs Baker the nurse will approach her with greater confidence if she knows that Mrs Baker is aware of her condition and her prognosis. For the patient who has been in hospital following a cerebro-vascular accident the district nurse would need to know how much the patient can do for himself. If she does not have this information the patient may regress in the stage of rehabilitation.

When the district nurse finds she has not sufficient *nursing* information about a patient who has been in hospital she should try

to visit the ward sister. Such a visit may well be helpful in clarifying the role of the district nurse and helping the ward sister to realise what information is necessary for a district nurse to carry out planned care. Personal contact with nursing colleagues is time well spent.

The first visit

The importance of the initial encounter between the nurse and patient cannot be overstressed since it may form the basis of a relationship lasting for years. The standard for care to be given is also set at this visit. If the patient has not got all the equipment required by the nurse such as separate towels and flannels the nurse needs to explain tactfully that these will be required on subsequent visits. The nurse should always remember she is the guest in the patient's home, albeit usually a welcome guest; but nevertheless there may be a conflict of roles and the nurse needs to be enough of a guest to enable relatives and patients to maintain the feeling that they are the master or mistress of their own home but at the same time she should remain a skilled professional and exert sufficient influence to establish her own authority in respect of nursing care of the patient.

It is important that the district nurse (SRN/RGN) who is accountable for the care of a particular patient makes a first visit to the patient. If for some reason this nurse is not available another district nurse (SRN/RGN) needs to make this initial assessment.

Interviewing

To collect a nursing history the nurse must be skilled in the art of interviewing, which is a goal-directed activity aimed at encouraging the patient to express ideas, feelings and facts that help to identify his immediate and long-term needs. The quality of the interview is partly determined by the climate the nurse creates, and if she seems to be hurried the patient will not feel free to explore his feelings. For this reason the timing of the interview is important. Depending on information she has received the nurse may feel it is preferable to leave a first visit until the afternoon when she is less rushed. On the other hand it may be that an initial visit is made in order to cope with an immediate nursing emergency, as when Mr Adams first had his stroke and became incontinent. Then the immediate nursing need for the visit would be life-preserving measures and dealing with his basic hygiene needs. Mr Adams would not be able to give informa-

tion and his wife would be anxious, so further information would have to be collected on a subsequent visit.

Interviewing is more than a question and answer session, it is also an observational technique. The interviewer should listen most of the time and watch for facial expressions and gestures as well as listening to the way the words are said. It is important to listen to what the patient is trying to tell you not just what he is saying, as the old jingle:

'A wise old owl lived in an oak
The more he saw, the less he spoke;
The less he spoke, the more he heard.
Why can't we be like that wise old bird?'

Many nurses have a tendency to talk too much and listen too little. When trying to find out what others think and believe the nurse should keep her questions and comments brief and to the point. She should not have to concentrate on her Kardex to the extent that she is unable to listen to the answers. This is why it is important to have a layout the nurse can memorise.

The nurse may use a series of direct or open-ended questions. Some information is factual and merely requires checking such things as the name and address and can be dealt with by the direct question. Other questions need to be open-ended such as 'how are you managing with your housework?'—and when open-ended questions are used the patient will usually feel freer to reveal what is of concern to him.

The interviewer must firstly clarify the purpose of the interview and explain why she needs the information. She also needs to maintain the momentum by such comments as 'you hadn't finished telling me that'; 'can we go back to that again?' To draw a line between redirecting tangential conversation, and not cutting off important elaboration is difficult. It is a skill which can be only acquired with practice. Above all the nurse needs to create an atmosphere in which the patient and his family feel free to talk. To do this she must feel at ease and this she may not feel if she is worried about filling up the information sheet or she feels is prying into the private life of the patient.

Barriers to communication

The patient's condition may militate against information giving and getting, and in some circumstances the relatives may not be co-

operative. The patient may have a preconceived notion of what the nurse needs to know and this may inhibit the giving of extended information. At the same time differences in age or in the experience of the nurse and patient, and differences in cultural, social and ethnic backgrounds, can all impose difficulties. Other difficulties include such things as other people in the room and the television or radio on. It is important in talking to the patient to use language he understands and this may well be linked with age, culture and social background. For example, 'How often do you pass water?' may be preferable to 'How often do you pass urine, or void?'

It must be remembered that people, particularly when anxious, may not understand what is said to them and there can be considerable distortion between what the nurse has told the patient and the message received by the patient. In a state of anxiety the patient often only hears what he expects to hear, the nurse should validate the answers: 'Is that how it seems to you?'—'Is that correct?'

The nurse may not be able to start her interview where she wants. She wants to gather information systematically but if visiting a patient suffering from constipation for example, she may find the first thing the patient wants to talk about is 'my bowels' so the interview starts there. She also needs to be aware of her own prejudices and values, as this may influence what she asks and how she interprets the answers. She needs to show understanding and acceptance, and refrain from making moral judgements.

Measurement

Accurate baseline measurements, from which progress or deterioration can be determined, are essential, and include the recording of temperature, pulse and respiration rates and blood pressure, and urinalysis. These should be recorded when making the assessment of the patient and thereafter should be recorded with discrimination. If there is a doubt about a patient's fluid intake and output, means of measuring and recording these must be found and this will probably involve the co-operation of relatives.

Accuracy in the assessment of the size of a pressure sore or varicose ulcer is necessary for the subsequent evaluation of progress. This measurement can be done by use of graph paper, drawing on a clear film held over the area, or a comparative description such as 'the size of a 10p piece'; but with the latter method it is necessary to remember that people's perceptions of size may vary considerably. The use of the Norton pressure sore rating scale[5] (Fig. 7.3) is a

Phys. Cond.	Mental Cond.	*Activity*	*Mobility*	*Incontinent*	
Good 4 Fair 3 Poor 2 V. Bad 1	Alert 4 Apathetic 3 Confused 2 Stupor 1	Ambulant 4 Walk/help 3 Chairbound 2 Bed 1	Full 4 Sl. limited 3 V. limited 2 Immobile 1	Not 4 Occasional 3 Usually/Ur. 2 Doubly 1	Total Score

Patients with a total score of 14 or less are liable to develop pressure sores and when the score is lower than 12 the risk is very great indeed.

Fig. 7.3 Patient Assessment Form (Scoring System)

tool all too rarely used by nursing staff, and although the study described was carried out in the hospital setting, the findings are equally appropriate for patients at home. By simply scoring using the scale it is possible to assess those patients most likely to develop pressure sores, but other factors such as availability of relatives to help the patient, and the provision of aids such as ripple bed or sheepskin, will also need to be taken into account.

Assessment of the environment

The district nurse as she approaches a dwelling will notice the type of neighbourhood and it is important that she gets to know the community in which she carries out the majority of her work. She needs to know of the resources available, the location of the Social Services' offices, any relevant voluntary organisations, and the location of the chemist's shop and post office may be essential in helping her with advice to patients and their relatives. The nurse needs to know the community sufficiently well to be able to assess the community atmosphere, because on this may depend how much she can involve neighbours if she is seeking help.

The type of dwelling in which the patient lives may be significant but it is important that the nurse does not jump to the wrong conclusions. Because Mrs Cray lives in a high-rise block of flats is

she necessarily lonely? Many people are so pleased with the modern facilities provided by a new flat that these may outweigh what seem to be disadvatages. Although in some cases the property may look neglected this is not necessarily due to apathy, but may be due to a variety of reasons such as a lack of finance, illness, or an unwilling landlord. Likewise an overgrown garden may not be a source of distress to the patient but, if it is, the district nurse may find a voluntary group to deal with this. Therefore, when making an assessment of the environment it is necessary to note not only the state of the environment but also how the patient interacts or reacts to this.

The observation of the immediate environment in which the patient is being cared for may give many clues to the nurse, and among questions the nurse should ask herself are 'Is it a suitable place in which to provide care?'; 'Is it adequately heated?'; 'Is it safe?'; and finally 'Will using it for nursing care disrupt the life of the rest of the family?' It should be remembered that although it is apparently a safe environment for the patient, it could be dangerous to others if drugs or equipment are left around. It may be that the room is not very clean, and with careful discussion and observation it should be possible to establish whether this is of recent origin because of the illness, or is the usual pattern. When washing her hands or collecting water from the kitchen the nurse should notice if there is food, how it is stored, and what are the cooking facilities and the general state of cleanliness.

The nurse should use her sense of smell. She may detect a smell of stale urine although the patient or relatives have not admitted that the patient is incontinent, or she may be aware of the smell of a discharging wound. Although the patient or his relatives may not mention these facts it is up to the nurse to try and find out as tactfully as possible if this is causing distress. If so, this should be noted under the appropriate assessment heading that deals with the patient himself.

Assessment of the patient

From her observations the district nurse will get a first impression of the patient's general state, and should observe whether the patient is thin, showing signs of recent loss of weight, or is overweight; whether he is pale or flushed; and, if the patient is up, his degree of mobility. At the same time she should notice the patient's general mental condition, and look for such signs as a furrowed

brow, the avoidance of eye contact, a reddening of the face and neck
or clasping and unclasping hands, all of which can be indications of
anxiety, embarrassment, or more serious mental disability.

Dependent on the reason for visiting, the amount of physical
assessment will vary. However if the nurse uses the structured
approach from head to toe she will ensure that she considers all
aspects of the patient's condition. The nurse does this more easily if
she is actually carrying out care for the patient, for instance when
she is with Mr Adams she will notice the condition of his eyes, ears,
mouth, skin, and movement of limbs, the degree of incontinence
and the level of his comprehension.

From what has been said it should be clear that at each visit the
nurse should observe any clues about the patient's mental state, his
physical condition and the environment in which care is being given.
She should do this by using her senses of sight, touch, smell and
hearing. Many of the patients being cared for by the district nurse
are long-term patients requiring daily visits and she should be aware
of the danger of familarity breeding contempt and of the need for
the same rigorous observation of patients whose condition is apparently static.

Assessment of the carers

The carers may be relatives, but quite often are neighbours or
friends. The contribution of such people to the care of sick people at
home is frequently not fully valued. It is therefore important that
the district nurse takes an interest in and encourages the care they
provide, for, if the carers become unable or unwilling to help, then
the district nurse will need to increase her visits or the patient may
require residential care.

Again, first impressions given by the relatives at a visit may give
much information. How Mrs Adams greets the nurse in the morning may indicate her degree of anxiety. If she doesn't look as smart
and is more curt than usual the nurse needs to find out discreetly,
whether this is because she has had a difficult night with her
husband, whether the caring is becoming too much, or whether she
just overslept. It is also important to observe the physical condition
of the relatives who are giving care, and to notice whether there are
signs of anxiety or signs of not being able to cope. Observation of
how the patient and carers interact with each other is also important, for example, the district nurse may notice that Mrs Baker's
elder daughter who gives every attention to detail in the care of her

mother is looking pale and tired herself and is irritable with the younger members of the family. This should indicate to the nurse that she must offer further help and it also gives her an opportunity for health teaching.

The first part of the assessment stage is complete when a comprehensive picture of the patient and family has been built up by interviewing, observation and measurement. The district nurse then has a nursing assessment on which to base her plan of care.

To summarise, a comprehensive assessment should:

1 Have a layout that allows the nurse to collect information systematically in a short time.
2 Include information that will help the nursing team plan a realistic programme of care for the individual patient and his family.
3 Provide a baseline of information from which subsequent progress can be measured.
4 Be concise, and not duplicate information collected by others in the health team unless the focus is different or that information is not available to the nurse.

The following chart gives an example of how a nursing assessment for Mrs Baker might be completed.

Page 1

PERSONAL DATA   Initial history taken by *J. Smith*   Date *6.9.80*
Surname: *Baker*   Marital Status: *Divorced*

Forenames: *Phyllis Ann*   Likes to be called: *Ann*

Address: *7 High Street*

Date of Birth: *8.5.32*   Age: *48 years*

General Practitioner: *Dr. Black* Hospital Consultant: *Mr Jones*

Referred by: *G.P.*   Reason for referral: *Pt. constipated Assess for other help required*

Medical Diagnosis: *Carcinoma of liver. Spinal metastases*

SOCIAL HISTORY   *Shorthand typist on leaving school*
Occupation: *Recently school meals supervisor*
                        Not worked for past 6 months

Family Composition: *Sarah—17yrs—shop assistant (not working at present)*
                            Paul—14 yrs—at St James school
                            Angela—12 yrs—at St James school

Next of Kin: *Sarah. Mr John Baker (brother) lives in Australia*

Other Carers: *Neighbour—Jane, 5 High Street—calls in at approx 8.0 am and in evenings—at work all day*

Environment: *Semi—well equipped—signs of recent neglect. Bathroom/W.C. upstairs. W.C. downstairs. Immersion heater*

Hobbies/Interests: *Knitting. T.V. Rarely has social outings since divorce.*

Religious Practices or Beliefs: *Non-practising R.C.*

Other Agencies Involved: *None at present. Home help offered but refused*

HEALTH HISTORY*(From G.P.'s notes) Nil of note until 1 yr ago—then sudden loss of weight.*
Relevant Medical History: *Jaundice—Nausea→hospital Metastases present Discharged 1 month ago*

Medications: *D.F. 118 1 tab 4 hrly.*   *7.9.80 Stemetil 5 mg 6 hrly.*
                Mogadon 10 mg bedtime

Patient/Family Understanding About Illness: *Pt. has been told diagnosis and given prognosis of approx 6/12 yrs. Ann does not wish children to be told yet.*

Patient/Family Reaction to Illness: *Ann 'accepts' illness but anxious about children—she thinks it will be longer than 6/12 yrs. Sarah realises mother is v. ill—tries to cope. Angela—does not seem aware. Paul—probably not coping—goes out a lot.*

ASSESSMENT   *Thin, frail lady.*
General Assessment on Admission: *Yellow tinge to skin and conjunctiva. Looks anxious. Up and dressed, sitting on settee.*

BASIC PHYSIOLOGICAL FACTORS

Activity/Movement: *Manages to get up and downstairs once daily. Inclined to stoop. Moves slowly around living room. Tires quickly.*

Rest/Sleep: *Board under mattress*
              Sleeps on 3 pillows
              Sleeps approx 6 hrs after Mogadon
              Naps during the day.

Nutrition: *Looks thin, obvious weight loss.*
            Eating v. little. Nauseated
            (?Sarah understands need for small tempting portions)

Elimination/Continent State: *Passes urine × 3/4 daily.*
                                         Urinalysis N.A.D.
Concentrated—no discomfort. B.N.O for 6 days—normal pattern daily. No menstruation for 1 year.

Fluids/Electrolytes: *Drinking 'small amounts'—poss. only 100 ml. 2 hly. Usually likes tea, coffee but these now nauseate. Looks a little dehydrated—skin dry—eyes sunken.*

Breathing/Circulatory State: *Respirations shallow No cyanosis Extremities cold to touch but pt not complaining. (T 36.6°C P88 R22)*

Sensory State: *Vision√ (glasses for reading) Smell√ Touch√ Speech√ hearing√ Pain— soreness in back sometimes 'like a knife' DF118 relieves. Finds hot water bottle comforting*

Skin Condition: *Dry. Slight reddening* Norton Score *16*
                  over sacrum. Heels√ Mouth dry, lips cracked.
                  elbows√   *Hair greasy, sparse. Nails brittle*

EMOTIONAL STATE   *Very talkative. ? frightened that we will talk about illness in front of Sarah.*

PROBLEM LIST

Date	No:	Date	No:
6.9.80	1. Pain due to metastases	6.9.80	3. Constipation due to
6.9.80	2. Inadequate fluid intake due to nausea		poor diet and inadequate fluids
		6.9.80	4. Anxiety re children
		7.9.80	5. ? children feel neglected

Where to keep the assessment

It is difficult to give specific advice regarding this as the organisation of district nursing varies from area to area. The nursing history may be kept at the group practice, the health centre, the district nursing centre or in some authorities the nurses may carry these with them on their rounds but the main criterion is that the history is available to whoever is visiting the patient. It is therefore important that histories are kept where there is ease of access but at the same time ensuring that they will only be seen by properly designated professional colleagues. However, if the patient has told the nurse something in confidence and expressly desired that it should not be repeated then it should not be written down.

Identification of problems

Collecting information about the patient and family is a means to an end. The nursing assessment is not an end in itself but an aid to identifying problems which are amenable to nursing care. The initial assessment should culminate in a mass of information from which the nurse must select that which indicates the patient's problems. In this book the term 'patient problems' is used to mean those problems with which the patient requires help. Other writers sometimes use terms like nursing diagnosis, nursing needs or nursing problems but the authors of this book feel that 'patient problems' is more explicit and focuses on the patient himself.

The most common classification of problems is into actual, potential and possible problems (Mayers 1978[6]). An actual problem is one that exists at the time of the assessment; potential problems are difficulties or concerns that a patient has an unusually high risk of developing or experiencing and identification of these problems enables the district nurse to take preventive action; possible problems are situations requiring more information before being ruled

in or out as actual problems. A clear statement of a problem is essential as this is the guide to the planning of care.

When attempting to identify problems the nurse may find that there is information she needs that is not available or there are inconsistencies in the information she has received from the patient and the family. For example Mrs Baker may say she has little pain yet her daughter is worried because she felt her mother did not sleep because of pain.

Precision in describing the problems is necessary, and it is important to establish where possible the cause of any problem, as this then indicates the nursing care required; for example, the patient's constipation could be due to a consistently low fluid intake, inadequate roughage in the diet, poor mobility, or haemorrhoids. The nurse must be aware of normal body development and functioning to be able to identify any deviations from the normal, and base her decisions on a sound knowledge of the biological and social sciences. If she is in any doubt she should seek advice.

Examples of the problems of particular patients are set out below:

Mr Adams

Actual problem:	Difficulty in communication due to slurred speech and confusion.
Potential problem:	Pressure sores due to immobility and incontinence.
Possible problem:	Inadequate finance due to extra money being spent on heating.

Mrs Baker

Actual problem:	Pain due to spinal metastases.
Potential problem:	Inadequate fluid intake due to nausea.
Possible problem:	Young children feel neglected because of mother's poor condition.

Mrs Cray

Actual problem:	Obesity due to life-time habit of over-eating and immobility.
Potential problem:	Lack of healing of ulcers due to excessive heat from fire.
Possible problem:	Social withdrawal and confusion.

John Davis

Actual problem: Urinary incontinence due to paraplegia.

Potential problem: Urinary tract infection due to inadequate fluid intake and poor mobility.

Possible problem: Sexual frustration due to his condition.

This list of problems is in no way complete, but is used to show how the nurse can analyse information gained during her assessment, and identify problems for which nursing intervention is required.

It is at this stage that the nurse recognises and rules out problems. For example, the district nurse is visiting Mr Fisher once a week to give injections of Cytamen and her initial impression is of a severely handicapped man who will need help in coping with his general hygiene needs, dressing and undressing. However, he and his wife have learned how best to deal with this, so these can be ruled out as problems at this stage, but as the disease progresses and the patient becomes more disabled these may become problems for which the district nurse will need to provide care. This shows the need for continuous reassessment of the patient and the family and it also emphasises the need to explore with the patient what the nurse and he see as being problems, because there may be different perceptions which could cause conflict.

Problem identification therefore needs to be carried out thoughtfully and where possible this should be done in conjunction with the patient and his family. When the district nurse has gathered the initial information she will need to share this with her colleagues, and together they will determine the problems for which they will need to provide care.

Conclusion

The assessment stage has two main phases, the drawing together of information from various sources, but particularly the patient, which the nurse then uses to identify the problems with which the patient needs help. Time spent at this stage is time well spent, as thorough and accurate assessment will mean that the nurse can realistically plan care for the patient and his family.

References

1. Henderson V. (1966). *The Nature of Nursing.* London: Collier Macmillan; pp. 16–17.
2. Maslow A. H. (1943). A theory of human motivation. *Psychological Review;* **50:** 370–96.
3. Wolff H., Erikson R. (1977). The assessment man. *Nursing Outlook;* **25** No 2: 103–107.
4. Shetland M. C. (1965). Teaching and learning in nursing. *American Journal of Nursing;* **9:** 112.
5. Norton D., McLaren R., Exton-Smith A. N. (1962). *An Investigation of Geriatic Nursing Problems in Hospital.* Edinburgh: Churchill Livingstone: 225.
6. Mayers M. (1978). *A Systematic Approach to the Nursing Care Plan.* 2nd ed. New York: Appleton-Century-Crofts; pp. 33–35.

Further Reading

Bower F. L. (1977). *The Process of Planning Nursing Care.* 2nd ed. St Louis: C. V. Mosby.

Crow J. (1977). The nursing process—2: how and why to take a nursing history? *Nursing Times;* **73:** 950–957.

Gebbie K., Lavin M., (1975). *Classification of Nursing Diagnoses.* St Louis: C. V. Mosby.

Kron T. (1971). *The Management of Patient Care.* 3rd ed. London: W. B. Saunders.

Little D., Carnevali D. (1976). *Nursing Care Planning.* 2nd ed. Philadelphia: J. P. Lippincott; p. 128.

Marriner A. (1979). *The Nursing Process.* 2nd ed. London: Y. B. Medical Publishers.

Owen G. M., ed. (1978). Skills of interviewing. In: *Health Visiting.* London: Ballière Tindall; Section II, Chapter 8.

Chapter 8

Planning Care

To ensure the highest possible standards of care, as well as economy of time and energy, it is necessary to plan skilfully and to provide an individual plan for each patient at the same time as organising the total caseload. Not only are there more patients to care for, but also, because of the higher survival rate, longevity and early discharge from hospital many are highly dependent. Not to plan is like exploring without a map. The intention of this chapter therefore, is to suggest ways of planning care for the individual and his family within the context of the total caseload of the district nurse. Tinkham and Voorhies[1] who give the principles to be borne in mind when planning care, emphasise that plans should be based on the identified desires, needs and interests of the patient, and those involved in carrying out the plan should be consulted. Above all the plan must be realistic and capable of practical implementation.

The nursing care plan

The assessment stage ends with a statement of the problems experienced by the individual patient and his family. The next stage involves making a nursing care plan which the nurse and patient should use to provide an answer to these problems. Just as in the assessment stage there are distinct phases in planning.

In the assessment of the patient's problems it was emphasised that the cause of the problem should also be stated, and this leads to the next step which is the setting of goals of care. Differing terms are used by the various authors, for example, aims, goals, objectives, expected outcomes. In this text the term desired outcome will be used as this implies a statement of the desired or realistically expected correction of the patient's problem.

The desired outcome of care

The desired outcome should be written in terms of the result expected in the patient, not in terms of the nursing action. The desired outcome needs to be brief, concise and specific; for exam-

ple, to state that a patient should have 'extra fluids' or 'be mobilised' does not clarify how much fluid is needed or the degree of mobility required, but to state that the patient 'will drink 1800 ml of fluid a day' or 'will walk to the front door using a Zimmer frame' gives specific detail of what it is hoped that the care will achieve. When, later, the nurse comes to evaluate care (Chapter 10), it will be clearer why it is necessary to state the desired outcome concisely. It is also important to state a date by which time the desired outcome should be achieved. This ensures that the nurse and other carers evaluate and re-assess the care given at specified times. With some patients a daily check is needed of such things as fluid intake or the degree of mobility, but with many of the long-term patients a weekly or monthly evaluation is sufficient.

Using some of the problems identified in the previous chapter, the plan at this stage would look like this:

MRS BAKER

Problem	A/P	Date	Desired Outcome	Check
1 Pain due to metastases	A	6/9/80	Pain free	at every visit
2 Inadequate fluid intake due to nausea	A	6/9/80	a) Nausea relieved b) At least 1000 ml fluid tolerated daily	Daily

JOHN DAVIS

Problem	A/P	Date	Desired Outcome	Check
1 Urinary incontinence due to paraplegia	A	5/8/80	Incontinence controlled	Daily
2 Urinary tract infection due to inadequate fluid intake	P	7/8/80	a) No infection b) 2000 ml fluid daily	Weekly (Thurs) Daily
3 Sexual frustration	Poss.	7/8/80		

In the above examples the problem is set out indicating whether it is an actual (A) or potential (P) problem and the date the problem was identified. The desired outcome is given and the date for checking the achievement. It should also be noted that whereas a desired outcome can be written for actual and potential problems this cannot be done for possible problems; these need to be identified and recorded but it is not possible to state goals because sufficient information is not available.

It takes time and practice to develop the skill of writing clear and concise goals for each patient but this is necessary if care is to meet individual needs. Kratz,[2] in a study which looked at the long-term care in the community for a group of patients suffering from stroke, showed that some care was given without goals. The aim of care for the seriously ill patient was usually known and this care was focused to meet the observed needs of the patient. At the other end of the continuum however, the aim of care was not known for the patient who was not getting better. Care did not correspond to the observed needs and was thus diffuse. Although a large proportion of the patients cared for by the district nurse can be put into the category 'not getting better' it is important nevertheless to focus care on clear goals rather than let it become aimless.

Priority setting

At the same time as setting goals for care it is necessary to determine if there is an order of priority for their achievement, and to decide on the best order for nursing care. Maslow's theory of a hierarchy of needs may guide the nurse in setting priorities (see Fig. 7.1, page 101); for example, until John's incontinence has been alleviated it will not be possible to attempt to restore his self-esteem and social contact with his peers.

Nursing action

Having set the goals the next phase is to plan the action required to achieve these; for example, if the desired outcome was that the patient should drink 1800 ml of fluid per day it might well be stated that in every two hours from 6.0 a.m. to midnight he should drink 200 ml of fluid. It must again be emphasised that the decision making must be based on a sound knowledge of biological and behavioural sciences, normal development, and the disease process.

Another consideration is who is available to provide the prescribed care. In the instance above it may be possible for the patient

to supply the drinks for himself, or if he cannot it may be necessary for the nurse to give drinks when she is present, the home help to provide a thermos flask of fluid, and possibly a neighbour to give drinks in the evening. There are numerous variations on this theme which need to be considered for the individual patient.

The plans for Mrs Baker and John will now look like this:

Mrs Baker

Problem	A/P	Date	Desired Outcome	Check	Action
1 Pain due to spinal metastases	A	6/7/80	Pain free	At each visit	Explain to pt. and daughter need for 4 hrly analgesic. Pt. to keep record of pain. Provide backrest
2 Inadequate fluid intake due to nausea	A	6/7/80	a) Nausea relieved b) at least 1000 ml fluid tolerated daily	Daily	a) See G.P. re drugs for nausea b) Explain to pt. and daughter. Suggest soda water

John Davis

Problem	A/P	Date	Desired Outcome	Check	Action
1 Urinary incontinence due to paraplegia	A	5/6/80	Incontinence controlled	Daily	Condom drainage
2 Urinary tract infection due to inadequate fluid intake	P	7/6/80	a) no infection b) 200 ml fluid	Weekly Daily	1 Urine test Fridays 2 M S U to lab monthly 3 Penile toilet 4 Stress importance of fluids
3 Sexual frustration	Poss	7/6/80			Male nurse to discuss

It should be noted that nursing action has been listed for the possible problem although the outcome cannot be forecast, and the problems have been numbered to save having to re-write when referring to them subsequently.

The patient's role in planning care

The patient should be involved in planning his care. How helpful he is will depend on his physical and mental state of health, his understanding of the current situation and his past abilities at problem solving. For example Mr Adams will have a limited role in planning his care but Mr Fisher should be a full participant in constructing his care plan. The nurse will need to help the patient to understand this problem solving approach to care, and together they will consider the assessment, identify the problems and formulate the plan of care. Involving the patient in planning his care is often seen as one of the most difficult parts of the nursing process as it is not traditionally a part of nursing, and so many patients are passive in their attitude to the nurse and do not expect to play an active role.

People who give care

When planning the nursing action it is important to know who will provide the care required, and to ensure appropriate referral or delegation it is necessary for the district nurse to understand the roles of the various care givers.

The patient and his family

The most important care givers are usually the patient and his family and so it is important for the nurse to assess their ability to cope with the care involved and to ensure that they have been taught how to carry out this care (Chapter 9). Other people closely linked with the family who often carry a considerable burden of caring are the friends and neighbours, and again the district nurse must not merely accept at face value that there are such people to provide care but must be sure of their ability, motivation and availability. Some of the complexity of family relationships has been described in Chapter 4.

Nursing staff in the primary care team

The primary care team was described in detail in Chapter 5. When deciding which member of the district nursing staff shall give care

to any particular patient it is necessary to consider the status and roles of the different members of staff, their previous experience, their training and education and the policies of the Health Authority. It is important for the district nurse to remember that she is responsible not only for the care she gives but also for the care she delegates to the State Enrolled Nurse or to the nursing auxiliary. She must, therefore, plan to make the first visit to the patient herself and then if she delegates care she must subsequently make periodic visits to ensure that the quality of care is all that she would wish, and if it is not, to give advice and guidance.

Referral to other agencies

Within the plan of care the district nurse should note care that needs to be provided by someone other than the immediate family or the nursing staff. The patient may be unable to get enough food of the right kind because he or she is unable to shop and cook. In such cases the nursing action may involve arranging for meals-on-wheels, arranging for a home help on days the meals are not delivered and possibly some arrangements whereby relatives or neighbours provide meals at weekends. The nursing action in this case therefore includes contacting the various agencies or people in order to obtain the equipment required. There are numerous voluntary and statutory agencies the nurse may need to contact and details of these are given in Appendices 2 & 3.

Liaison between hospital and community

Skeet, in her study of the home care needs of recently discharged hospital patients, *Home from Hospital*,[3] says that 'care must be planned, and planned before discharge, if it is to be continuous . . . ' and she highlights the inadequancies of care occurring because of poor planning. The most glaring fault was lack of communication; not only did the hospital fail to communicate with the community services but in a high percentage of cases no letter was sent to the general practitioner. The patients' greatest need was advice about activity or drugs, many of the elderly having a multiplicity of drugs with no instructions for taking them. Some patients were struggling to do their own dressings and most knew little about the various services to which they were entitled. Many patients needed more help than they could get and two patients spent their day sitting on commodes waiting for relatives to return in the evening to get them off. In many instances the district nurse or other members of the

primary care team were not aware that the patient had been sent home from hospital, but it must also be said that district nurses were sometimes at fault. One of the case studies in the book described 'Mr M., age 69, married, subarachnoid haemorrhage, deaf, almost blind, doubly incontinent, sent home to wife . . . a district nurse called once and delivered incontinence pads'.

To avoid such situations from occurring it is important that transfer should be as smooth as possible whether the patient is being transferred from hospital to home or vice versa. The channel through which information should be sent will vary depending on whether there are liaison officers and if there are what is their function. Whether a liaison officer is available or not, when a patient needs to be transferred from one area of care to another the nurse must ensure that sufficient information for the continuity of care is sent to the next person responsible for the nursing care of the patient.

Where to keep the plan

As with the assessment, practice will vary from authority to authority. If the plan has been determined with the patient, and the patient is aware of his role in the care, it would seem appropriate to leave it at the patient's home. However in some cases there will be problems, particularly when the patient is unaware of his diagnosis, and in such a situation it may be preferable to keep the records at the district nurses' place of work. But no matter where the plan is kept, it must always be available to any nurse who may be called upon to give care to that particular patient.

In summary, therefore, the good care plan is specific to the individual patient, it states the problems and causes of the problems and sets the desired outcome of care for each problem and the nursing action necessary to achieve this goal. The nurse will need to decide between choices of action and she should make her decision by using her assessment, her knowledge of the patient's condition and the use of research. The plan must be realistic and whenever possible should be made and discussed with the patient, and where appropriate the family. Deadlines should be set for achieving goals and evaluating the progress made.

Some patients will have only one problem with which they need nursing help; others will have many. In the examples given only a

few patient problems have been identified but all these patients have other problems for which care would need to be planned.

Planning work for a group of patients

Having devised a plan for each patient it is next necessary to consider the care of individual patients within the context of the total workload of the district nursing team. The term 'workload' is used here rather than 'caseload' because there are many factors other than the actual number of patients to be considered.

It should by now be obvious that a clear assessment and plan of care gives a better indication of the degree of dependence of the patient and the approximate length of time required for the visit than a statement such as 'general nursing care' indicated. McIntosh and Richardson,[4] in a study which included looking at the workload of district nurses, showed that designation of tasks is not a good indicator of the time taken. For instance they found that the time taken for bathing a patient ranged from 11 minutes to 84 minutes. To give Mr Fisher his injection of cytamen may only take a few minutes but to make a re-assessment of his physical and psychological status will take considerably longer.

By identifying the problems it is possible to sort out priorities of care. There is no absolute rule as to the order in which patients should be visited. Most district nurses like to visit their diabetic patients as early as possible but it may well be that a patient who has an early hospital appointment or one who is in considerable pain needs to be visited first.

While it is not generally advisable to give patients an exact time for visiting it is often helpful to give an approximate time—particularly, for example, if the nurse requires water heated for bathing a patient. It may be decided that the appropriate nursing action for cleansing Mr Evan's wound is a daily saline bath prior to the district nurse's visit to pack the wound; he therefore needs to be given a reasonably precise time for this visit. It is also important that the patient's day is not disrupted too much because this overemphasises the sick role. If patients are able to get out of the house to do their shopping this contributes toward their feeling of well-being, and they should not be kept waiting all day for the nurse; of course, both the nurse and the patients must be prepared for emergencies to occur and for the well laid plans to go astray. If this does happen every attempt should be made to contact the patient and to explain and if necessary apologise for the delay.

The number of visits the patient requires during the twenty-four hour period needs to be taken into consideration; the timing needs to be specific for the patient requiring six hourly analgesic injections and in such a case should be planned in consultation with the night staff. Often the number of visits required will depend on the availability of relatives; for example, Mr Adams will need to be visited twice a day because of his incontinence and dependence and the fact that his wife is elderly and has arthritis. With some patients two nurses will be required to give care because of the weight or ill condition of the patient, and in such situations both nurses need to plan their work and arrange to meet at an agreed time.

In planning the day's work, consideration needs to be given to the number of staff available and to their experience, status and training. Apart from selecting the most suitable nurse for a particular patient, account must be taken of the transport available to each nurse, their hours of work and the policies of the Health Authority concerning the use of the State Enrolled Nurse and nursing auxiliary. The district nurse, however, must never forget that she is accountable for the proper delegation of the work (Chapter 18).

For reasons of economy it is necessary to keep the amount of time spent on travelling by each member of staff to a minimum. One of the disadvantages of group attachment for district nurses may be an increase in travelling time since all general practitioners do not zone their practice areas.

One of the privileges in district nursing is the building up of long-lasting relationships with the patients and their families some of whom will be visited for many years. On the other hand this can mean long-term contact with the difficult or unpopular patient. One advantage of team-work and the discussion of plans enables some rotation of staff to such patients. This can be as helpful to the patient as it is to the nurse; communications and relationships operate in two directions and it may happen that a patient dislikes a particular nurse for some reason that is arbitary or unrelated to her professional role. These situations do not occur frequently but it is important to be sensitive to the possiblitiy, and to try to intervene before a crisis situation occurs.

The nurse needs to plan her day throughout the span of duty and to be sure of regular coffee and lunch breaks to preserve her own health. If she is tired and hurrying to get the maximum work done in the morning this can adversely affect the patient. Besides visiting the patient at home the nurse may carry out some work in the

general practitioner's surgery or at the health centre and time should be allowed for this. It is important to ensure that time in the surgery is also well planned. An appointment system for patients to see the district nurse can be a help in saving the time of both the nurse and the patients and it is worthwhile spending time thinking this out in order to save time in the future. The amount of time and the period of the day spent in the surgery work needs to be carefully thought out. For example, if the district nurse continually finds she cannot carry out necessary care for ill and incontinent patients prior to surgery time, perhaps the allocation of work needs to be re-negotiated with others in the health care team.

Meeting other members of the team face-to-face is important. Some members of teams rely mainly on informal meetings and as long as the necessary contact with one another is made this may be satisfactory; in other teams formal meetings are arranged. Whichever system is in operation it is important to plan time for these meetings.

Referral of patients to other agencies can be time-consuming but the time spent in meeting other personnel face to face will usually pay dividends by easing future telephone conversations, and will ultimately save time. An understanding of the roles of others and their problems and restrictions is necessary to ensure proper referral. It may be helpful to visit a patient in hospital before he comes home. This not only facilitates continuity of care but it also helps to reassure the patient that his care will be continued when he goes home. It enables the district nurse to check that the appropriate services and aids have been organised. The district nurse needs to be selective in deciding which patients to visit prior to discharge but this can be time well spent and needs to be programmed into a days work.

Increasingly, district nurses are required to have student nurses and other personnel accompanying them on their visits. Time for teaching needs to be allowed and this must be seen as an integral part of the district nurses workload.

A final demand on time, to be considered when planning work for the district nursing team, is the need for all nurses to keep abreast of current knowledge. This means allocating adequate time for attending study days, for demonstration, refresher courses and reading (Chapter 18).

References

1. Tinkham C. W., Voorhies E. F. (1977). *Community Health Nursing: Evolution and Process.* 2nd ed. New York: Appleton-Century-Crofts; Chapter 8.
2. Kratz C. R. (1978). *Care of the Long-term Sick in the Community.* Edinburgh: Churchill Livingstone.
3. Skeet M. (1974). *Home from Hospital.* 4th ed. London: Macmillan Journals; p. 28.
4. McIntosh J., Richardson I. M. (1976). *Work Study of District Nursing Staff.* (Scottish Health Service Studies No 37). Edinburgh: Scottish Home and Health Department.

Further Reading

Gilmore M., Bruce N., Hunt M., (1974). *The Work of the Nursing Team in General Practice.* London: Council for the Education and Training of Health Visitors

Hockey L. (1968). *Care in the Balance: A Study of Collaboration Between Hospital and Community Services.* London: Queens Institute of District Nursing.

Hockey L., Buttimore A. (1970). *Co-operation in Patient Care: Study of District Nurses Attached to Hospital and General Medical Practice.* London: Queens Institute of District Nursing.

Kron T. (1976). *The Management of Patient Care: Putting Leadership Skills to Work.* 4th ed. London: W. B. Saunders.

Mager R. F. (1962). *Preparing Instructional Objectives.* California: Fearon.

Marram G., Barrett M. W., Bevis E. O. (1979). *Primary Nursing—A Model for Individualised Care.* 2nd ed. St Louis: The C. V. Mosby Co.

Parnell J., Naylor R. (1973). *Home for the Weekend Back on Monday.* London: Queens Institute of District Nursing.

Roberts I. (1975). *Discharged from Hospital.* London: Royal College of Nursing.

Skeet M. (1974). *Home from Hospital.* 4th ed. London: Macmillan Journals.

Skeet M. (1981). *Discharge Procedures: Practical Guidelines for Nurses.* London: Macmillan Journals.

Stockwell F. (1972). *The Unpopular Patient.* London: Royal College of Nursing.

Chapter 9

Implementation

The third stage of the nursing process is the implementation of the plan, in other words the actual provision of care. Here the interlinking and overlapping of the stages of the nursing process are obvious, for although implementation is the carrying out of what has been previously planned the district nurse must constantly re-assess the situation and modify the plan accordingly. For example, when visiting Mr Fisher she may find that his wife is unwell and has been unable to assist him with washing and dressing. The district nurse, therefore, will need to help with this basic care and assess whether the plan needs to be revised in the long-term. She must ask herself whether Mrs Fisher is now finding it too much of a strain to cope with her husband and her job or whether this is just a temporary set-back.

If the patient and family have been actively involved in planning care they will be more inclined to help with the actual delivery of care. The professional nursing input may be minimal but if this is so it means that a good deal of care must be provided by the relatives, other carers and the patient himself. Thus it is important to consider the teaching role of the district nurse. The family may be very willing to learn and able to cope but the inevitable burden must not be underestimated, and the district nurse needs to give support and counselling to the patient and his family.

The planned nursing action may have involved the district nurse in contact with other personnel to arrange for services or equipment and this will require communication skills and a knowledge of services available (see Section IV). The actual delivery of nursing care by the district nurse frequently requires adaptation of the practical skills learned in hospital such as aseptic and lifting techniques and the administration of drugs. The principles of these remain the same but the execution may require considerable adaptation for the home situation.

Returning again to the philosophy for care and the belief that the district nurse should be assisting the patient towards self care. This

will involve not only teaching the patient, co-ordinating the services for his care and carrying out nursing tasks for him but also using skills required to promote his rehabilitation. Therefore it is important to consider the skills of teaching, counselling, communication, adaptation of nursing techniques and rehabilitation. Development of these skills will help the district nurse to implement care that is best fitted to the patient and family.

Practical procedures must be adapted to the particular situation, but a text book such as this can consider only the principles. A principle is a general law that acts as a guide to action. Principles serve as guides for future investigation and give practical direction for present action. It is not enough to know and state a principle; it is necessary to be able to apply it in varied situations. In her discussion of the principles of asepsis Hunt[1] gives some guidelines that could be applied to any nursing procedure. She suggests that: 'one should be able to assert confidently that the nurse's actions will never endanger the health and safety of the patients and . . . that nursing procedures are always carried out in accordance with the principles on which they are based'.

Learning and teaching

The district nurse is only available for short periods in the patient's day. Many patients are able to cope entirely with their needs for the rest of the day, but others need some care provided by other people; Mrs Adams will need to be taught the best way to care for her husband between the district nurses' visits; John and his parents together need to be taught aspects of his care such as how to use the hoist; although Mr Evans does not require assistance with care once the district nurse has redressed his wound she may take the opportunity while she is there to teach him and talk about the amount of lifting he will be able to do and give advice about his diet and the care of his bowels.

Teaching opportunities in nursing are boundless and it is important that the nurse recognises and uses such opportunities. However, the person to be taught must also be ready and willing to learn. Learning is a process by which changes are brought about in an individual's response to the environment. The changes may be in knowledge, skills or attitudes. For example, the district nurse may need to increase, and thus change, the diabetic patient's knowledge of his dietary needs, his skill in giving his injections and his attitude to the disease. If these planned changes do occur the patient

can be said to have learned. Learning and teaching go side by side, and a useful maxim to remember is that 'telling isn't teaching and listening isn't learning'.

Redman[2] links the learning and teaching process to the nursing process. She identifies 5 stages:

1 Assessment of the need to learn.
2 Assessment of the readiness to learn.
3 Setting objectives.
4 Teaching and learning.
5 Evaluation and re-teaching if necessary.

This process can be used for any teaching situation the district nurse encounters, including teaching patients, relatives, other carers and other nursing staff. These stages will be considered in relation to the patient and his carers. The teaching of students will be looked at separately.

Assessment of the need to learn

When making the initial assessment of the patient and his family the district nurse should have assessed their degree of knowledge and skill, and the attitudes they hold. It may be obvious in discussion that the patient and his family have detailed knowledge of the illness and its implications but on the other hand they may have totally misconceived ideas. They may have had previous experience of caring for a sick person at home or it may be an entirely new experience and the patient and his family may be resentful of a situation that changes the family's lifestyle. In her assessment the nurse needs to help the patient and family identify their learning needs because the learner must perceive a need to learn.

Assessment of the readiness to learn

The nurse may realise that the patient and his family lack knowledge but unless they are willing, learning will not take place. Various factors affect the readiness to learn, and sometimes the person may not be unwilling but simply too anxious to pay attention and retain the knowledge. A low level of intelligence does not necessarily mean that a person is unwilling to learn, and in fact the reverse may be true.

Setting objectives

The objectives or goals of teaching must be realistic and achievable

since success is more motivating than failure. Once determined, the objectives need to be discussed with the learner, and the nurse needs to determine what the patient and his family must, should and could know. For example the diabetic must know the amount of insulin to inject, he should know the relationship between diet, insulin and activity and he could know the pathology of the disease. Teaching needs to proceed from the simple to the complex, from known to unknown, to be broken down into manageable parts and objectives should reflect this.

Teaching and learning

The learning environment affects the rate, amount and quality of learning. Sometimes in the home it is difficult to achieve the ideal learning situation; for instance, it may be difficult to find a quiet place away from the distractions of family activities to obtain the learner's concentration. Interest and motivation increase when the learning experience is seen to have relevance but it may be difficult to demonstrate that relevance. For example, it is easy for the nurse who has seen pressure sores and contracted limbs to realise the need for pressure area care and passive exercises. However patients and relatives who have not seen such complications may have difficulty in understanding the need to be taught these activities and indeed they may feel they are actually cruel to the patient.

The learner has certain expectations of the teacher. The nurse is generally regarded by the public as a person knowledgeable about health matters and her opinion is respected. While she must live up to this reputation she can also capitalize on it as it often means she has a willing learner. An important teaching principle is that learning is more meaningful when the learner is actively involved as summed up by the maxim, 'What I hear I forget, what I see I remember, what I do I know'. Much of the teaching given by the district nurse concerns the learning of practical skills and such teaching, particularly, demands the involvement of the learner. For example, to change the drawsheet of an incontinent patient with the patient in the bed may have become a simple task for the experienced nurse but will be difficult for the relatives to carry out. To tell them how to do it would be meaningless, to show them would be a good introduction to their learning but the only way they will learn is by doing it for themselves.

Feedback is an essential component of learning. The learner needs to know whether he is performing a skill well or poorly and

this is particularly crucial early on so that bad habits are not formed. The district nurse herself should always act as a role model in the care she gives, the organisation of her work and the attitudes she displays to the patient and the family. Teaching the patient self-care may be initially time consuming but in the long term it will save time and increase the patient's independence.

Evaluation of teaching

Evaluation should be continuous during the learning-teaching process. The district nurse may need to pick up clues as to whether a person understands, and also she may use questions and answers, and get the learner to repeat the information. Some people are able to tell the teacher what they do not understand but others have difficulty in perceiving that they don't know. If learning has not taken place there is a need to reconsider the teaching and it is necessary to question whether the goals were realistic and whether the method of teaching was the best.

Health education

The principles of learning and teaching have so far been linked with the care of the sick person, but the district nurse has a unique opportunity to contribute to the promotion of health and prevention of ill-health on an individual basis. Patients and families are particularly conscious of their health when the nurse is around. Caplan[3] describes three different levels of prevention; primary, secondary and tertiary. The district nurse has a contribution to make at each of these levels.

Primary prevention is when specific and identifiable measures are taken to forestall disease and injury, and during her visit to a home the district nurse has the chance to observe for health hazards. Many of the patients the nurse visits are elderly and a home that was once considered safe may now be potentially hazardous, so the nurse should observe the physical environment and look for such dangers as poor lighting, frayed flexes, inadequate storage of drugs and unguarded fires.

In teaching relatives, the nurse can prevent illness or injury by stressing the importance of their having an adequate diet and sufficient rest to prevent them from becoming ill or too tired to cope. In this connection the nurse should also teach the relatives about the correct methods of lifting. The district nurse constantly needs to observe relatives and other carers for any signs of break-

down in their health, because excessive tiredness and anxiety may lead to the occurrence of accidents. Again, the nurse should set an example in such matters as handwashing, careful disposal of soiled dressings and storage of drugs.

Whilst visiting an elderly person at home the nurse may observe friction within younger members of the household, she may notice unexplained bruising on a child leading her to suspect non-accidental injury. In this situation she should immediately report her suspicions to the health visitor.

In *secondary prevention* measures are taken to limit or stop the progress of an already established disease or injury, to prevent complications and sequelae and to limit disability. For example, whilst visiting Mrs Cray the district nurse should teach her about the need for a sensible diet and the need for exercise and rest in order to maintain her general health and to promote the healing of her ulcer.

An increasing need for health education by the district nurse is in the prevention of hypothermia. This is a particular problem with the elderly although other groups such as young babies, patients with lowered thyroid function, the poor housebound and those taking certain drugs are also susceptible. Again the important function of the nurse is to look for signs of susceptibility to hypothermia and to look at possible means of preventing its occurrence. Inadequate heating, clothing, nutrition and exercise may all be contributory factors and these may be due to ignorance, apathy or sheer lack of finance. The nurse through her teaching may be able to make improvements or she may well need to seek the provision of other services and extra finance.

Tertiary prevention involves taking measures to maintain an incurably ill person at the optimum level of activity and to forestall unnecessary suffering. The district nurse is now increasingly involved in caring for the chronically sick, the disabled and the terminally ill at home, and she needs to know how to assist these patients and their families achieve the best quality of life in the time left.

Most of the health education given by the district nurse will be with individuals and their families, but she may also be involved in group health teaching in a field of particular interest, for example slimming groups or, because of a particular expertise in something such as first aid measures or promoting keep fit groups. Group teaching uses the same principles of identifying a need to learn,

setting objectives, planning teaching and evaluating the results. Particular points that need to be considered are the size and composition of the group to be taught, the previous knowledge of the group, the time allowed for teaching and the setting in which the session is to take place.

Teaching other personnel

Increasingly, students and staff from other health and social services, as well as student nurses, are required to gain some experience in the community. Under EEC regulations (see Chapter 19) the student nurse is required to spend at least two weeks in the community as part of her basic training although some of this time may be spent with members of the team other than the district nurse. The district nurse has a unique role in sharing her knowledge and skills with these learners and she must ensure that the time spent with her is a true learning experience. To do this she must know at what stage on her course the student is and what previous teaching about district nursing and the community services she has received. The district nurse must define the objectives of the student's experience and remember that the student is gaining an *insight* into district nursing, not learning all about it. To achieve this insight the district nurse must identify the aspects the student needs to experience in order that she may relate her experience when she returns to the hospital. It is often difficult while in a house to highlight the points the student should note, and adequate briefing before entering the house and discussion afterwards are therefore essential.

Although a one-to-one teaching situation can be an ideal, it can also be tiring for both the teacher and the learner. Nevertheless there may be advantages of having a visitor accompanying the district nurse on her rounds as she may be able to help with the lifting and the care of patients. However the privacy and dignity of patients must be respected and their permission sought to bring a visitor into the house, for although another person is usually welcome, occasionally a third person may break a developing relationship or inhibit a patient from sharing confidences with the nurse. In such a situation it may be preferable to ask the student to wait in the car, and this can then be used as a positive teaching point on the importance of confidentiality and development of relationships.

As well as nurse-learners the district nurse may be asked to take with her on her rounds health visitor students, social work students,

general practitioner trainees or other community workers. The district nurse should use this as an opportunity to teach other workers something of her role and such teaching and understanding should eventually help to improve working relationships and communication between members of the community health team.

Counselling

The district nurse increasingly has a role as a counsellor, a means of giving support to the patients and their carers which may be in the form of a discussion or an interview to help people with their difficulties. Problems for the patient associated with his illness may include a change in life style, limitations in his activities or the need to accept a poor prognosis. The relatives too may have similiar anxieties and may need help in sorting out their priorities; for example, there may be the conflicting demands of a young family and a sick elderly relative.

Nurse[4] gives some clear guidance for nurses about their role as counsellor and the use of professional counsellors. She says that counselling differs from teaching in as much as it helps the person to become aware of alternative courses of behaviour and it is the function of the counsellor to assist the individual to make his own decision among the choices available to him. Counselling requires a non-judgemental attitude on the part of the nurse, an empathetic approach and a relationship in which the person being counselled can express his thoughts and feelings in such a way as will clarify his problems and his attitude to them.

Counselling takes time and nurses must make time available for this, and be alert to cues from patients and relatives that they need to talk. In order for counselling to be effective there must be a relaxed atmosphere and this is probably best achieved by sitting down with the person or persons concerned and having a cup of tea. Sometimes it may be difficult to find the right environment, particularly if it is the relatives who need the help and they cannot talk within the hearing of the patient. In such cases counselling may have to take place in the kitchen or garden. The district nurse therefore needs to create an atmosphere where the family feel free to talk about their worries and help them to find the means of coping with their problems. Counselling does not necessarily mean that the problems themselves can be resolved but that problems can be faced with less anxiety and tension. Sometimes the value of counselling simply involves getting the patient to ask the right question; for

example, 'How am I going to adapt my living style?' rather than
'When am I going to get better?'

The need for understanding listening is as important as the
giving of actual information and advice. At the same time it may
involve elements of comforting, consoling, teaching and correcting
or giving information. The nurse should beware of giving false
reassurance to a patient and his family for this implies there is little
cause for anxiety, and they will mistrust a nurse who says 'don't
worry' when they are obviously concerned. To give false hope
shows a lack of understanding and sensitivity. The reassurance the
nurse can give with conviction is that the patient and family will
receive all possible support and that the patient will be kept as free
from pain as possible.

Collaboration, co-ordination, communication

Frequently the nursing action planned for the patient will include
contacting other personnel for services or equipment. This involves
the use of skills of collaboration, co-ordination and communication.
Collaboration means working with other persons to plan, provide
and evaluate aspects of care; for example, to ensure that Mrs Baker
remains as free from pain as possible the district nurse, the general
practitioner and Mrs Baker together should be planning and
evaluating the drug regime. John and his family should agree
together with the nurse and the physiotherapist, his programme of
exercises.

The district nurse's role in co-ordination is rather like that of the
conductor of an orchestra, bringing together the many parts to
function harmoniously as a whole. The district nurse may assess the
need for the patient to have meals on wheels and a home help but if
the patient also attends a day hospital one or two mornings a week
she needs to co-ordinate the provision of the services on the other
days to avoid gaps and overlaps. Co-ordination also requires the
collaboration of the various personnel.

Communication, which may be written, verbal or non-verbal, is
an integral part of collaboration and co-ordination. There are three
components to any process of communication, the communicator,
that is the person sending the message, the message and the recipient of the message. To be sure that communication is effective it is
essential that the message is received and understood and this can
be difficult if the message has been sent as a written communication
or a telephone message to a third person. Whenever possible direct

communication with the person concerned is preferable because personal contact means that alternative approaches can be discussed. For example, if the district nurse is unhappy about the present treatment for Mrs Cray's ulcer it would be helpful if she and the general practitioner met at the patient's home to discuss together with the patient possible changes in treatment. In providing the best care for Mrs Baker it will probably be helpful to have a team conference involving the district nurse, general practitioner, health visitor and social worker.

Collaboration, which implies freely sharing information and working with other people, is essential in providing a co-ordinated approach to achieve mutually acceptable goals. To work well with other people requires an understanding of their role and function as well as being able to convey one's own role and function to other people. The quality of communication between the nurse and the patient, and the nurse and other workers, has direct bearing on how well the patient's needs are met.

Adaptation of nursing techniques

The district nurse needs to use her previous knowledge of principles of techniques and any new knowledge gained in the community and has a responsibility to remain a safe practitioner. Nurses in the home have fewer technical resources than they would have in hospital, more ambiguity to deal with, and they are also in the anomalous position of not having a clearly defined authority. The district nurse will be called upon to carry out a whole range of techniques ranging from the simple to the complex but it is merely the intention here to describe the adaptation of known principles to a few techniques that are considered by many to be the more difficult to adapt.

Aseptic technique

In a discussion of aseptic techniques in the community, Davison[5] says that 'as long as nurses understand those underlying principles, adjusting to individual circumstances should present no difficulties'. He believes that nurses should develop an aseptic conscience arising from this understanding. Maurer[6] whilst stating that infection is not a common problem at home, does stress in the case of wounds that no risks should be taken and no microbes should be allowed into an open wound. In addition she says that equipment which is used to pierce or cut the skin or cover a wound should

always be sterile. Therefore, although the person may have acquired immunity to the micro-organisms commonly present in his own environment it is important the district nurse takes steps to avoid introduction of new organisms.

It is now easier for district nurses to adhere to these principles because they usually have available to them dressings and equipment from a Central Sterile Supplies Department (CSSD). If this is not so, dressing packs can be obtained on prescription and alternate means of sterilising instruments will need to be used. Boiling of instruments before and after use is an acceptable means of sterilisation and even if disposable forceps are provided it may be necessary to boil ancillary instruments such as scissors and probes. Some authorities provide an antiseptic solution for sterilisation but to soak instruments before and after treatment is time consuming. Hampshire dressing packs which incorporate sterile gloves rather than instruments are convenient for use at home and are increasingly being provided.

The district nurse has to adapt her technique from that learned in hospital where frequently there were two nurses to carry out the procedure; now she needs to act as her own 'dirty nurse', pour out the lotions herself, remove the dressings and complete the whole procedure unassisted. To do this she must work out the best method for use in each situation which enables her to adhere to the principles of asepsis.

Handwashing may be difficult in some households. Broome[7] showed that use of a Hibitane impregnated tissue was at least as effective as handwashing, or solutions such as Hibiscol or Hibiscrub may be used instead. The guiding principle is that hands should, at the least, be cleansed before commencing a procedure and afterwards, and it is up to the district nurse to determine the best way of achieving this. Before commencing a technique it is important that the nurse prepares a clean working surface. She may be offered a clean formica topped trolley or a rubbish strewn table and it may need considerable tact to get the latter cleared. In choosing the room in which an aseptic procedure is to be carried out a number of things need to be considered. Whilst the kitchen may seem ideal in terms of availability of running water and working surfaces it is not appropriate when there is a discharging wound to be exposed. The nurse must at all times respect the patient's property and protect the furniture used, and pets should be removed from the room. Nursing bags vary in size, style and

contents but it must be remembered that the contents must be kept clean and that the nurses hands need to be cleansed prior to removing articles from the bag. The bag should never be put on the floor but a suitable protected surface found for it. In the majority of households the nurse will find that the patient and/or family are most anxious to make arrangements to suit the nurse.

Disposal of dirty dressings and used instruments is the final consideration when carrying out aseptic techniques. Dressings should be well-wrapped and burned if possible, although this is less easy now that few open fires exist. If there are large amounts of offensive dressings to be destroyed, arrangements can be made for their collection by the environmental health service. Disposable forceps should be broken to avoid their re-use and when possible wrapped and put in the dustbin. If the nurse is in doubt about the safety of disposal it may be better for her to wrap the articles concerned and take them back to her work base for destruction. Some instruments need to be returned for re-sterilisation, and again it is important to ensure these are wrapped to avoid cross infection.

Carrying out an aseptic technique in the home may call for considerable ingenuity on the part of the nurse but if she bears in mind the principles of asepsis taught in her training it should be possible to do this even in an unsavoury environment.

Use of equipment

Equipment may be obtained from various sources and to arrange for its provision in the home frequently takes time in communicating with the various services. As part of her planning for care the nurse must determine which equipment is required and be realistic in this and not order unnecessary items. One very necessary item is frequently a commode or chemical toilet for the patient with particular elimination needs. For some of the aids to daily living it may be useful for the nurse, physosotherapist and occupational therapist together to work out with the patient, the most appropriate device, but it must be remembered that equipment costs money and once it is no longer required it should be returned. The district nurse has a responsibility to make sure equipment is used correctly, maintained and returned.

The district nurse needs to use much imagination in finding the best means of caring for the patient at home, and frequently it is the patient or his family that devise the best adaptations. Equipment is not always readily available and there may be a waiting list for

delivery, but in the meantime patients need care, so household objects may have to be used temporarily as a substitute. For example, an upturned dining chair or a suitcase well padded with pillows or cushions can be used as a backrest, a coffee table or cardboard box can act as a bed cradle and newspaper under a sheet will help to protect the mattress of an incontinent patient until incontinence sheets and laundry can be provided. Economy and thoughtfulness in the use of equipment is necessary, for while it may be ideal to change the patient's clothes and bedding each day the district nurse must consider who is doing the washing. Sometimes aids such as incontinence pads will need to be used to protect the bedding although this is not the treatment of choice. The use of aids also needs to be determined in the light of help available, for example, if it is not possible for a patient's position to be changed frequently it may be necessary to provide a ripple bed or sheepskin to help prevent pressure sores occurring. Mr Adams may need such a bed or a ripple cushion in the chair as his wife cannot move him between the nurse's visits, whereas another patient with a similar degree of disability may not need such equipment because there are enough carers to move him regularly.

The organisation of the nursing environment is important and it is necessary to plan with the patient and family in which room care is preferable. This means taking into account such factors as toilet facilities, stairs and the family activities. The arrangement of the room is crucial; for example, if a patient needs lifting in bed it is obviously easier if the bed is not against a wall, but it is all too easy to concentrate on the sick person and forget the normal family activities. In some households this may be acceptable but in others it can cause resentment. The organisation of the home for John obviously took considerable time and consultation between members of the family, health and social services before he was transferred home from hospital. Time spent planning before discharge from hospital can be of great value in such instances.

Sometimes the nurse needs to find a compromise between the ideal equipment and that preferred by the patient. A notorious problem with district nurses is that of caring for patients in a double bed. Whilst this is obviously not ideal for nursing the psychological comfort to the patient may be preferable to some physical discomfort caused to the nurse and other carers. However, if the patient is heavy, and needs lifting and nursing care while in bed, it may be necessary to move him into a single bed. One of the chief considera-

tions is the height of the bed, and a hospital type bed is preferable to a divan although it may be possible to raise the latter on blocks. On the other hand the hospital type bed will tend to emphasise the sick role, but this may be inevitable. Many would argue that Mr Adams should not be in his double bed but if a single bed was recommended where would the double bed be put? Where would Mrs Adams sleep? And how much would it upset both Mr and Mrs Adams to sleep separately after all these years?

Lifting

Lifting is an important area in which the district nurse has to adapt her known skills. She is at particular risk of back injury because she may not have help with lifting; beds and chairs are often low and a large proportion of the patients requiring lifting are elderly and can do little to help themselves. The district nurse will have been taught lifting methods in her nurse training and will need to adapt these methods in the home. The principles of good, safe lifting however remain the same and are:

1   The weight to be moved should be as near the workers hip level as possible, and therefore the height of bed and chair need to be considered.
2   The lifter(s) should stand near the weight to be moved in order to maintain balance and use the large muscles.
3   Legs should be apart to get a broad base and to enable the lifter to shift the weight of her body as the particular object is moved.
4   The weight should be moved toward rather than away from the lifter.
5   The lifter should keep the back as straight as possible, flexing the hips or knees rather than bending the back. This ensures that the large muscles of the thigh and trunk are used rather than those in the arm.

These principles should be applied when lifting any patient and when teaching others to do so.

If possible the nurse should get help with lifting and to do this she will need to assess the ability and physical strength of other carers. Not infrequently the carer may also be elderly or disabled; for example, Mrs Adams could not be expected to help with lifting her husband. If the nurse has any doubt about her own ability to lift a patient unaided because he is heavy, very ill or awkward, she should

arrange for another member of the nursing team to meet her at the house. This in the long term saves time and energy and prevents injury to nurse and patient. If a relative or other person is to help with the lifting it is important that the nurse teaches that person the best way to lift. Besides being lifted in and out of bed, patients may need to be put into and out of chairs and baths. The latter can cause considerable difficulty as most bathrooms are small with the bath fixed to one wall and with no handles.

Aids for lifting should be used when possible; hoists can be invaluable as long as there is room to manoeuvre them and the nurse can instil the necessary confidence in the patient and the relatives in their use. Lifting poles may be provided to fit some beds and sometimes heavy furniture or a bar fitted to a wall can be used to help the patient lever himself; a rope tied to the foot of a bed can be used for the patient to pull himself into a sitting position. The nurse, patient and family together must work out the best methods of lifting to preserve the health and strength of not only the patient but of all the carers concerned.

Administration of drugs

After the stringent rules in hospital the district nurse may feel the storage and administration of drugs in the community is very relaxed. Drugs are the property of the patient for whom they were prescribed but also they may be taken irregularly and haphazardly stored. The district nurse has a responsibility to try to ensure that drugs are taken correctly, that they are effective, and that they are stored safely, and at the same time she must observe for side effects.

When interviewing the patient the district nurse should check the drugs the patient is taking with the medical notes, and ensure that the patient knows when and how to take the drugs. Drugs should be stored in their proper containers, kept in a safe place and clearly labelled. Patients, particularly the elderly and the confused, should be advised not to keep drugs at the bedside as they may forget they have taken them and then on waking in the night take further drugs, leading to accidental overdosage. The nurse needs to check that the patient understands the need to take a full course of drugs and obtain a further supply when necessary. Drugs, are the property of the patient but the district nurse should advise the patient or his family that any unused drugs be destroyed by burning or flushing down the lavatory.

Except where the patient is giving his own injections or having regular injections administered by the nurse, as in the case of a diabetic patient, syringes should not be left in the house. The district nurse should make sure that a used syringe is destroyed in order to avoid any chance of re-use or of its falling into the hands of a drug addict. Teaching regarding the taking of drugs, their storage and disposal is another important aspect of health education.

The district nurse has further responsibilities pertaining to the administration of drugs and the effectiveness of drugs taken. For example if a patient is having diuretic drugs she should observe whether the oedema is reduced and urine output increased as well as checking if the patient is taking necessary potassium supplements. Side effects should also be looked for, for example by the regular test-in of urine for glycosuria when patients are taking corticosteroids.

Many patients have a multiplicity of drugs to take and this is a particular problem with the elderly. They may have difficulty in opening the containers, reading the labels and remembering when to take the various tablets, not to mention the reason for each medicine, so it may be helpful for the nurse to label the drugs in a manner understood by the particular patient. For example, a diuretic may be labelled 'Water tablets, take on getting up'. With some patients the district nurse may need to visit to organise the day's supply or arrange for a neighbour to do this.

If the nurse has actually to administer drugs she should take the usual precautions of checking that she has the correct drug dose and observe for any incipient side effects. When possible the nurse should have written instructions from the doctor but if these have been given verbally she should make sure they are clearly written on the patients records as soon as possible. Verbal or telephone messages should be repeated back to the doctor to be sure they are interpreted correctly.

Administration of controlled drugs

The patient and family may be responsible for administering oral drugs which fall into the category of controlled drugs as defined in the Misuse of Drugs Act 1971. In these cases the district nurse should be particularly vigilant in ensuring they are aware of the correct dosage and frequency, and the importance of safe storage. Specific rules apply for the administration of controlled drugs by district nurses. The person administering must be a trained nurse. (Trained nurse according to the Act can be SRN or SEN but some

health authorities may have a policy for it to be SRNs only). As this is different from hospital policy, where a second nurse always checks the drug with the trained nurse, special care must be taken.

In the giving of controlled drugs there must always be a written prescription from the doctor available in the house, and careful records must be kept. Exceptionally one dose may be given following verbal instructions but this must be one dose only and must be written up by the doctor as soon as possible. The records must include the stock provided, the amount given, amount left and the signature of the nurse, and most authorities have special forms for this. Disposal of any controlled drugs remaining when the course is discontinued or the patient dies is of particular importance. Again the patient or family need to be consulted, but the nurse must make it her responsibility to try to ensure the drugs are destroyed. Usually the relatives are only too willing for the nurse to do this herself, and she should then record the amount of drugs destroyed and if possible get a witness to sign the record.

Patient's drugs are ordered on a prescription which should be collected from the chemist by a responsible person, and this is particularly important in the case of controlled drugs. Occasionally the district nurse may need to collect prescriptions on behalf of the patient if there is no-one else to do so. It is difficult for any nurse to keep up to date with the constant changes in drugs available. If the nurse does not know of the drug, its action or side effects she needs to find out by looking it up in MIMS (Monthly Index of Medical Specialities) available at the surgery or by asking the general practitioner or chemist.

Concept of rehabilitation

Rehabilitation is often viewed as a speciality with a focus on long-term chronic conditions when in fact it should be an integral part of all patient-centered care. Mitchell[8] defines rehabilitation as 'the process of restoring persons to their previous capabilities or helping them make the most of their existing capabilities', which ties in with Henderson's definition of nursing,[9] '. . . helping the patient gain independence as rapidly as possible . . .', and the philosophy of assisting towards self-care. Returning also to the World Health Organisation's definition of health as 'a state of physical, social and psychological well being, not merely the absence of disease', it can be seen that rehabilitation needs to include the social and psychological aspects of disease as well as the physical. A major

objective is limiting the extent to which a disability becomes a handicap.

Any person who becomes ill or injured needs to be rehabilitated to some extent. There may be only a temporary disability, as for example with Mr Evans, where it should be possible to return the patient to his previous job and capabilities. On the other hand disability may be permanent as in the case of John where he must be helped to make the most of his remaining capabilities. A third category of disability is progressive disability as in the case of Mr Fisher, whose condition can be expected to deteriorate progressively although there may well be periods of remission. His existing capabilities will vary at different stages of the illness and will need to be re-assessed constantly. Because a diagnosis of a terminal illness has been made this should not detract from rehabilitation. For example, Mrs Baker needs to be helped to make the most of her capabilities, helped to remain the mother figure and to get the maximum fulfillment in the life that is left to her. Throughout any care there should be an emphasis on prevention of the occurrence of secondary disabilities such as pressure sores and contractures.

With the trend for patients to be discharged from hospital early, few have reached the optimum point of recovery when they return home, so it is important for the district nurse to start a programme of rehabilitation as soon as possible. To do this she needs to bear in mind the principles of rehabilitation as described by Boroch[10] which can be summarised as follows. Rehabilitation:

1 Requires the co-operation of patient and family.
2 Is patient-family centered.
3 Is a continuous process with varying degrees of emphasis on physical, social and psychological needs.
4 Is goal directed.
5 Requires collaboration of all health team professionals.

The district nurse is fortunate in knowing the home where she makes her assessment. She actually sees and experiences the social setting, the family network, the immediate environment in which the patient is being cared for, and she can discover how the family interacts without having to rely on hearsay. It is necessary to have a clear picture of the patient's previous health status and way of living if the aim of rehabilitation is to be to return the patient to his previous state as nearly as possible. Physical, social and psychological rehabilitation need to be carried out concurrently, for it

would be fruitless to spend time and effort on producing maximum physical function with John if he is not helped at the same time to accept the limitations of his disability and to feel socially acceptable and economically independent.

The changes patients and their families are able to make in their life styles in order that they may adjust to altered levels of health will depend on their individual ability to cope and adjust as well as their general resources. It is important that the nurse helps families to maximise their strengths in this respect and minimise their weaknesses.

Rehabilitation therefore is a complex operation and to say simply that the goal is 'to rehabilitate a patient' is being too vague. Specific goals need to be set and rehabilitation must be an integral part of total care.

Progress notes

During the implementation stage of the nursing, progress records should be kept, but they do not necessarily need to be made at each visit. If the plan of care has clearly identified what the nursing action should be, the nurse does not need to record that she has carried out what was planned. For example, there should be a clear plan detailing treatment for Mrs Cray's ulcer, and if the treatment has been carried out as planned and there is no obvious change in the state of the ulcer or the patient herself, records need not be made. Repetitious, meaningless recording such as 'dressing renewed', 'general care given', have no place in the progress notes, the purpose of which is to communicate a current situation to someone who is not present and to create a record of that situation.

The frequency with which these notes are written depends on the stability or otherwise, of the problem and the relevance of the observations. Progress notes for some patients should be written weekly or monthly, as for example for Mr Adams and John, whereas Mrs Baker's progress regarding pain, nausea and fluid intake should be recorded at each visit. Record keeping is an important component of each stage and a summary of the major points is included in the next chapter.

References

1. Hunt J. M. (1974). *The Teaching and Practice of Surgical Dressings in Three Hospitals*. London: Royal College of Nursing.

2. Redman B. K. (1976). *The Process of Patient Teaching in Nursing.* 3rd ed. St Louis: C. V. Mosby; p. 24.

3. Caplan G. (1961). *An Approach to Community Mental Health.* London: Tavistock Publications.

4. Nurse G. (1975). *Counselling and the Nurse—An Introduction.* London: H M and M.

5. Davison V. (1971). Current dressing techniques. *Occupational Health* (London); **23:** 287–292.

6. Maurer I. M. (1973). Disinfection and sterilisation in domiciliary nursing. *Nursing Mirror;* **136,** 17: 46–47.

7. Broome W. E. (1971). *Dressing Techniques.* London: Butterworth.

8. Mitchell P. H. (1977). *Concepts Basic to Nursing.* 2nd ed. New York: McGraw-Hill.

9. Henderson V. (1966). *The Nature of Nursing.* New York: Macmillan Publishing Co; p. 15.

10. Boroch R. M. (1976). *Elements of Rehabilitation in Nursing—An Introduction.* St Louis: C. V. Mosby; p. 7.

Further reading

Learning and teaching.
Anderson D. C., ed. (1980). *Health Education Practice.* London: Croom Helm.
Hinchliff S., ed. (1979). *Teaching Clinical Nursing.* Edinburgh: Churchill Livingstone.
Pohl M. L. (1978). *The Teaching Function of the Nurse Practitioner.* 3rd ed. Iowa: Wm C Broom.
Mager R. F. (1962). *Preparing Instructional Objectives.* California: Fearon.

Counselling.
Royal College of Nursing Institute of Advanced Nursing Education (1978). *Counselling in Nursing* (Report of a working party). London: Royal College of Nursing.

Nursing Techniques.
Chartered Society of Physiotherapists (1975). *Handling the Handicapped at Home.* Cambridge: Woodhead-Faulkner.
Jacka S. M., Grifiths D. G. (1976). *Treatment Room Nursing: A handbook for nursing sisters in general practice, schools and industry.* Oxford: Blackwell.
Queen's Institute of District Nursing (1965). *Safer Sterilisation of Equipment.* London: QIDN.

Communication.
Ashworth P. (1980). *Care to Communicate:* London: Royal College of Nursing.
O'Brien M. J. (1978). *Communications and Relationships in Nursing.* 2nd ed. St Louis: C. V. Mosby.

Collaboration.
Gilmore M., Bruce N., Hunt M. (1974). *The Work of the Nursing Team in General Practice.* London: Council for the Education and Training of Health Visitors.
Roberts I. (1975). *Discharged from Hospital.* London: Royal College of Nursing.
Skeet M. (1974). *Home from Hospital.* 4th ed. London: Macmillan Journals.

Rehabilitation.

Field M. (1967). *Patients are People. A Medical-social Approach to Prolonged Illness.* 3rd ed. New York: Columbia University Press.

Johnstone M. (1976). *The Stroke Patient. Principles of Rehabilitation.* Edinburgh: Churchill Livingstone.

Johnstone M. (1980). *Home Care for the Stroke Patient.* Edinburgh: Churchill Livingstone.

Chapter 10
Evaluating Care

The nursing process is incomplete without the stage of evaluation. This is the means by which the care given to the patient and his family is checked. Evaluation can lead to re-assessment, and may thus be seen as re-starting the cycle which emphasises the dynamic and cyclical nature of the nursing process. Reilly[1] defines evaluation as 'a process concerned with the quality of a substance, action or event'.

The provision of high quality care must be the goal of all nurses and it is essential that they have a reliable means of measuring the standard of care given. Evaluation is unfortunately often neglected but it is necessary if the nurse is to know whether care should be continued as planned, whether goals and subsequent action need to be changed, or if more information is required. Of course, a thinking nurse is continually evaluating the results of her care while she is actually nursing the patient and helping the family, but a more formal evaluation that is written down is needed. The very process of putting the evaluation on paper encourages critical thought and, once written, the evaluation can be shared.

The skills required for evaluation are the same as those used in assessment: observation, interviewing, communication, analysing, judging and inferring from the clues given by the patient and his relatives. The main difference between assessment and evaluation is that evaluation is undertaken in retrospect after the plan of care has been implemented.

Evaluation has three elements: the evaluation of the outcome of the planned action for the patient and his family; the evaluation of the actual nursing performance and whether nursing tasks have been performed satisfactorily; and finally the evaluation of the system of care. Evaluation therefore is an attempt to identify the quality of care received by individuals and the quality of care provided by the care givers. These three elements will now be considered in greater detail.

Evaluation of the goals of care for individual patients

The primary function of nursing care is the resolution of patient problems. In the planning stage the desired outcome of care was precisely set out; now, the goals that were enumerated must be checked. For example, in the case of John Davis, one goal set was that he should drink 2000 ml of fluid a day, and whether this goal has been achieved can be seen simply by checking the record which the family have kept of his intake. If the goal had merely been 'extra fluids' it would be impossible to evaluate whether it had been achieved because definitions of 'extra fluids' vary. Similarly, unless the actual size of Mrs Cray's ulcer has been stated it will be impossible to determine by how much it has decreased or increased. Evaluation, therefore, emphasises the need as far as possible to set goals in measurable terms.

Although the desired outcome is set out for actual and potential problems (see chart, page 118) it is also necessary to evaluate the 'possible' problems that were noted in the planning stage and decide whether further information is necessary and whether these problems should now be ruled out, or included as either actual or potential.

Evaluation will not always show positive results, but it is just as important to determine if and when care is *not* producing the desired results, and to ask the reason why. It may be that the assessment was inadequate in the first place and the problems were not clearly defined, or that the information on which the plan was based was either inaccurate or insufficient. On the other hand, the goals set for a patient in that condition or in those circumstances may have been unrealistic, and insufficient regard may have been paid to the available resources for care. Sometimes the failure to set clear and realistic aims is found to be due to the fact that the patient and his family were not sufficiently involved in the plan of care; or for some reason they did not understand; or they misinterpreted what was expected of them. Finally, and often sadly, the patient's condition or the availability or ability of other carers may change radically, in which case, of course, plans that were once realistic cease to be so.

Changing the plan

There are therefore several reasons for changing the plan of care. Firstly, the goals may have been achieved and the patient's problem

solved. If this is so a line should be drawn through this part of the plan and the date by which the problem was resolved should be recorded. It should be remembered that a 'patient problem' is a problem with which the patient requires help; therefore when nursing help is no longer needed and the patient can cope for himself this requirement can be removed from the plan. For example, it is hoped that many of John's initial problems will ultimately not be problems once he learns aspects of self-care and independence. Following nursing advice and teaching he and his parents should be able to cope with the urinary drainage and observation for signs of infection and to inform the district nurse if they have any worries. Similarly, the plan for a diabetic patient, who with the help of the nurse is learning how to manage his own care, will need to be changed as he achieves independence.

Another reason for changing the plan is that information is now available that was not revealed at the assessment. This may include new information about the patient's condition, his lifestyle or his relationships with his family and due to the fact that this information was not originally available the wrong goals may have been set. In some cases the nurse and the patient are too optimistic and this can lead to frustration, while in other cases the nurse, or the patient, as both may have made a wrong assessment of the resources that would be available; they may, for example, have been over-optimistic about the provision of meals on wheels or the supply of home helps.

However, although evaluation may indicate the need to change the plan, one hopes that in most cases it will show that the plan was adequate. For many patients visited by the district nurse the plan will remain the same for a long time. However these cases too must be evaluated periodically; for example, Mr Adams will have a continuing potential problem of pressure sores due to his poor mobility and incontinence. If at the time of evaluation he remains free from sores the plan would be considered appropriate and care would be continued as before.

Evaluation of the carers

If in the initial assessment it was decided that relatives and others could carry out certain aspects of care it is necessary to monitor their ability to do so. For example, the district nurse needs to watch each day how Sarah is coping with Mrs Baker. At each visit to Mr Fisher the nurse needs to evaluate the plans they made, in which he and his

wife were to cope with the majority of his care; if they can no longer manage she must reconsider the plan. It may be that the goals remain the same but the plan will need to be changed.

Responsibility for evaluation of nursing care

The definition of the district nurse (DHSS[2]) stated that she is 'professionally accountable for assessing and re-assessing the needs of patient and family, and for monitoring quality of care'. Evaluation of care, therefore, is the particular responsibility of the district nurse although she may have delegated the giving of care to the State Enrolled Nurse or nursing auxiliary who have a responsibility to make observations while carrying out care and to report their findings to the district nurse. The district nurse must herself visit patients whose care has been delegated to others and ensure that the quality of care is good and that the plan is still appropriate. If, for example, the bathing of frail elderly patients is delegated to a nursing auxiliary the district nurse herself must visit these patients at least monthly to evaluate the care and to re-assess the patient. An ideal way of carrying out this evaluation is for the nurse to perform the bath herself and make a systematic re-assessment of the patient, his family and environment.

Care conferences

It is sometimes difficult for the nurse to evaluate care alone, particularly in the case of the patients she is seeing almost every day, because subtle changes in the patient, his family or his environment may easily escape her notice. It is therefore important to involve the other people who have been concerned with the patient to whom the patient may have expressed quite different fears and anxieties. If plans have been formulated clearly at the daily meeting of the district nursing team it should be possible to discuss these plans and to change them if necesary. Although the district nursing team should meet daily, the timing of the meeting will depend on the working conditions and the travelling distance for different members, and on the staff available. Many teams seem to prefer the early afternoon. The purpose of such meetings should be to discuss the progress of patients, highlight problems and plan subsequent care, and also to set aside a definite time for those patients whose care needs to be evaluated on a weekly or monthly basis.

Sometimes it will be beneficial to use the meeting of the team as an opportunity for a wider care conference involving general prac-

titioners, health visitors and social workers. It may be useful to discuss with the whole primary care team whether plans for particular patients are realistic and to gain further information and advice. For instance it will be important to involve the social worker in discussions regarding the Baker family, for when Mrs Baker dies the care of the children will be her concern. Although such meetings do take time, it is time well spent if it produces better care.

Criteria for discharge and termination of visits

Mayers[3] suggests that the criterion for discharge is the achievement of the long term goals that were set on admission. It is not always easy, however, to know when patients no longer need nursing help.

One reason for discharging a patient from the care of the district nurse may be that the patient has reached a state of health in which he no longer needs professional help; this may well be the case with Mr Evans. With some patients the needs and problems may be partially resolved and the resources within the family mobilised in such a way that the nurse can withdraw; this situation may eventually be reached with John, with the district nurse remaining available if the family run into any difficulties. Other patients may have been referred to another health or social worker, and unless there are nursing tasks to carry out the district nurse can withdraw her services; for example the district nurse's involvement with Alison will be intermittent while that of the health visitor may be continuous. It is a waste of manpower to duplicate care unnecessarily.

Other reasons for discharging a patient are that he has moved to another area or has been transferred to hospital. When this happens good liaison is important to ensure continuity of care. Finally the patient may die, but this does not necessarily mean that the district nurse's involvement in that household has ended, for she may need to visit the bereaved family to offer continuing support.

Terminating care in some cases will mean breaking a long-standing relationship between district nurse, patient and family, and the patient may be reluctant to 'let go' of the nurse, and vice versa. The patient needs to be prepared for discharge by encouraging his independence and if other workers are to be involved it may be a good idea to introduce them before the district nurse leaves. The patient needs to be assured that if he encounters any difficulties the nurse can be contacted again.

The district nurse (SRN) has the responsiblity for admitting and discharging patients, and before discharge she must decide whether

the desired care has been achieved and if necessary the right referrals have been made. It is, of course, not enough to say that the treatment has been completed or the wound healed, but the nurse must be assured that the patient can cope with his continuing care.

Actual discharge

When it has been agreed that the patient should be discharged, the district nurse should remove the records and take away or arrange for collection of any equipment; however some patients will need to retain certain equipment and they should be told whom to notify when it is not needed. Drugs should be destroyed as described in the previous chapter. The patient and relatives will feel more secure if the nurse leaves a telephone number for them to contact her if necessary.

When a patient dies the district nurse needs to be sensitive to the needs and wishes of the bereaved, and if she has formed a long trusting relationship with relatives such as she would with Mrs Adams she may well visit several times before saying goodbye or introducing the health visitor. Once Mrs Baker dies, Sarah and her brother and sister will need a great deal of support but this may be best given by the social worker. If Mr Fisher's condition deteriorated and he died his wife might gain her support from work colleagues and friends but because she is articulate this does not mean that she does not need, and would not value, professional support. There is not, therefore, any definite rule about bereavement visiting but the district nurse needs to assess the needs of the bereaved and should plan to visit or to refer to others as appropriate (see Chapter 9).

Observational visits

Periodic visits may need to be made to patients who do not require any nursing intervention but need evaluation of progress. Such visits may be made to a patient who has had care in the past and is coping satisfactorily with the help of his family, but who may be expected to suffer a recurrence of his original condition or perhaps some general deterioration of his circumstances. Visiting such patients may be useful as a preventive measure and will help to support and reassure the relatives in a time of doubt. Another reason for making an observational visit is to establish a trusting relationship with a family with whom nursing needs are anticipated, the obvious example being where a patient has been diag-

nosed as having a terminal illness but who is at present coping adequately and does not yet require practical nursing help. On such occasions the nurse can act as a general guide in helping the patient to get the best out of life while he can.

Although 'observational' visits may appear 'social', and they should of course appear that way, it is important that they have a clear purpose so the nurse should identify goals and make a systematic re-assessment.

Recording the evaluation of nursing care

Progress notes explain the progress of the patient in achieving the stated goals; the frequency of recording these details depends on the condition of the patient, for example Mrs Baker's condition will change on a daily basis and progress notes will be written at each visit, whereas for Mr Adams a full evaluation will be recorded only monthly unless significant changes occur.

Numbering of problems saves repetition and unnecessary writing when recording progress. For example two of Mrs Baker's problems for which goals were set and care planned were (see page 118):

Problem 1 Pain due to spinal metastases.

Problem 2 Inadequate fluid intake due to nausea.

The progress notes will read:

7.7.80 1. *D.F 118 taken every 4 hrs. Pain less but patient drowsy.*

2. *Stemetil 5 mg prescribed by G.P. Occasional nausea. Tolerating approx 50 ml fluid hrly. Sarah not yet got soda water.*

Similarly two of the problems identified for John (page 118) were:

Problem 2 Potential urinary tract infection due to inadequate fluid intake.

Problem 3 Possible sexual frustration.

Progress notes for John will read:

7.7.80 2. *Urine tested. N.A.D. M.S.U. sent.*

Father coping with penile toilet. At least 2000 ml fluid per day.

Family aware of signs of infection — will report if any. Review ¹/₁₂

3. *Male nurse visited. John not concerned at present but will ask to see male nurse again if he wishes further discussion.*

The check date for Problem 2 has now been made for one month's time so unless the family report any changes further pro-

gress notes will not need to be written for one month. Problem 3 can now be crossed off the problem list and plan.

Evaluation of nursing performance

Linked with the monitoring of care for individual patients is the evaluation of the quality of care given by the nurses. Such evaluation is necessary for nurses wherever they work but it is especially important in district nursing where so much care is carried out in isolation and where it is easy to develop a ritual approach guided by habit rather than the best interests of the patient.

Assessment of nursing performance is frequently thought to be limited to the appraisal of a learner by a trained nurse. While this is important, it is also necessary to monitor the quality of care provided by the trained nurse. The most important person to assess the care given by the district nurse is the nurse herself. During much of her time the district nurse will be her only examiner and thus she needs to be a severe and reliable judge. Reilly[4] makes some suggestions about the way the nurse should behave if using the nursing process as the method of care, and provides a useful checklist for self evaluation, but as it uses American terminology and relates to the American care system it has been adapted here.

The district nurse should assess her own abilities in the following areas:

Assessment—
1 Forms good relationships with patient and family.
2 Makes relevant observations.
3 Conducts purposeful interviews.
4 Elicits appropriate information from patient and family.
5 Uses other sources of information gathering e.g. records, other personnel.
6 Shows understanding of the patients response to health/illness/environment.
7 Accepts the right of families to their own beliefs, moral code and life style.
8 Seeks to avoid interference of own biases when interpreting information.
9 Identifies family resources that can be used in meeting health needs.
10 Identifies patient problems from information gathered.

Planning—
1 Involves patient and family in planning care.
2 Identifies short and long-term goals for care.
3 Selects appropriate nursing care measures.
4 Refers to other members of the health and social services.
5 Determines priorities in care.
6 Organises a caseload.
7 Communicates plan of care to other nursing personnel.

Implementation—
1 Performs nursing care procedures adapted to the home environment.
2 Uses technical skills competently.
3 Cares for and uses equipment appropriately.
4 Encourages patient to use his/her capabilities to the maximum.
5 Preserves the patient's privacy.
6 Helps patient and family to accept realistic limitations imposed by illness.
7 Instructs the patient and his family in relation to identified learning needs.
8 Utilises opportunities for health education.
9 Initiates appropriate referrals to other personnel.
10 Records significant information accurately.

Evaluation—
1 Measures the results of nursing action in terms of the outcome of care.
2 Modifies care plan as appropriate.
3 Communicates with others in the primary health care team.
4 Examines individual care planning within the context of the total workload.
5 Evaluates the district nurses role within the local setting.

This checklist can also be used to assess the abilities of others, but peer evaluation happens whether it is intentional or not; another nurse visiting a patient will inevitably notice the standard of care by observing the availability of equipment, the plans of care, the involvement and attitudes of patient and other carers. Patients and families will often make comparisons between different nurses and this must be accepted; patients too have their favourites. Because a

nurse carries out care differently it does not necessarily mean it is worse than that of another nurse but different methods can cause confusion and conflict for the patient—hence the importance of the clear plan which enables continuity.

Superior and subordinate evaluation

The district nurse who is accountable for the nursing care of a group of patients will need to make assessments of other members of the nursing team and be aware of their strengths and weaknesses.

The nursing officer has responsibility for the standards of care provided by the nursing teams responsible to her and she, too, will visit with the various members of the district nursing team and discuss problems and look at records.

Evaluation is not however confined to the experienced nurse looking at her subordinates; the student visitor will also evaluate care as she sees it. The student may well challenge the district nurse about aspects of her care which may sometimes appear less professional than that given in hospital. While it is right that the student should make such an evaluation it is important that she understands the principles of the caring in the home and remembers that the nurse is a guest and can work only with the patient's consent.

It is important to remember that the purpose of evaluation is not to find fault but to assess the quality of care; if the quality is good then praise should be given as this gives encouragement and helps to maintain motivation and high standards.

Evaluation of the system of care

A nursing audit may be carried out by members of the district nursing team in association with nurse managers and possibly other members of the primary care team in order to evaluate the effectiveness of the whole system through which care is given in a particular locality.

A paramount problem is, inevitably, the way the district nursing team fits in with the primary care team as a whole and a number of problems, some of which have legal consequences, may arise because different members of the team are accountable to different authorities and the doctors are virtually independent. The nurse will look to the doctor for authority in clinical matters, such as the prescribing of medication, but the nurse is employed by the health authority and responsible to them through her nursing officer. The authority may lay down rules about what the nurses should do or,

more often, should not do, or the circumstances in which they may perform certain tasks, but with which the doctor may disagree.

The doctor, used to having structural authority over practice nurses, may be genuinely confused about his role and the extent of his authority while, the nurse, anxious to please, and seeing no harm in extending her duties, may all too easily carry out the doctor's wishes without realising the confusion and conflict this can create for the team as a whole. Examples of such areas of conflict are the performance by the district nurse of procedures such as immunisation, ear syringing, venepuncture, electrocardiography and assessment visits. Conflict is not necessarily caused by any doubt as to the district nurses' ability to carry out the tasks, but more likely by doubt about the appropriateness of these tasks to the work of the district nurse. This problem must be tackled, not by surreptitiously doing one thing and saying another, but by a frank discussion with the team as a whole and it may well be that at the audit the two viewpoints can be reconciled. If nurses are needed to undertake extended duties, the nursing management can arrange for those selected and willing to do them to have proper training, and the necessary changes in their employment contracts.

The nursing audit can be used to identify the various problems that may arise within the primary care team due to lack of harmony and consultation between members, lack of resources or poor management and planning. The research of Goldstone and Worrall[5] has confirmed the earlier findings of Hockey[6] and suggests that in the intervening years the planning and work of the district nursing team has not been rationalised. The work load for district nurses varies widely both in the actual caseload and the number of high-dependency patients alloted to each nurse and there still appears to be no agreement in practice as to which duties are best done by enrolled nurses and which by registered, and which nursing duties can be delegated to auxiliaries. Furthermore, many district nurses still spend too much time on travelling and on non-nursing duties.

The whole subject requires more research, but in the meantime the nursing audit can pin-point local difficulties and by consensus management can try to rectify them. It is, however, up to each nurse to question and analyse how she spends her time and reflect why the help given to one patient is defined as 'nursing' and the same help given to another is defined as 'non-nursing'. For example, when is getting the patient a cup of tea part of nursing and when is it not? The balance between the 'It's not my job' attitude and

simply doing tasks to save bother, or because the doctor said so, or there was no one else on hand, is delicate and in the end each nurse must make her own decision. However, the decision is likely to be sound if the nurse remembers to ask, 'Why am I doing this?', 'Could it be done just as well by someone else?' and 'Am I doing it at the expense of my true nursing function?' She might even ask 'Does it need to be done at all?'

Finally the nursing audit audit will look at comments and complaints from patients or from team members about difficulties with other agencies. Some of these may be resolved on discussion, but if they cannot be overcome then at least an explanation for the difficulty or complaint should be given to all members of the team involved.

Record keeping

Throughout this section record keeping has been mentioned in relation to the planning of patient care but as each health authority has its own system and design of records no hard and fast rules can be given. Some general principles will, however be considered.

Patient care records

For each of the stages of the nursing process the type and content of the record to be kept has been discussed and suggestions made as to where these records should be kept. To be sure the records are meaningful it is important that the nurse bears in mind their purpose which can be summarised as follows:

1 To ensure continuity of patient care.
2 As a means of communication between team members—not only nursing staff but with general practitioners and health visitors as well as with the patient and family.
3 To provide a means of monitoring efficiency of the services by checking the outcome of care.
4 To provide useful information for research into patient care, use of equipment, or use of the services.
5 For legal purposes—which is why it is important that they are accurate and say something meaningful.

Other records to be kept

The district nurse will have to keep a variety of records other than those relating to individual patients. Facts will be required for

statistical purposes and possibly for local and national research. The statistical information required will generally include the number of people visited by each nurse, the age group of the patients, the treatment given by the nurse, the medical diagnosis, the source of patient referral, and the outcome of care. The actual information required will depend on the current survey but nurses must recognise that the completion of these details is an important part of their function to ensure that accurate statistics are available about patients' needs and the provision of care so that any overlaps or gaps can be highlighted.

Apart from records about patients and their care it is also important to keep accurate records of any equipment loaned and services requested from other health and social services. Finally the district nurse will be expected to keep certain records of her personal activities; for example, depending on her duty hours she may need to record evening or weekend duties, and she must also keep accurate records of mileage covered during her working day if she has a car; in some authorities telephones are provided for the nurse at home and calls made for the purposes of her work need to be recorded. Accuracy in record keeping is crucial and all records must be signed; the signature means 'I take responsibility for what precedes my name'.

References

1. Reilly D. E. (1975). *Behavioural Objectives in Nursing: Evaluation of Learner Attainment*. New York: Appleton-Century-Crofts; p. 2.
2. Department of Health and Social Security. (1977). *Nursing in Primary Health Care;* CNO (77) **8:** 2.
3. Mayers M. G. (1978). *A Systematic Approach to the Nursing Care Plan*. 2nd ed. New York: Appleton-Century-Crofts; pp. 16–17.
4. Reilly D. E. (1975). *Behavioural Objectives in Nursing: Evaluation of Learner Attainment*. New York: Appleton-Century-Crofts: 2; pp. 141–143.
5. Goldstone L. A., Worrall J. (1980). The problems of variations in work patterns of district nurses. *Nursing Times;* **76,** 11; pp. 45–51.
6. Hockey L. (1972). *Use or Abuse? A Study of the State Enrolled Nurse in the Local Authority Nursing Services*. London: Queens Institute of District Nursing.

Further reading

Kron T. (1976). *The Management of Patient Care. Putting Leadership Skills to Work*. 4th ed. Philadelphia: W. B. Saunders Co.
McIntosh J. (1978). Record keeping: a boon or a bind?
   —1 Record content. *Nursing Mirror*. July 6 1978: 43–44

—2 Nurses' views. *Nursing Mirror.* July 13 1978: 39–40

—3 The Way forward. *Nursing Mirror.* July 20th 1978: 36–37

Phaneuf M. C. (1976). *The Nursing Audit: Self regulation in nursing practice.* 2nd ed. New York: Appleton-Century-Crofts.

Rowntree D. (1977). *Assessing Students: How shall we know them?* London: Harper and Row.

Yura H., Walsh M. B. (1978). *The Nursing Process: Assessing, Planning, Implementing, Evaluating.* 3rd ed. New York: Appleton-Century-Crofts.

Section III

Special Groups for Care

Systems of health care management have been altered to accommodate changes in the treatment of patients. The turnover of patients in acute hospitals is continually increasing bringing many pressures to bear on all the health and social services and in particular the community health services. The increase in the number of elderly people as a proportion of the total population has brought added pressures especially in relation to patients over 75 years old. Continued development of day facilities for patients, especially the elderly and the mentally ill, together with day-surgery and five-day wards is particularly encouraging but these trends also have their effects on members of the primary care team.

Report on the Education and Training of District Nurses 1976.

Although the principles governing the nursing process laid down in Section II are applicable to all patients wherever they are nursed, there are nevertheless groups of patients whose special needs cannot be dealt with within the generality of nursing care principles. Therefore, at the risk of some overlap, it was decided that the special aspects of care for the groups most likely to be seen by the district nurse should be the subject for separate short chapters.

The groups selected are to some extent arbitrary, and some patients will fall into more than one group, but by separating off the special needs for groups like the young disabled it is hoped that students will appreciate that the particular may be contained within the general.

Chapter 11
The Sick Child

The care of the sick child constitutes a minimal part of the district nurse's caseload as the majority of such care is provided by the parents. However, although she may care for few sick children, the district nurse needs to be aware of the special needs of this group when the occasion arises. The children who will require care can be divided into those with acute, short-term illnesses and those with long term or handicapping conditions.

In the 1920s much of the district nurse's work was involved in caring for children with infectious diseases but with the advent of immunisation and antibiotics such diseases are less prevalent. Unfortunately, however, with the recent fall in the 'take-up' of immunisation against whooping-cough this disease is once more becoming more common and it can be fatal, particularly for young babies. Similarly, while measles is less prevalent, the complacency of some parents about vaccination has led to the inevitable increase in this disease, which can lead to complications such as otitis media, bronchitis and encephalitis; again the district nurse may need to help in the early stages of the illness. The general practitioner or health visitor may also refer to the district nurse children with other acute illnesses such as upper respiratory tract infections or gastro-enteritis. Planned early discharge from hospital of children following surgical treatment will involve the district nurse in dressing wounds, removing sutures or caring for the child in a plaster of Paris splint.

Children born with physical and mental handicaps are living longer and parents may need practical help with the long-term care, or in the short term when the child develops one of the childhood illnesses. Others, like Alison, have progressive diseases such as cystic fibrosis and the parents may normally cope with the child's care but during an acute exacerbation of the illness may need help with physiotherapy and administration of antibiotics. It is sometimes possible and preferable to care for the child with a terminal

illness at home and the district nurse may be involved in this inevitably distressing situation.

The district nurse therefore may be called upon to care for or advise parents on the care of sick children with any one of a whole range of illnesses and she cannot be expected to have knowledge of all the diseases, their implications or the care required; if in doubt she must consult hospital staff or a colleague. In a few authorities specialist paediatric district nursing schemes are available for providing care or giving advice and such schemes will be discussed later.

Reasons for keeping the sick child at home

Research into the effects of hospitalisation on the young child (Bowlby[1], Robertson[2], Hawthorn[3]) shows that this can psychologically harm the child, and have long-term effects such as future delinquency and job instability. Hospitalisation frequently leads to other more immediate problems such as regression in walking, feeding and language development, and bed wetting; it has also been found that wound healing may be delayed and there is always a risk of cross infection. A further problem for the parents may be that many specialist children's hospitals are regionally based and this can involve considerable travelling which is costly in both time and money.

Because of great publicity in the 1950s of the National Association for the Welfare of Children in Hospital (NAWCH), and subsequent Government recommendations, most hospitals now have free visiting arrangements and many have living-in facilities for the mother. Some mothers cannot avail themselves of these facilities because of other children at home and this can cause conflict. Other improvements include an increase in play and educational facilities in hospital (as recommended by the Platt Committee[4]) and a policy that children should not be nursed in adult wards but in children's wards with a Registered Sick Children's Nurse in charge; but these improvements are not enough and unless it is absolutely necessary hospital admission for the child should be avoided.

Having said that the child should be cared for at home it is important to recognise that this can cause considerable stress to the parents. Harrisson,[5] in her study *Families in Stress*, highlights the anxiety incurred by parents caring for two different groups of children at home, those with Perthe's disease and those with cystic fibrosis like Alison, and although the pattern of these illnesses is

very different, both cause great stress for the families. This would apply equally to families with any sick child and while it may not be possible to avoid stress it is important to recognise that it exists and to give the parents support.

Assessment of the child

Firstly, the district nurse needs to assess how much information the child is able to give and what is his reaction to her as a nurse. The degree of fear or co-operation will depend on the child's previous experience of nurses, on what he has seen on television, or on the nurse's particular task; for example, if she is to give him an injection and he understands what this means, she will be unlikely to get much co-operation before this has been carried out as any friendly approaches will be treated with mistrust. Even a toddler can be involved in giving some information such as his name and age, likes and dislikes, and it is important to encourage him to talk; the information can be checked with the mother afterwards. However, the nurse's best ally in assessment will usually be the child's mother as she is most likely to notice any changes in the child's physical condition or behaviour.

Assessment of the child needs the nurse's acute skills of observation since, for example, the child may not be able to locate or describe pain, although the position in which he holds himself may be an indicator. Accuracy in measurement of temperature will be important with the acutely sick child because many children are prone to febrile convulsions and the district nurse should aim at prevention of such a distressing occurrence. Another crucial assessment particularly with the baby is the fluid intake and the nurse must observe for any signs of dehydration.

Assessment of the carers

The most significant person providing care will invariably be the mother, although the father and possibly other children may be involved. The ability of the mother to cope needs to be assessed and this ability may be hampered by her anxiety, sleepless nights, other children to care for, or other commitments such as the fact that she normally works.

Assessment of the environment

An important consideration is where to nurse the child. If he is to stay in bed it may be preferable to have a bed made up on the settee

downstairs to avoid the mother going up and down stairs. In this way the child does not feel isolated and can be constantly observed. The heating, ventilation and safety of the room in which the child is to be nursed are further areas to be assessed.

Most of the information the nurse will gain from the child and the family, and from her observations and measurements, but she should also get information from others who know the family. In particular, the health visitor may be able to give some idea of the family's strengths and weaknesses and their ability to cope in a crisis. It is important that the district nurse refers back to the health visitor anything she feels is of importance.

From her assessment the district nurse needs to identify the problems with which the family needs help. Paramount may be the parents' anxiety, and alleviating this may be the nurse's first priority.

Planning care

Goals of care need to be set and the nursing action determined, and this will include teaching parents how to give care. For example, for the child with a raised temperature the desired outcome will be that 'the temperature will subside' and the action to this end may involve tepid sponging of the child. The mother should be advised to wash him in tepid water and change his clothes. Care given by the mother will be less likely to make the child fretful than care from a stranger.

An important part of the care plan is ensuring an adequate fluid intake; the amount will depend on age, size of baby and his normal intake. The plan may include mother giving clear fluids if the baby is reluctant to feed, or is vomiting or has diarrhoea. The mother must be given specific instructions about making up these feeds. For example, a 5% sugar solution can be made with one teaspoonful (just over level) of sugar to each 100 ml of water; if the baby is vomiting or has diarrhoea a pinch of salt should be added.

The district nurse may need to help the mother plan the giving of the child's medications in relation to feeds and suggest means of overcoming an unwillingness to take drugs.

When planning care for the child with a long-term illness it is necessary to consider the child's daily routine; for example, it is important to establish a routine for the diabetic child that fits in with his normal school day so he does not constantly feel 'different'. An important fact to bear in mind when planning care for the child at home is that it invariably takes longer to carry out any specific

procedure such as an injection than it would with the adult, and time needs to be allowed for this.

Special schemes for care

Some urban authorities have a specialised service for the care of the sick child at home. The first such scheme started in Rotherham in 1954 and the next in Birmingham in 1955, and others have since evolved. Some schemes are organised for all sick children in an area, others are for special groups such as post-surgery or children with spina bifida. These schemes usually employ Registered Sick Children's Nurses, who are also qualified district nurses, working in close liaison with paediatric units and hospitals and the health visitor. The schemes vary in their organisation but the aim is to give specialist high quality care at home to the sick child, and support to the family. In some areas a night nursing service has been introduced because this is often the time when parents most need support.

The advantages of a specialist service are that there is a nurse available with a wide knowledge of childhood illnesses and the specialist care required; invariably the caseload will be numerically smaller and this means she can plan to give the time required to each child. The nurse can form close links with the hospital units and keep up to date with current treatments. However, a disadvantage of such schemes is that it involves considerable travelling for the nurse. Such a specialist service is at present only feasible in urban areas. Another disadvantage is that the specialist nurse is not attached to a group practice as her colleagues but with planning this problem can be overcome.

The Court report[6] recommends the formation of paediatric teams including specialist child health visitors and child health nurses to provide a range of child care at home. The roles and relationships of these personnel would need to be more clearly defined but the principle of providing specialist care for this group is clearly spelt out.

Implementation of care

In implementing care the district nurse's role will be primarily that of a teacher but she will also need to counsel and to co-ordinate services. She must teach the parents how to give the care she advises and frequently she will learn hints from the parents on how best to carry out certain aspects of their child's care; for example, the

easiest means of bathing the severely handicapped child or washing and cutting the hair of the child with cerebral palsy who cannot sit still. While it is preferable in the majority of cases for the parents to carry out care the nurse must constantly be aware of the need to relieve the mother to give her a rest. Sometimes nurses have guilt feelings because they are not doing the care themselves and they have to learn that the counselling and supporting role must be seen to be of great importance as this helps the mother to keep going.

The district nurse's co-ordinating role is again important. She needs to be sure that the family are receiving all the help to which they are entitled. Links with the appropriate voluntary association can be supportive to the parents, such as the Cystic Fibrosis Society, the Spina Bifida and Hydrocephalus Association or the British Diabetic Association. Through such societies families can get help with baby sitting and holidays and get ideas about equipment and services available. The district nurse needs to liaise with the health visitor and possibly the school nurse who may arrange for treatment to be carried out at school.

Evaluation of care

A child's condition may quickly change for better or worse and therefore a basic rule of thumb is to overvisit rather than undervisit. Acute skills of observation are required for the degree of dehydration, temperature and activity but above all the opinion of the mother should be sought, as she will notice the subtle changes with her child.

The nurse needs to evaluate her own and the team's ability to cope with the child and she also needs to consider how to fit the child's care into the total caseload, she must evaluate the quality of her relationship with the child and family and she will need to consider carefully when she should terminate her visits. In some cases as for example with Alison it will be helpful to visit periodically even in her 'good' phases to maintain the relationship with the child and family.

References

1. Bowlby J. (1965). *Child Care and the Growth of Love.* 2nd ed. Harmondsworth: Pelican.
2. Robertson J. (1970). *Young Children in Hospital.* 2nd ed. London: Tavistock Publications.
3. Hawthorn P. J. (1974). *Nurse I want my Mummy.* London: Royal College of Nursing.

4. Ministry of Health (1959). *Welfare of Children in Hospital* (Platt Report). London: HMSO.
5. Harrisson S. (1977). *Families in Stress.* London Royal College of Nursing.
6. Department of Health and Social Security. (1976). *Fit for the Future.* Report of the Committee on Child Health Services; (Court Report). Cmnd 6684. London: HMSO.

Further Reading

Atwell J. D. (1975). Paediatric day case surgery in Southampton. *Nursing Times;* **71,** 22: 841–3.

Department of Health and Social Security (1976). *Fit for the Future: Report of the Committee on Child Health Services* (Court Report). London: HMSO.

Duncombe M., Weller B. F. (1979). *Paediatric Nursing.* 5th ed. London: Bailliere Tindall.

Hawthorne P. J. (1974). *Nurse I Want my Mummy.* London: Royal College of Nursing.

Jenkins S. M. (1975). Home care in Paddington. *Nursing Mirror.* **140,** 9: 68–72.

Robottom B. M. (1969). The contribution of the children's nurse to the home care of children. *British Journal of Medical Education;* **3,** 4: 311–2.

Robottom B. M. (1978). Care of the child with whooping cough. *Journal of Community Nursing;* **1,** 8.

Chapter 12

The Young Disabled

For the 15–19-year-old age group, the rate of road traffic accidents is nearly twice the rate for the total population, and society is now experiencing an upsurge in the sale of motorbikes and mopeds to young people. Teenagers are more prone to athletic injuries because of their high degree of participation in sports by comparison with other age groups. The growing problem of residual disability in sportsmen is reflected in the advent of the Association of Sports Medicine which advises on, and researches into, the specialised prevention and management of sport injuries; and its work is increasing.

Cystic fibrosis and spina bifida are no longer conditions confined to children and the thalidomide victims are now young adults. Improved treatment techniques have increased longevity, so 'new' handicapping conditions present themselves to those caring for young adults. It must also be remembered that the process of ageing itself affects the course of disease and disability, for example in diabetes and asthma. The diabetic regime and the occurence of asthmatic attacks may be affected by menstruation, especially at the menarche, and later, by the menopause; the effects of long-term drug treatment in these two conditions, which may itself bring about disabling changes, are well documented.

There is a great deal of evidence to suggest that the young adult is disadvantaged in terms of medical provision—and this occurs at the time of the difficult transition from childhood to adulthood, from dependence to independence and self-sufficiency. There are paediatricians for children, and surgeons and physicians for adults, but there are children's wards in which a well-developed 15-year-old would be out of place, and adult wards in which an immature 16-year-old would be equally misplaced; the existing district handicap teams cater only for the needs of children of school years.

Thus, while children and adults can rely upon specialised care, the young adult often cannot. At around 16 years of age the transfer of responsibility for care passes from a child-orientated

service to an adult-orientated service and the fact that this transfer is itself inadequate is highlighted by the Warnock[1] and Court[2] Reports. The Court committee noted that:

... physical and mental handicap predispose children to psychiatric disorder and in this and other ways may aggravate and prolong the developmental problems facing all adolescents. The constraints to living imposed by handicap affect the adolescent's life at home, at school, in employment and in society. Additionally he is subject to all the stresses of accelerated physical, sexual and emotional development and to the prospect of change in environment and occupation. For the handicapped, adolescence is a period of crisis, yet at the moment of leaving school, there is the danger that they are less supported than at any time hitherto.

The Court Report goes on to discuss the need for continuity in care, and stresses time and again the importance of close liaison between all those workers involved in the care of disabled young people. The Committee accept that the team will include specialist and primary care medical and nursing services, remedial services, social services and volunteers, and also welfare and employment agencies and careers services.

The Harris Report[3], commissioned by the Department of Health and Social Security, showed that out of a population of 54 million, 1 129 000 people were sufficiently handicapped to require support and 157 000 required specialised care, and whilst most were people over 75 years of age, a substantial number were young people. *The Chronically Sick and Disabled Persons Act*, 1970, requires that special and separate units for chronically handicapped young people should be provided locally, but the growth of such units is slow and in some areas the chronically disabled adults remain the responsiblity of the geriatrician irrespective of age.

Assessment for care

The initial assessment of the disabled will centre upon the activities of daily living—the ability to eat, wash, dress and use the toilet. With the young disabled, the majority of the needs in these areas will have been met, either because the disability has existed through childhood or, as in the case of John Davis, they have been dealt with by the hospital service, and involved doctors, remedial therapists and social workers. Nothing should be taken for granted

however, and the best laid plans may be incapable of implementation once the patient is discharged. Preparations were made for John, and the primary care team were involved with the family prior to discharge, but, as the work of Skeet[4] and Hockey[5] demonstrates, there is often a sad lack of preparation for hospital discharge and an even more common exclusion of the primary care team from that preparation.

No assessment can be contemplated without the total involvement of the family of the young disabled person for, as the case histories of John Davis and Mr Fisher illustrate, the contribution of parents or wife to the daily care is immense. The relatives will bear the burden of looking after the young person on a constant day-to-day basis and will thus hold a responsibility for noting behaviour and for monitoring progress or otherwise. In order to do this, the level of ability and the strengths and the weaknesses of the patient must be understood and accepted by the carers. In addition, an awareness of any association between the handicapping condition and existing behavioural problems, or anticipated ones, is essential if change is to be noted or potential problems prevented or detected early. Bearing the burden of care, the parents or the young spouse must be participants in the process of assessment and decision-making, not only in formulating the nursing care plan but in discussions with the doctors, the remedial therapists and the Disablement Resettlement Officers. The relatives must not be seen merely as welcome 'caretakers'.

The teaching and counselling role of the district nurse is of paramount importance here, as is her ability to sit and listen and to accept the advice and the knowledge of the relatives. The teaching role may not only include instructing relatives in therapeutic procedures to be continued at home, such as nursing care, but also advising on physiotherapy and speech therapy. The nurse will need to determine such needs before entering the home, so contact and liaison with all who have been involved in care is essential. Domiciliary physiotherapy services are still few, even though the need is tremendous for such disabled people as John Davis. While the nurse will assess the need for continuing physiotherapy and do what she can, she needs help; the written exercise sheet for the use of both nurse and relatives is invaluable, and, is absolutely essential when physiotherapy is concerned with active treatment as well as prevention: care must be therapeutic.

Assessment of relatives must include an assessment of their

ability to cope and to cope continuously. Parents are more often than not anxious to care for handicapped children at home and special schools are available, as are paediatric services and financial support. As adolescence and young adulthood supervene, the 'child' becomes bigger and heavier, the demands, including the financial demands, become greater, the relatives become older, and service provision alters. The burden of caring becomes difficult and even impossible, yet relatives are often reluctant to admit to the burden, and feelings of guilt may be experienced. Where the disability has existed from childhood, such occurences can to some extent be anticipated and prepared for; for example where a father has previously carried the child up and down stairs to bathroom and bed, alterations to the home can be made in readiness for adulthood, lifts installed or a downstairs toilet added to the home. The knowledge that the patient can be admitted to a holiday home or hospital once or twice every year can do much to relieve the stress experienced by relatives who will know that they can have a break whilst their loved one is being cared for.

The nurse will need to find out about local provisions for holiday accommodation and social services generally, and further assessment will identify particular problems. John, for example, is bed and chair bound, he can go outdoors but will only venture into the garden in sunny weather because he worries about his condom drainage. Although he seemed to have accepted his changed bodily image while in hospital among people in a similar condition to himself, or worse, now he is at home he is not really ready to accept the stares of other people. He likes to read and gets through a thriller a day most days, his parents visit the library for him but keep bringing back books he has already read. He used to like the cinema and always attended the home matches of his favourite football team but he cannot go to these places now because of his concern over his incontinence and anyway the cinema does not accommodate wheelchairs. Dad would push him to the football ground but it's unfair to ask him every Saturday when usually he goes down to the allotment, and anyway, there are also all those people at football matches.

Apart from the counselling role that will centre upon John's involvement in the assessment and the decision making, the nurse will need to be familiar with the following:

Other safe urinary drainage units;

The availability of a travelling or voluntary services library;

Local facilities to accommodate the disabled at libraries and in
other public buildings;

The availability of volunteers to transport or push the patient to
libraries, shops and football matches and/or football supporter
clubs,

The existence of self-help groups where patients and/or relatives
can meet people in similar circumstances to themselves.

Mobility remains a problem for the disabled, in spite of the
responsibility of Local Authorities to ensure that public buildings
are accessible, and the availability of the mobility allowance. A
number of voluntary organisations try to help by making available
drivers and volunteers.

Any assessment of the needs of the disabled will include financial
considerations. Finances are not always considered by the hospital
team because sickness benefit is forthcoming from the state and the
employer for some time if the patient has been employed. The
financial burden of caring for someone in the home is great: for
example the immobility of the patient means that heating must be
adequate, and John's parents' heating bill will become much
higher as John and his mother spend all day in the home. Thought
needs to be given to applications for financial assistance, and the
relevant DHSS leaflets, available also from health centres and
larger post offices, include:

NI 16A	Invalidity Benefit.
NI 212	Invalid Care Allowance.
NI 211	Mobility Allowance.
H 11	Your Hospital Fares.
M 11	Free if you're on a low income. (Dental treatment, glasses and prescriptions.)
NI 6	Industrial Injuries, Disablement Benefit.

Planning care

The future for the disabled can be forbidding, and honesty about
any prognosis is usually advocated, but nursers will need to know
how much the patient and the family know before they enter the
home. Honesty about the future can assist in laying the foundations
of the nursing care plan in which patient and family can be involved.

John, for example, is going to remain largely immobile and very
little can be done about that, but he still has some movement which
can be exploited, and new skills can be learned using what is

available. A start should be made by ensuring that the good muscles are kept in prime condition and even strengthened with a view to doing more with them. The useless parts of the body cannot be ignored however, because pressure sores will cause weakness, vulnerability to infection, and cosmetic disfigurement; exercise and movement of the whole body is therefore important. This involves planning, and planning together, and the emphasis should be on encouraging the patient to concentrate on what he can do and achieve rather than on what he cannot do—on the positive rather than the negative.

The nursing care plan will therefore focus mainly upon preventive measures such as avoiding pressure sores, prevention of further disability, the early detection of indicators to ill-health and early treatment, the maintenance of continence, prevention of accidents and provision of a diet that will prevent obesity where there is immobility.

A district nurse who is suddenly asked to visit a John Davis who is a tetraplegic, recently discharged from hospital and is in need of a daily bath and dressing, might well find herself completely at sea and unable to plan care because she does not know who is doing what with the family. Where then does the nurse begin? John has obviously had a hospital based social worker working with him and the family since the home has been adapted to meet his needs. Responsibility for continuous assessment for financial benefits, home adaptations and aids for daily living may be referred to a community-based social worker. The team of health care workers surrounding John now includes the hospital specialists, the GP, the social worker and the district nurse; between them they will possess a great deal of information about John, but this will be utterly useless if it is left uncoordinated. Teamwork is essential to avoid the risk of individual team members working to conflicting ends, each having different priorities.

A case conference is one way of ensuring that activity is coordinated and that realistic targets are set. With patients such as John, there is special value in a case conference prior to hospital discharge, but any team member should be able to initiate the case conference if there is a need, be it patient need or the need for information and co-ordination by health care workers themselves.

Some psychological problems can be anticipated when caring for the disabled and their families. An enforced change of job can lead to loss of earnings and an inability to support the family in the

manner to which it has become accustomed. To have no prospect of a job at all is worse still and goes against the work ethic on which our society is based. The inability of a husband and father to carry on working can lead to a reversal of roles where the man stays at home and the wife goes to work. This is discussed in more detail in Chapter 14. Employment Resettlement Centres enable persons who have lost work skills to undergo assessment and re-training. The Disablement Resettlement Officer (DRO) is trained to undertake assessments and to advise disabled people about the possibility of returning to work or the need for re-training. The DRO often recommends registration as a disabled person because, by law, firms who employ more than 20 people must employ a 'quota' of registered disabled people. Many DHSS financial benefits are also dependent upon registration. For those who are unable to work, diversional and occupational therapy is important, but, as in the case of the elderly, activities should not be designed merely to fill in time. The participant must also experience a sense of achievement. John can read, go to football matches and has his own television and cassette recorder, but where is the sense of achievement and contribution? For him a workshop might be an answer, or encouragement to achieve proficiency in a sports group for the physically disabled.

A particular feeling experienced commonly by relatives is that of isolation—they feel that they are alone in caring, that they are the only couple (or spouse) within their neighbourhood and social group who have a disabled son or wife. Participation in existing self-help groups and involvement with voluntary bodies can be of value in enabling such feelings to be shared, as well as actually providing support and assistance. Nurses should know what organisations are available locally and the community physician, the local library, the Community Health Council and Citizens Advice Bureau can usually provide relevant information. The relevant voluntary organisations are listed in the Appendix 2, but those of special interest to the young disabled include:

Central Council for the Disabled, the Disabled Alliance, the British Council for Rehabilitation of the Disabled, British Sports Association for the Disabled and Sexual Problems of the Disabled (SPOD).

Sexual problems can be anticipated; John will never experience a normal sex life but his desires and needs will remain. The arthritic

patient, the person with only one useful arm, the cosmetically disfigured, will all experience problems. These problems are now acknowledged and widely discussed, and further reading is recommended. The counselling role of the nurse is important here, as is her ability to discuss sexual needs and to recognise that the available ways of meeting them are normal and therefore acceptable activities, and do not represent perversions or inadmissable behaviour patterns.

Guilt is a feeling that can be experienced by both patient and family. The patient feels guilt because he cannot contribute to the family life as before, physically or financially. The relatives feel guilt when the realisation dawns that they no longer want, or are physically unable, to continue caring.

John's mother has given up work to care for her son, but she may eventually resent his intrusion on her lifestyle only to feel guilty about this very feeling later on. John may feel guilt over his mother actually making changes just for him. The nurse must be sensitive to changes in family dynamics, and where possible prevent disharmony by promoting the continued discussion of problems within the family.

Lifestyles should not be drastically changed if it can be avoided. Mrs Davis could continue in her part time job if John's independence was encouraged and care was planned. For example, if the district nurse visits John in the morning, washes him, gets him up and dressed, changes the urine bag and generally meets his needs, surely Mrs Davis would not be missed? If John were to attend a workshop, sports or OT group, or if the home help called in towards lunchtime too, Mrs Davis's continued work might become a realistic possibility. Equipment to assist John in his independence when alone would be important and might include remote control for the TV, a mechanical hand for retrieving items from the floor, a nearby telephone, an intercom system to the front door and even a flask of coffee and a novel on the bedside table.

Relatives who can no longer cope need careful and sympathetic understanding. A holiday break should not be offered unless the answer is that a break is all that is necessary, and if it becomes necessary for the patient to leave home the family should have the reassurance that suitable residential care is available.

Implementation and evaluation

The attitudes of the whole family must be considered and evaluated

as any nursing plan is put into practice. Siblings for example may seem fully involved in planning care and express commitment, even excitement, yet in practice jealousy over the disproportionate amount of time spent on and with the disabled family member is almost inevitable.

Dislike of the disabled sibling can arise when his frustration at being disabled and different is converted to anger, which is of course vented on those nearby and those who are really most loved.

The disabled are in need of care but not to the exclusion of all else and of all other people. Overprotection and overindulgence are common but families should be urged to avoid this, and to share themselves and material things as equally as possible. The benefits of the nursing plan, as implemented, should be conveyed to the family so that they are encouraged to recognise their own dispensibility and the potential of the patient for a degree of independence.

Evaluation will determine when the needs of the patient have been met and district nursing intervention is no longer required. Complete discharge from care may of course never occur because the immobility of the patient and the lack of family involvement mean that nursing care must be continuous, and in this case the nurse may decide to undertake continuous preventive health care and so remain involved with the family. This type of case could be passed to the health visitor, but whatever the course of action, patient and family should always have access to professional advice and support when needed. Every effort must therefore be made to ensure that self-referral will occur in case of future need.

References

1. *Report of the Committee on the Education of Handicapped Children and Young People*. (Warnock report) (1978). London: HMSO.
2. Fit for the Future. *Report of the Committee on Child Health Services*. (Court Report) (1976). London: HMSO.
3. Harris A. I. (1971). *Handicapped and Impaired in Great Britain*. London: HMSO.
4. Skeet M. (1974). *Home From Hospital*. 4th ed. London: Macmillan Journals.
5. Hockey L., Buttimore A. (1970). *Co-operation in Patient Care*. London: Queens Institute of District Nursing.

Further Reading

Arthritis and Rheumatism Council. *Marriage, Sex and Arthritis*. Free from the Arthritis and Rheumatism Council, London.

Blaxter M. (1976). *The Meaning of Disability—A Sociological Study of Impairment.* London: William Heinemann Medical Books.

Consumer's Association. *Coping With Disablement.* London.

Disabled Living Foundation. *Dressing for Disabled People.* London.

National Fund for Research into Crippling Diseases. *Sex and the Physically Handicapped.* London.

Chapter 13

The Mentally Ill

Throughout history, attitudes to people whose behaviour has deviated from normal has varied widely. At times fools and madmen have been regarded as 'inspired' and endowed with special sight, but on other occasions they have been connected with evil spirits and witches. To the confusion of the historian there have been times when both attitudes co-existed.

Because mental health is relative it is often difficult to tell where health ends and disease begins, for what is regarded as mental illness varies, not only from period to period, but also between different groups in the same period. Eighteenth century rural England tolerated eccentrics like Squire Western or bizarre poets like John Clare more readily than would people in the new industrial towns of that time. On the other hand, the wayward genius of men like Van Gogh and Blake—whether in town or country—today would probably be treated by tranquillizers, group therapy and social rehabilitation. Mass production and the computer age require conformity.

By these tokens it is impossible to say whether mental illness is increasing; some illness, especially that due to infection, has declined. For example, at the beginning of the century one in five admissions to mental asylums was due to syphilis, now it is less than one in 200. Also, due to better living conditions, it is likely that the incidence of schizophrenia has decreased.[1] But mental illness associated with ageing is increasing, for the simple reason that there are now more old people, and the proportion of elderly with mental infirmity rises rapidly over 75 years.[2] Although it cannot be proved, it seems likely that there is an increase in stress-related diseases and psychoneurotic illness due to the pressures of modern urban life. This begs the question, however, of whether these illnesses have become more common, or is it just that we better recognize them? And has stress really increased? Living through Tudor inflation and the Reformation, with the Age of Faith crumbling, must also have been quite stressful.

From time to time the district nurse will come across patients, their relatives, or other carers whose behaviour 'interferes with their ability to lead a life acceptable as normal within the context of their social surroundings'[3] and this will impede the nurse's efforts to give total care. She is unlikely to encounter cases of overt psychosis, which comprise a small part of the sum of mental illness, but there is a wide range of deviation from what we call 'normal', ranging through mild paranoia, delusion, amnesia, cyclical depression, aggression and other manifestations of disturbance that do not call for the whole gamut of the psychiatric services, but nevertheless, if the nurse does not make a sound assessment, can cause suffering and untold trouble to the nurse herself later.

Since few district nurses are trained as psychiatric nurses, what can they do to ensure that they are safe practitioners when they encounter mental illness? Above all they should have some basic knowledge of the characteristics, predisposing factors and aetiology of the various groups of psychotic and neurotic illnesses. For example, Mr Adam's disorientation at the age of 85 years is hardly likely to indicate incipient schizophrenia, but a sudden manifestation of delusion or paranoia by John Davis would be cause for alarm. Depression in Mrs Cray would not be surprising; she lives in a high rise flat and we know that such dwellers consult their doctors with psychoneurotic symptoms more frequently than people who live in houses, and she is in fact already obviously socially withdrawn.

All the cases mentioned in Chapter 1 could be candidates for different forms of stress and each could show different signs and symptoms. However, to be a safe practitioner the district nurse must not only be able to differentiate the signs and signals that may indicate an impending breakdown, she must also recognize at what point she needs help and at the same time know where to get that help.

Assessing the need for care

Mental illness is associated with a temporary or permanent disturbance of the mind characterized by disorders of behaviour and reasoning, and generally occurring in adult life. These disturbances are usually associated with endogenous factors but sometimes the origin is exogenous as with alcohol, drugs or the effect of toxins. It is important that the exogenous factors are excluded before considering psychological factors.

Firstly, it is important to exclude the effect of drugs as a cause of a

patient's apparent disorientation. It is well known that patients have been described as suffering from 'senile confusion' when in fact the confusion was due to the injudicious prescribing of sedatives, or that the multiplicity of drugs being taken were interacting in such a way as to cause mental disturbance. It is important to check that the patient is taking the right drugs, in the right doses, at the prescribed times, and, since elderly patients tend to treasure all drugs like a valued rosary, that they are not taking 'pain killers' or 'stomach pills' prescribed by some previous doctor—or not prescribed at all—now hoarded in the bathroom or on the mantlepiece.

Secondly, because severe infection is comparatively rare and the 'delirium of fever' largely confined to Victorian melodrama, it is often forgotten that infection can cause mental disorder. After all, the 'wandering mind' was a symptom of the typhoid state. Infection that is being held at bay by antibiotics may still manifest itself in 'light-headedness', as can a variety of other conditions—including constipation.

Apart from drugs, other poisons may affect the mental facilities, the most important being alcohol. According to E. M. Jellinik, 'alpha alcoholism' is due to an underlying personality defect, but this only accounts for a minority of cases, whereas it is estimated that probably two per cent of the population suffer from health effects due to alcohol.[4] To become alcoholic all that is necessary is the availability of alcohol and the incentive. Some occupations are particularly prone; for example, journalists, public relations men and publicans, and alcoholism tends to be a problem of the extremes of social class, being comparatively low in the middle classes. Alcohol depresses the function of the brain and makes the subject more accident-prone, and it must be remembered that it can lie at the root of otherwise unexplained aggressive behaviour such as battering and violent family quarrels.

Finally, though rare, a sudden change of behaviour may indicate a brain tumour or presage a cerebral accident, and this possibility should not be ruled out without investigation. Moreover, because a patient already has a personality problem or is thought to be mildly alcoholic, this is not to say that he is not developing a brain tumour. A wise surgeon once asked: 'If a man says he has a pain in his stomach who am I to say he has not?'

Most of the mental disturbance encountered by the district nurse will, however, be endogenous, and if she is to pick up the danger signals she must learn to assess vulnerable personalities and situa-

tions. Some patients and carers are as stable as the Rock of Gibraltar, but others have personalities that are potentially 'at risk'. These include the introverted and withdrawn, the immature and insecure, the over-aggressive and those with poorly developed powers of ratiocination and communication skills. The latter are vulnerable because they are denied the catharsis of 'talking things out', and the former cannot be helped by appeals to reason. Unfortunately it is often the vulnerable personalities that create, or somehow find themselves in, risk situations, which may include trouble with the boss, minor law breaking, marital quarrels and broken homes. When a number of these factors combine the storm cones might well be hoisted.

Apart from the 'at risk' personalities, there are situations of vulnerability that are the common lot of most people. For example, there are the crisis points in life mentioned in Chapter 3 which include a sudden change in the life-style such as marriage, parenthood, redundancy or retirement, bereavement or exposure to some external disaster. With regard to the latter it must be remembered that the effect may be delayed for some time, as was seen with men who had been prisoners of war—a point worth remembering when taking a nursing history.

Since endogenous depression is widespread the district nurse should be alert to its signs and dangers. Most people show some cyclical movement between elation and depression, and when the peaks and troughs are violent this may indicate manic depression. Some people, however, have long depressive phases not warranted by circumstances. This proviso is important. If Mr Fisher's wife leaves him, he loses his job and his sclerosis gets worse, his subsequent depression is not pathological—it is justified. Indeed when people do *not* get depressed or anxious when circumstances warrant it they may equally be displaying a personality disorder. However, if Mr Evans, with no obvious worries, starts sitting with his head in his hands, refusing to speak to his family and complaining of insomnia, the nurse would be right in regarding these as sinister omens for which she needs further advice.

Besides the distress that depressive patients cause to themselves and those around them, the possibility of suicide must be kept in mind. Throughout the world something like 1000 people commit suicide every day, and although in terms of actual numbers the age group over 55 years is most heavily represented, in terms of deaths per 1000 for a specific age group the figure is highest for those

between the ages of 24 and 35 years.[5] In England there are over 4000 suicides recorded each year and of course not all suicides are recorded as such. The upper classes seem more likely to kill themselves than the lower, with doctors having a particularly high rate. Predisposing factors seem to be the availability of the means, such as access to dangerous drugs, highly competitive job situations, and domestic stresses such as marital break-up and divorce proceedings. In women the premenstrual syndrome is important: Strindberg's Miss Julie characteristically cut her throat with a razor when 'her monthly was coming on'. Similarly, of course, hormonal swings are linked with puerperal depression, once the cause of many suicides in comparatively young women.

An important factor in the histories of suicides and attempted, or parasuicides, is a disorganised life pattern—possibly a disorganised marriage, a broken home or unsettled housing, and, all too often, heavy drinking and drug taking. While young adolescents are the most vulnerable group and the district nurse should be vigilant for danger signs among the young carers, numbers of lonely old people take their own lives either because they are confused or because life has become meaningless, or, tragically, because they feel that they have become a burden to those around them. Finally, in this elderly depressive group, is the train of events that so often occurs with bereaved people, where, particularly after the death of a spouse in what has been a long and happy marriage, a surprising number of surviving partners die (sometimes called 'heartbreak death') within a year of their partner's death.

Planning care

Each patient is an individual, and unique. Where the nurse feels that the mental state of the patient, or the carer, is such that those around him are at risk, the doctor should be consulted and probably a case conference called. In an emergency the machinery for compulsory admission can be invoked but it must be remembered that an 'urgency order' is only valid for 72 hours.

Hospital admission will be the exception, and with emphasis on care in the community the patient is likely to be returned home comparatively quickly. In these circumstances the district nurse can get support from other members of the team one of whom has probably had some psychiatric experience. However, the nurse's most valuable ally in such cases would be a community psychiatric nurse if such a nurse were available in the area. This group of nurses

had their origin in the work of far sighted psychiatric hospitals in the 1950s, and they grew in numbers and in scope after the Seebohm Committee recommended the virtual abolition of the psychiatric social worker. In 1974 the Joint Board of Clinical Nursing Studies approved a course for psychiatric nurses working in the community and by 1979 five polytechnics were providing courses. There are now over 1200 such nurses, who for practical reasons are still attached to psychiatric hospitals, but the time may well come when psychiatrists, instead of being appointed to hospitals, will be attached to health centres, and then the community psychiatric nurse will be part of the primary care team. Experiments have already shown that where such nurses are used there are fewer referrals to hospital and the whole primary care team has benefited by the opportunity to learn.

The type of help planned for patients with psychological problems will depend on the patient's age, condition, potential and the suspected primary reason for his breakdown. For example, the school nurse might well be consulted about so called 'problem' children who may be worrying the patient or his carers; illness in the house sometimes has a disturbing effect on children and it may be necessary to seek help from the child guidance clinic. Social workers with particular experience with youth work may be able to help with difficult adoloscents and Mrs Baker's children may well need considerable help in this respect both before and after their mother dies, for, being fatherless as well as watching their mother die, they are at risk and may be prey to all sorts of fantasies.

However, while problems concerning children are generally only likely to come to the district nurse in her capacity as 'guide, philosopher and friend' her main concern will be about the psychological overlay that is likely to exist in patients like Mr Fisher, Mrs Baker and John Davis, and their carers. A watchful eye must be kept lest the strain imposed on such families tips over into real depression. Planning care therefore involves prevention; ideally the stress placed on carers should not be more than they can bear, but if it is, then there must be intervention and this will inevitably involve other members of the team, particularly the health visitor, and then probably other agencies.

Implementing the plan

Unless the mental disturbance is such that it overshadows all other aspects of the patient's illness, the plan to meet the psychological

needs of the patient, or his carers, will be integrated into the main plan and probably much of this will be actually implemented by other people, such as social workers or the community psychiatric nurse. Although the causes of mental illness are usually multiple and defy tidy diagnosis there are ways in which mild and temporary disturbances can be mitigated.

It may be that such problems as insomnia and depression or other stress symptoms can be dealt with by drugs; sometimes a short, sharp course will break a bad spell. However it goes without saying that such courses must be properly monitored for patients react in a variety of ways and for some 'the dreams that come' are worse than the insomnia. For the most part however, the causes of mental disturbance lie outside the realm of mechanistic medicine, and help must come from elsewhere. How effective that help is depends on how accurately the assessment has been made, how severe the disturbance and, of course, what resources are available and how easily they are mobilized.

If the primary cause 'seems' to be marital breakdown—'seems' because there is always a cause beyond the cause—then it is possible that help can be obtained from a marriage guidance counsellor. If, on the other hand, disturbance or depression seems to have its roots in a sense of uselessness and social withdrawal—sometimes the accompaniment of retirement—then it is possible that help can be provided from the Social Services Department or through the vocational training services of the Department of Employment, but it must always be remembered that social withdrawal is a symptom as well as a cause. The patients and their carers who serve as models in this book all have different needs and each must be helped as an individual. Mr Fisher may prove himself very useful, and therefore much wanted, as a treasurer to various voluntary societies. John Davis might be helped by some educational course tailored to his capacity which gives him a series of hurdles to overcome—and therefore a purpose to life. Mrs Adams needs a break if she is to continue caring, but her idea of a holiday will not be the same as that of Mrs Davis. Planning this type of care needs imagination, co-operation with other agencies and knowledge of what is available.

Evaluating the plan

In caring for people with mental or emotional problems the best laid plans are more likely to go astray than in almost any other branch of care. Alas, patients and clients do not always respond to occupa-

tional therapy, diversional activity, visits to day centres or courses in music and drama, and some, obstinately, do not respond to drugs in accordance with the claims made by the manufacturers. Because so often the problem resides in the patients themselves rather than in external circumstances, the plan may have to be re-evaluated many times. Success may only be partial, and since from time to time anxiety and depression must be the common lot of man, the nurse must be thankful if she is instrumental in preventing real, and damaging, breakdown when people are exposed to stressful conditions over a long period.

Mental handicap

The district nurse will not be asked to plan care for the mentally handicapped as such, but she may meet the problem tangentially; maybe there is a mentally handicapped person in the house, and alternatively of course as handicapped persons achieve longevity they will themselves succumb to the normal degenerative disease processes. When a patient has such a handicap it must be taken into account when planning care, for the patient can only be involved in his own care plans to the limit of his intelligence. In such cases, however, the nurse would do well to consult her health visitor colleague.

As with mental illness the nurse should possess some knowledge about the main groups of mental handicap and know something about such problems as Down's syndrome, autism, epilepsy and spastic manifestations and, of course, the normal milestones to be expected in children. In fact the nurse should know enough to know when further advice is necessary.

Apart from this the district nurse should know how the services for the mentally ill and the mentally handicapped are organised in the National Health Service bearing in mind that after the reorganisation of the health services in 1981 these services will be the responsibility of the District Health Authorities. Equally important is some acquaintance with the various voluntary organisations like MIND and the Society of Mentally Handicapped Children, and the many organisations that deal with specific problems such as the British Epilepsy Association, and familiarity with the local activities of these societies.

Although the concept of 'hospitals' for the mentally handicapped is changing and there is a tendency to keep people in the community as long as possible with community supporting services, it must be

remembered that some handicapped persons have no stable family to go home to and some need protecting from the community. With a higher survival rate among the less well endowed and the long term mentally ill this problem will grow and will be made worse by a mobile society in search of jobs.

The Greeks saw the needs of the mind and the body as inseperable, and in planning total care for her patient the nurse needs to return to this concept, bearing in mind that the generalist nurse cannot know all the answers but should at least know where to find them.

References

1. McKeown T., Lowe C. R. (1974). *Introduction to Social Medicine* 2nd ed. Oxford: Blackwell Scientific Publications; p. 329.
2. Department of Health and Social Security (1978). *A Happier Old Age*. London: HMSO; p. 7.
3. McKeown T. and Lowe C. R. (1974). *Introduction to Social Medicine* 2nd ed. Oxford: Blackwell Scientific Publications; p. 325.
4. Lewin D. C. (1978). Care of the dependent patient: Alcohol addiction. *Nursing Times*, 6 April; p. 570.
5. Lock S., Smith T. (1976). Harmondsworth: *The Medical Risks of Life*. Penguin Books; p. 30.

Further Reading

Better Services for the Mentally Handicapped (1970). London: HMSO.
Carr P. J., Butterworth C. A., Hodges B. E. (1980). *Community Psychiatric Nursing*. Edinburgh: Churchill Livingstone.

Chapter 14

The Long-term Sick and Handicapped

People who are subject to disease and disability over a long period of time are usually referred to as being chronically ill or disabled. But, how long is long-term, what is chronic illness and, indeed, what is handicap? Handicap is associated with a loss of function. Short-sightedness is a loss of function, but if glasses are available no handicap is experienced by the individual or noticed by society. Wheelchairs replace limbs but those in them are perceived by society as handicapped people and when society makes kerbs too high, steps too many and ramps and wide doorways to public buildings too few, handicap is experienced and imposed. Society itself often determines whether any loss of function will be a handicap or not.

The blind and the deaf are severely handicapped but many learn to cope adequately with life and become independent; they will then call upon the health service no more often than the rest of the healthy population. Diabetics who require insulin replacement are going to be diabetics for life, yet they can learn to cope well with their diet and treatment regimes—even to the extent of anticipating imbalances and meeting emergencies while maintaining a life of quality. However, many diabetics tend to require care as the years advance when eye and other bodily changes occur. Many people with long-term illnesses, and/or residual handicap, can be assisted to at least partial recovery, but there is a second group composed of those chronically ill with no prospect of recovery, for example, sufferers from multiple sclerosis which usually first affects people in their thirties and is a progressive disease.

Definitions of chronic illness are numerous but surprisingly recent, first appearing in the 1960s and corresponding with the growth of the concept of 'whole patient care'. Even then the first definitions were hospital or medically orientated; for example, Wessen[1] defines a patient as chronically ill if he stays in hospital for

more than 30 days. Gerson and Strauss[2] accept that diseases do not make the patients and state that chronic illnesses are, 'long-term, multiple, disproportionately intrusive and expensive, as they require large effort and a wide variety of services including ancilliary services'. They also state that chronic disease care is primary care. Further definitions centre upon the characteristics exhibited by the chronically ill. Bogdonof[3] notes that there are disturbances of one or more bodily systems, changes in usual behaviour patterns, changes in usual activity patterns, limitations on social interaction and swings in emotions from anxiety and despair to acceptance or to guilt.

One characteristic of these definitions is that they do not concern themselves with specific diseases and are no longer medically orientated. A common theme is the presence of disability, and the long-term effects of the disability on bodily systems and functions, for which long-term care must be considered. A definition of long-term care is given by Hammerman et al.[4] as:

> . . . the sustained and prolonged health, social and personal care given to individuals who are chronically ill and/or disabled . . . a type of care given to those whose chronic conditions and accompanying problems have affected their daily functioning.

Diabetics come to require long-term care, for example, when they are no longer able to deal with a medical crisis or carry out prescribed treatment regimes.

Most nurses will agree that long-term care should be achieved, whenever possible, within the home. This view arises partly from the need to maintain a life within as normal an environment as possible, but also from well documented and publicised literature about the effects of institutional life on the chronically ill and especially those who are elderly. Studies show that transfer to an institution is accompanied by increased morbidity and mortality rates. Attention is therefore now centred upon the provision of community based services, but nurses will know that many of the chronically ill will eventually require the level and intensity of care that only the institution can provide. Such patients, and their relatives, will need the assurance that adequate residential care facilities will be available as physical disability and/or social problems intensify. Bigot and Munnichs[5] are concerned that the opposition to institutional care is unfortunate and unrealistic. They state:

... the opposition has tended to limit efforts to develop a more positive stance towards institutions, as well as constructive advocacy to improve institutional life, especially in relation to social and psychological quality of life supports for the residents. Realistically, both community-based services and institutional care services are required now and in the future ... gradual, continued deterioration in the state of health cannot be totally prevented. One of the tasks of community-based service should appropriately be to prepare the person for that eventuality.

This statement becomes more acceptable with the knowledge of studies showing that when transfer to an institution is accompanied by individual care and attention and supplemented by continuing 'good' care, the detrimental effects of institutionalisation can be largely avoided. Good care is seen, of course, to be whole patient care.

Assessment for care

By virtue of the process of disease, a chronically ill patient is likely to be, or to have been, transferred from community care to institutional care and back again. The health history is likely to be complex and the health care workers involved will be numerous. Any assessment for care must be an individual one, but the approach must be multi-disciplinary. As was highlighted in Chapter 12 the family must be participants in the health care team if only because they often bear the burden of care.

If the chronic illness is such that there is no chance of complete recovery, for example, multiple sclerosis in the case of Mr Fisher, the approach of the nurse to the assessment, and her teaching and counselling role, will be different from the approach to the patient who hopes to experience partial recovery and stability. When confronted with his diagnosis, Mr Fisher probably asked, 'Why me?', a question the terminally ill also ask. Although Mr Fisher is not catergorised as being terminally ill, he has no hope of recovery, unless medical research finds the cause and cure. He is likely to present the same psychopathology as the terminally ill—denial, anger, depression, bargaining and finally acceptance. These problems were described in Chapter 3. For the nurse to encourage such a patient to look on the 'bright side' all the time, and to deny the needs of the patient to consider the future and beyond, would be inappropriate. Assessment must be based on the knowledge of the

psychological effects of progressive illness, the mental mechanisms involved (Chapter 3), and the reality of the prognosis. This is not to say that encouragement and reassurance are always out of place when caring for the chronically ill, but that the encouragement should be positive and realistic. Mr Fisher for example, should most certainly be encouraged to work for as long as possible at his normal workplace and then to work from home. The positive aspect is the recognition of his abilities and contribution, and encouraging him to use them; the realism is acceptance that disability will eventually alter his activity patterns and limit his social life.

The consideration of limitations on social interaction is important when assessing the needs of the chronically ill. It is marvellous that Mr Fisher can work from home, can continue to use his skills and can, therefore, experience a sense of achievement and contribution. One major problem is solved. The working from home means, however, that his normal activities are curtailed; gone are the pub lunches with colleagues and clients, gone is the membership of the work group and probably the sports or other recreational club; less easy is the trip to the theatre or the sports club dinner-dance with friends. Mr Fisher is actually one of the lucky ones because as a professional man he is able to continue earning and contributing to the household budget and can continue to satisfy his own and society's expectations in this respect. But what of the unskilled or skilled factory worker or the building-site craftsman? There chances of continuing work from home are slight. They experience the loss not only of income but also of the social contact that the working group brings. Social interaction is important, and here a long-term patient's friends can be of tremendous value, if they are able to come to terms with and face his disability themselves.

Re-training is appropriate for some of the chronically ill, and should always be considered, as should membership of self-help and voluntary groups. Occupational and diversional therapy is essential and, as with the elderly, past skills should be used to advantage and should determine the type of therapy to be undertaken and promoted. An assessment of the financial situation and a knowledge of benefits available is also important (see Appendices 2 and 3). A reversal of roles is often seen when caring for the long-term ill; the husband cannot work so the wife goes out to work to supplement the family income while the husband stays at home. However much housewives may deny it, housework *is* seen to be non-contributory and to be the appropriate role of women with

children, supported by the husband. The role reversal is therefore difficult for the average man to accept, and the psychological effects can lead to conflict within the marriage itself—in spite of the willingness of the wife to accept change. If such problems are evident, referral to a marriage guidance service might be useful but the patient must of course be willing to accept help.

It must also be remembered that home life is not easy, that housework involves a great deal of physical effort and that caring for young children is hard work. Role reversal may not be satisfactory even when accepted by both partners. When it is the wife who is disabled it is important that her concern about her ability to care for the home and the children, in spite of her disability, is recognised and understood. The home help service is important, as is the involvement of the health visitor if there are young children, because she can give information about local nursery and play school facilities and she understands the problems of children that are likely to arise when there is a disabled or ill family member.

Planning care

Consciousness of disability will be increased by daily encounters with the outside world; in both small and major ways the chronically ill are reminded that life is not what it used to be. Major changes include admission to hospital through illness and the sudden inability to catch the morning train to the City, but there are also many small reminders like the sudden reflection of the changed bodily appearance in the hall mirror. The existence of disability or illness cannot be ignored even when a brave front convinces all around that disability has been accepted and the problems of change overcome. The care plan will need to include assisting the patient to make realistic assessments of what he can and cannot do; in fact, to set new boundaries.

Mr Fisher has lost an entire world; he may respond by trying to keep that world alive, in memory if not by physical action, and to ignore the reality of his new situation. Alternatively he may react by doing the exact opposite, and shut out his past life completely by concentrating on the immediate environment; he may deny that there are any limitations to, or losses in, his life, and struggle to carry on as normal with perhaps damaging or dangerous results. Honesty about the diagnosis, the likely course of the disease and the prognosis will form the basis for establishing a nurse-patient relationship within which fears, feelings and beliefs can be discussed

and advice given concerning which aspects of daily living must be confined to the past.

As there are limitations to daily living, there will be gaps—time to fill. New activities can replace old ones, and much joy and fulfilment can result, but the past can offer help in meeting new challenges. As is discussed in more detail in Chapter 15, the carpenter can be encouraged to make models and the gardener to 'pot' at home. Mr Fisher is however a man of figures and he may have few practical skills and interests; he is also rather isolated because he moved to his present home from the North and has not had the time to make friends locally because of the demands of his job and commuting. What can he do when confined to the home and yet still experience a sense of achievement and contribution? Here local self-help groups can be of tremendous value, as can the advice from the voluntary organisation, but a look at the needs of the community can often bear fruit. Mr Fisher might be a tremendous asset to the voluntary groups, advising clients on tax problems, and helping those who cannot read and write, or by helping school children with their maths O-levels. Thoughts of basket making, painting and jigsaw puzzles are surely too limiting for those who remain alert in mind even if the body will not co-operate.

Aids that enable and assist the chronically ill to continue occupational and diversional activities, together with necessary adaptations to the home, are of obvious and essential importance. Here the occupational therapist can offer advice if she undertakes home visiting. The Disabled Living Foundation has a wealth of knowledge and experience, and if their 'showrooms' cannot be visited they can supply leaflets and catalogues. It is often the charities and voluntary organisations that can be most useful because of their involvement in and experience of the needs of smaller, specific groups. Many of these organisations provide news-sheets and even newspapers to members, from which information about new aids can always be gleaned by the patient himself. A list of such organisations is included in Appendix 2. For nurses, all the nursing journals carry information about new aids and ideas and the local hospital's occupational therapy department could always be visited.

Care should also of course be planned to meet the needs of the family of the long-term sick. Mrs Fisher has a good job that will keep her away from the home most of the day but she will still need to do some housework. A common feeling of such spouses is guilt—guilt about leaving her husband and enjoying social and

work contacts, guilt about needing more than he can give her. Common problems within such marriages concern the sexual life, or lack of it, the enforced role reversal, and financial pressures; and, of course, fear about the future. The family require support and, as participants in the caring plan, involvement in the decision-making, which must be dependent upon their knowledge of the diagnosis and the prognosis.

Any care plan for the long-term ill must focus upon prevention—prevention of unnecessary disability, the early detection and treatment of change and prevention of physical and mental strain in the caring relatives. One factor that is often forgotten because of the pressing nature of physical and psychological problems is the immediate environment in which the family live. Think of the family who have always prided themselves on the decoration of their house and their tidy, attractive garden. Disability intervenes and the house cannot be redecorated or the spring bulbs planted. To see a previously cared-for garden become overgrown and ugly can be soul-destroying, especially when tidiness is a feature of the neighbourhood and 'keeping up with the Joneses' is important. Some people will be able to pay for help in the garden but many will not, and in this case, local volunteers can be invaluable, especially school children and scout groups.

Implementation and evaluation

It is likely that if the original illness was diagnosed in hospital or if hospital admission has taken place at some stage, the more severely disabled will have been assessed within the occupational therapy department, an estimate made of their abilities to cope with daily living activities, and plans made for the home accordingly. The plans may not have been implemented however, and in any case an earlier assessment may be misleading in the case of progressive conditions. The nurse must note continuously the abilities of the patient to cope with making tea, lighting the gas fire, using knife and fork, negotiating steps and reaching into cupboards. Many patients may not readily admit to increasing disability, and this can often result in accidents. Reassessment by the occupational therapists may be needed or the social workers may need to become involved to discuss further home adaptations.

This highlights the necessity to be prepared for change whether it be insidious or sudden. The change can be so sudden and drastic as to bring about a whole change of approach—Mr Fisher may suffer a

relapse and go into hospital, never again to be independent enough to return home, or he may return home but with a far greater degree of debility. Preparation for hospital has already been mentioned and contact with the hospital caring team is essential so that information about any changes is forthcoming. Only then will the nurse be able to consider her present care plan, evaluate it in the light of new information and begin to replan in preparation for the return home or in preparation for the continuing care of the family if no return is to be achieved. Such an evaluation may reveal a need to visit the hospital to discuss problems with the patient, occupational therapist and doctor. This would allow for easier reassessment, in readiness for the implementation of the changed plan on discharge—probably far better planning than can be achieved by the receipt of notes from the doctor or phone-calls from any liaison nurse.

References

1. Wessen A. F. (1961). Sociological characteristics of long-term care. *Gerontologist*; **4**: 7–14.
2. Gerson E. M., Strauss A. L. (1975). Time for living—problems in chronic illness care. *Social Policy*; Nov/Dec.
3. Bogdonoff M. D., Nichols C. R. (1960). Perspectives of chronic illness. *Journal of the American Medical Association*; 174.
4. Hammerman J., Friedsham H. H., Shore H. (1975). *Management Perspectives in Long Term Care Facilities*. New York: Spectrum Publications.
5. *The Aged in Residential Homes: Integration or Apathy?* (1975). London: HMSO.

Further Reading

*British Medical Association Family Doctor Publications No. 65. (1971) *Strokes and How to Live With Them*. London: BMA.
Brocklehurst J. (1977). *Geriatric Care in Advanced Societies*. Lancaster: MTP Publishers.
Brocklehurst J. ed. (1978). *Textbook of Geriatric Medicine and Gerontology*. 2nd ed. Edinburgh: Churchill Livingstone.
*Disablement Income Group. *An ABC of Services and Information For Disabled People*. London.
Griffith V. E. (1970). *A Stroke in the Family*. Harmondsworth: Penguin.
Isaacs B., Neville Y., Rushford I. (1976). The stricken: the social consequences of stroke. *Age and Ageing;* **5**: 188.
The Aged in Residential Homes: Integration or Apathy? (1975). London: HMSO.
Wallis M. G. (1970). *A Guide to Activities for Older People*. London: Elek.

*Can usefully be recommended to patients and relatives.

Chapter 15

The Elderly

In 1951 approximately four million people in the United Kingdom were receiving retirement pensions; by 1961 the figure was just under six million and by 1976 it had risen to eight and a half million.[1] The United Nations[2] reported that, as a consequence of the falling birth rate and the increased life expectancy, the average age of the World's population was going up, and they went on to forecast that the figure of 291 million people in the world over the age of 60 years in 1970 would double by the year 2000. Many factors contribute towards this growth including a better diet and housing, improved social services in many parts of the world, and, of course, recent advances in medical knowledge and technology. In Britain, as elsewhere, this growth of the elderly population is socially and economically important because many of the elderly have stopped work and are dependent on social, health and other services for support for a longer period than ever before. Moreover, occupational pensions and State pensions are paid to more and more people for a longer time, a situation which is especially complicated in a time of high inflation.

The growth of the population over 65 years old has led to an increased demand for, and an expansion in, the health and social services. Demand continues to rise as the size of the group increases and, as a result, society—and especially the caring professions—have come to think of the elderly as a 'special group' and of old age as a 'problem.' Added to this is the fact that the label 'Old Age Pensioner' is attached to all those over retiring age, which distorts perceptions and leads to stereotyping. The old may be seen as sick, senile, old-fashioned, cantankerous or a nuisance, regardless of individual mental and physical abilities which in some cases continue unimpaired to a late age. However, 'age' is the criterion by which the advent of 'old age' is determined and, since retirement in industrial societies is imposed at about 65 years, chronological age alone determines when the useful working life is at an end. In a society based on the work ethic, in which productivity and self-

support equate with social acceptability, is it not a fact that society imposes this problem on itself?

The French philosopher, Jean Paul Sartre, when himself an octogenarian, said at an interview:

> I dont feel my age—so my old age is not something that in itself can teach me anything. What does teach me something is the attitude of others towards me. Old age is an aspect of me that others feel. They look at me and say 'that old codger' and they make themselves pleasant because I will die soon and they are respectful. My old age is in other people.[4]

Some authorities can find no scientific evidence to support retirement at 65, stating that political and economic reasons are responsible for the age-based practice. It has been argued[3] that the age link is unsatisfactory because:

Within a particular individual, the rate of age related changes can differ greatly;

There are important differences between individuals in the rate and pattern of age related changes;

There is no sharp drop-off in either physical or psychological functioning at or around the age of 65;

The worker at the age of 65 may be slower in physical actions but actually quicker in other actions because of a background of experience to guide his perception;

Each aged individual has unique capacities and limitations regarding his ability to fulfil his demands for self care.

The focus of nursing is to take action in a planned, organised and therapeutic manner in order to:

(a) strengthen self-care capacities,
(b) eliminate or minimise self-care limitations,
(c) provide care when self-care demands cannot be fulfilled.

The elderly have their needs as do all other individuals, and when the elderly person becomes dependent on care the nurse must always ask herself whether she is enhancing the quality of the patient's life. As an example, Mr Adams may find that eating fish and chips from a spoon is a degrading experience, yet be unable to communicate that feeling or express the desire to try and use his good hand to feed himself. The nurses and the family have taken over; individual need is not determined nor is independence promoted.

When assessing patients and their families nurses are apt to concentrate on their recent social history and on societal norms, but it must be remembered that to elderly people the past can be equally important. The age in which the patient grew up and the social conditions he experienced will have influenced his attitudes; for example, many elderly people are reluctant to divulge information about personal finances because of memories of 'means testing' and the treatment of the poor under the Poor Law system. This fact illustrates a principle of the application of the nursing process, namely that use must be made of knowledge derived from various fields including psychology, biology and other physical and social sciences when assessing the patient.

Finally, the nurse must remember that she has a preventive role to play in helping people to adjust to change and to prepare for retirement and changed life styles. Unfortunately, although the value of preparation is well known and well documented, the attitudes of others to the elderly often colour the perceptions the elderly have of themselves. Therefore, since stereotyping is common, preventive health practices must include discussions with young children and the teaching that ageing is a natural process and than an old man remains a unique individual.

Psychogeriatric care

In October 1980 the Secretary of State for Health and Social Security said that there were some 70 000 psychogeriatric patients in the United Kingdom of whom only 13 500 were in hospitals or other institutions—the vast majority are therefore at home. Professor J. Brocklehurst claims that the psychiatry of old age is now a specialty in its own right and he expects to see more psychiatrists with a responsibility for running psychogeriatric services within the next decade, and the recognition of dementia as a condition for care in its own right.[5] The need for such a service is demonstrated by recent studies which have shown that over one third of the people over 65 years now receiving nursing care at home or elsewhere have psychiatric problems.[6]

There are now suggestions that a psychiatrist should be appointed to co-ordinate the services for psychogeriatric cases within a defined area, who would be able to plan hospital and community care and liaise with Local Authorities. However, the role of the primary care team will remain of the greatest importance as a preventive service especially in the detection and assessment of

mental disease in old age. In the meantime experimentation continues into assessment based on the hospital, into small assessment units, and into home assessment.

The segregation of those with dementia from the mentally agile creates a need for separate day-centres and residential homes for psychogeriatric patients. Resources are limited, however, and the burden on relatives in caring for a mentally disturbed member of the family is inevitably heavy (Chapter 13).

Assessment for care

Ageing should be accepted as a normal process even though the separation of the elderly as a group in need of special attention by the health and allied services is welcomed. Although age brings a slowing of the heart rate, a loss of elasticity in the lungs and blood vessels and a replacement of muscle and fibrous tissue, this is normal and the elderly still look like, and share, the desires of all ages. This must be the principle that guides the application of the nursing process to the elderly. Eliopoulous[7] places great emphasis on this and is concerned that the principle is not always practiced. She says:

'Ageing is not a crippling disease and although some limitations may be imposed as the body systems lose efficiency in function, ageing itself does not reduce the opportunity for happiness, fulfilment and independent function. An increased understanding of the ageing process may promote a more positive attitude towards old age.'

The same author lists several other important principles of geriatric nursing practice:

'Ageing is a natural process.
'Heredity, nutrition, health status, life experience, environment, activity and stress are factors which influence the normal ageing process and demonstrate unique effects on each individual. Scientific data related to normal ageing and the unique characteristics of individuals are combined with nursing knowledge in the application of the nursing process to the aged.
'Aged individuals share similiar universal demands for self-care with all individuals.'

In making an assessment it is important to take into account the past working life of the patient; for example the carpenter who has

no form of recreation and is depressed because he experiences no sense of accomplishment might well be persuaded to use his old skills to meet these needs. In order to promote communication skills in Mr Adams it will be important to introduce a subject immediately interesting to him, and, something related to his past experience, such as what he did in the Second World War, is more likely to promote a response than trying to talk about the weather or the state of the economy. Knowledge of the patient's past occupation or war-time activity is sometimes essential when assessing his present financial situation and entitlements as well as his physical condition. Examples of the importance of this are miners with lung disease or ex-service men with war wounds or disabilities.

When assessing an elderly patient the nurse must be aware of her own values and beware of imposing them. Mr Adams is old, handicapped, constantly wet and often difficult to manage because of his confusion. Being confused, he does not seem aware of his condition nor wish to seek improvement. Mrs Adams is not fit and there are no relatives to help; the house is old, facilities are poor—even squalid—and the environs are dangerous. The nurse who values modern living and who uses only her own preconceptions when making her observations might well want to try and remove the Adams's to a new house or even get Mr Adams into hospital. But, she should ask, is the house really dangerous? The 'clutter' constitutes a carefully built, cherished and familiar home environment. The paraffin heater is familiar, cheap and sensibly used, and although there are no relatives, villagers and friends abound and the couple have lived this way for over fifty years; they would hate separation and their attitude to it must be determined before any action is taken.

The observational skills of the nurse when dealing with the old are particularly important. For reasons of pride the elderly may not answer questions quite truthfully; for example they may deny incontinence out of shame or embarrassment, or they may claim that their heating arrangements are adequate when in fact the fuel bills cannot be met and heat is only turned on when someone comes. The nurse's sense of smell and a suspiciously low room temperature may help her detect such problems. At the same time she must be alert to hazards in the home; accidents in the homes of the elderly are commonplace and the nurse must remember that hallways, bedrooms and bathrooms are as dangerous—or potentially dangerous—as are the kitchens and living areas.

Possibly as a legacy from the days when medical care was costly, many elderly patients are confirmed 'home doctors' and the nurse should try to be aware of self-prescribing. Some remedies are harmless, like hot water to aid digestion, but some can be harmful like the prolonged use of laxatives especially when there are problems of dehydration. 'Do you take laxatives?' may get a negative answer when in fact senna pods are grown in the back garden, picked, stored and soaked and taken daily as a matter of course. 'Do you use anything to keep your bowels regular?' would be better understood.

As has been stressed in previous chapters the emotional needs of the patient and the family must not be overlooked. In Chapter 7 the need to discuss with John Davis his enforced lack of sexual activity was emphasised; this was not said of Mrs Adams even though the lack probably exists. There is now a great deal of literature about sex and the elderly and no better resumeé can be found than that of Kastenbaum[8] who says 'the intimacy of two people who have shared years of joys and sorrows together is an excellent buffer against a world that looks at old men and women but does not really see them. In each others arms they continue to be themselves rather than society's impoverished image of the aged. The small intimacies, the quiet conversation, the sense of togetherness, remain both precious and life-affirming.'

Although there is no validated research to confirm this it has recently been suggested that some elderly patients are subjected to abuse or neglect. After reports about this had reached the Royal College of Nursing an attempt was made to gain more concrete information from nurses. Evidence was scant, but while some nurses substantiated the occurrence of ill-treatment others found no evidence, and still others, while suspecting such occurrences, could not offer evidence[9] (see also Chapter 19 on confidentiality). Instances included actual physical and verbal abuse, and elderly patients being kept in a cold room, often in isolation, and being given an inadequate diet. There were also reports of relatives using pensions and social service grants for their own use. Most nurses making reports were of the opinion that relatives received inadequate counselling and support and that they often cared for relatives under such pressure that they themselves began to suffer from depression or even actual physical disability. The solution to this problem would seem to lie in the provision of more nursing and other support services including more home helps, day centres and holiday places.

(The nurse's responsibility in dealing with violence in the family is discussed in Chapter 19).

Planning care

The problems of the elderly are frequently multiple and may embrace medical, social, psychological, financial and emotional needs. A multidisciplinary approach is therefore required but this has dangers in itself. The list of persons and agencies dealing with Mr and Mrs Adams could be lengthy and, without good liaison, each worker could be aiming at a different goal and giving different advice. This could lead to confusion not to mention the sheer annoyance of having so many visitors in the home often asking repetitious and seemingly impertinent questions. The nursing care plan must take into account the number of agencies to be co-ordinated and the nurse must be prepared for the role of co-ordinator to fall on her because of her continuous and intimate involvement in the household.

When planning care for elderly patients some medical and nursing problems can be readily anticipated; a possible checklist would include:

1 Deficiencies in communicating abilities—sight, hearing, speech—and loneliness.
2 Management of constipation.
3 Management of pressure areas.
4 Management of diet—including fluid intake.
5 The need for chiropody.
6 The adequacy of heating in the home.
7 The safety of the home.

Commonly met problems such as these can be anticipated but it does not mean that once met they should be accepted. It is normal for older people to lose the ability to hear high-pitched sounds but deafness is not part of normal ageing; usually there is some loss of mobility of the joints with advancing years but arthritis and rheumatism are not inevitable. Another problem that could be added to the list is the need to prepare for seasonal changes because of the susceptibility of the elderly to respiratory problems and, of course, the well-documented problems of hypothermia.

The district nurse is well aware of the important contribution of relatives caring for patients at home, and particularly in the case of the elderly, for 95 per cent of people over 65 years old who require

care live in the community. It is, however, important that the nurse determines the abilities of relatives to lift, fetch and carry, and that she is also aware of their attitudes to performing such intimate tasks as washing and giving skin fold care to patients. Some relatives feel that they cannot give this intimate care and their feelings must be respected.

Problems often arise when an old person is brought into the younger generation's family home. Some difficulties can be anticipated in advance and the nurse should help and encourage families to discuss the problems and plan carefully. Agreement should be established from the outset about such things as money, the running of the home, the bringing up of the children and, the cause of many a family squabble, radio and television programmes. The old person should not be pressurised into moving in, nor the young family excluded from the preparations and discussions. The old require solitude as well as care and if possible they should have their own room in which they should be encouraged to entertain friends and to continue with old interests. The life-style of the family should change as little as possible; for example, if the mother works she should continue to do so and family holidays should not be stopped but rather a holiday arranged for the elderly relative at the same time.

Planning diversional therapy is important for elderly patients if they are to avoid being lonely and to retain a sense of achievement, but 'filling time' is not sufficient; the occupation must have a recognisable purpose. Here a knowledge of the patient's past life is important, the gardener can be encouraged to garden and grow tomatoes for the family, or at least to do indoor potting; those with practical skills like knitting or basket-making can make a contribution to the family—many a grandmother is fully occupied knitting for children and grandchildren. But not all patients have practical skills; some have intellectual gifts and training which they should be encouraged to continue and possibly to share with the less fortunate; for example, retired school teachers are often invaluable in giving individual coaching.

Implementation and evaluation

Whatever the reason for nursing intervention and for however long the need for direct care continues, when caring for an old person the nurse must concentrate on prevention as well as on active treatment. Since the older age groups are likely to require more and

more health care a case can be made for retaining the patient over the age of 65 years 'on the books' instead of discharging him. Surveys have shown that this group are conditioned to accept bodily deterioration and may well fail to report a lump in the breast or frozen shoulder either through fear or because it is something they 'must accept'. Relatives and patients need to be educated that ill-health is not normal and they should be encouraged to report any change. The same positive attitude must be encouraged towards those vital ancillaries to health as people grow older: the provision of the correct spectacles, regular dental care, hearing aids if necesary, good shoes and chiropody services. As the Royal College of Nursing said in evidence to the Royal Commission on the Health Service, 'It is more important to keep the elderly on their feet, with their shoes on, than to provide geriatric beds'.

Although it is helpful if the nurse can discharge an elderly person to a regular screening clinic, the continual teaching of good health care to the elderly remains an important component of any health care plan.

Evaluation is dependent upon continual assessment and the constant examination of the carer's own attitudes, prejudices and beliefs. Although nurses and social workers may express delight in the provision of such facilities as day centres, clubs and organizations for the so-called 'lonely and socially deprived' they are not necessarily a panacea for the problems many old people encounter. It has been suggested that people who have never had close friends at other stages of their lives, or single persons, are less likely to be unhappy or lonely in old age: what they have never had they do not miss. One study found that the elderly did not consider that communication with their own age group was of much value. One lady said 'it is not good to stay in one age group, but to make friends with people younger than yourself as well as people who are older.' Another study showed that enforced family gatherings such as at Christmas time could be conducive to mental trauma.

As we reach even higher survival ages with the likelihood of more patients over the age of 85 years, we must accept that we have not only pushed back the frontiers of death but also that wavy line that denotes old age.

References

1. *Facts in Focus* (1978). London: Penguin Reference Books in association with HMSO.

2. United Nations Fund for Population Activities (1979). *State of the World Population.* United Nations.
3. Kastenbaum R., Derbin V., Sabatini P., Artt S. (1972). The ages of men. *International Journal of Aging and Human Development;* **3:** 197–212.
4. Nicholson J. (1980). *Seven Ages.* London: Fontana.
5. Brocklehurst J. C. (1978). In: Brocklehurst J. C., ed. *Textbook of Geriatric Medicine and Gerontology.* 2nd ed. Edinburgh: Churchill Livingstone.
6. Pasker P., Thomas J. P. R., Ashley J. S. A. (1976). The elderly mentally ill—whose responsibility? *British Medical Journal;* **3:** 164–8.
7. Eliopoulous C. (1980). *Geriatric Nursing.* London: Harper and Row.
8. Kastenbaum R. (1979). *Growing Old* (a Life Cycle book). London: Harper and Row.
9. Royal College of Nursing (1976). *Neglect and Ill-treatment of the Elderly at Home.* London: Royal College of Nursing.

Further Reading

Brearly C. P. (1975). *Social Work, Ageing and Society.* London: Routledge and Kegan Paul.
Comfort A. (1976). *The Process of Ageing.* London: Weidenfeld and Nicholson.
Isaacs B. J. (1972). *Survival of the Unfittest.* London: Routledge and Kegan Paul.
Joint Board of Clinical Nursing Studies (1974). *Outline Curricula: Courses No. 296 and 940. Geriatric Nursing.* London: Joint Board of Clinical Nursing Studies.

Chapter 16

The Terminally Ill

There are two major considerations when discussing the problem of the terminally ill: firstly, the prevailing attitudes to death, and secondly, whether or not a dying patient and his relatives should be informed.

In a secular society few people contemplate death and few prepare for it. In the nineteenth century death was talked about freely but sex was a taboo subject: now the topics have been reversed. Nor are nurses immune; hospitals, particularly training hospitals, are there to 'cure', death somehow represents failure, and the chances are that nurses witness death comparatively rarely. Moreover, when on the district the nurse is unlikely to be present when death occurs, so with the low death rate and the small nuclear family it is quite possible for the nurse to have little acquaintance with death, and yet, 'death, a necessary end, will come when it will come.'

Before a nurse can give support to families where a patient is terminally ill she must come to terms with her own attitude to death and her own particular prejudices and convictions. A purely academic approach is not enough; the nurse must face up to her own acceptance of mortality. Because of the 'treatment and cure' model of much of nurse training, in the past all too frequently the trainee nurse was given little support in this sensitive and personal realm. Using the nursing process as a system of nursing should help to change this attitude.

On the question of whether the patient and his family should be informed of his condition, nurses tend to leave the decision to the doctor and to plan nursing care accordingly. Some patients are not told and the reasons why they are not told should be analysed objectively; all too often the patient is aware that something is being withheld from him, and this can be 'a cruel absence of care' because the patient needs to be able to communicate his fears about pain, solitude and death itself. By not telling the patient, the carers may be protecting themselves from facing up to an embarrassment that they would rather deny. Moreover, it is increasingly realised that

the separation of the terminally ill from their family and familiar surroundings is inhumane and that people deserve to die as they themselves choose. However, unless patients are given all the facts how can they choose? If they are fobbed off with being taken into hospital for the wrong reason there is no choice. The way people are told—or not told—often reflects the carer's own attitude to death. Kubler-Ross[1] comments that 'the manner in which the news is broken depends on the doctor's own ability to face terminal illness and death.'

It is one thing to cope with the patients who know their own prognosis, but it is even more difficult to deal with the terminal patient who does not know. Before entering the home the nurse should always ask the question, 'Who knows the diagnosis?' and then plan her care accordingly. If the continued assessment of the patient and his family lead the nurse to decide that the patient would benefit from knowing his condition, the doctor should be told and new care plans agreed on to meet with the situation, if and when the patient and his family are told the prognosis.

Most deaths still occur in some kind of institution and death is rarely witnessed by the family and friends. However, recognition of the inhumanity of removal to hospital for terminal care, the advocacy of the right of the individual to choose where to die, and the comparative decline of the number of hospital beds, mean that the primary care team, and especially district nurses, are more and more frequently meeting patients who will die at home.

Assessment for care

Dying is unique for every individual. Though people die 'the death of their disease', and the course the disease will follow can be anticipated and care planned accordingly, there are also other factors to be taken into consideration such as the patient's religious beliefs, or absence of them, his age and previous health, his acceptance or not of mortality, and his family commitments. Nursing care must be unique for the individual and the assessment must take into account all these facts. Knowledge of the religious beliefs of the patient is essential for two reasons. The first is, of course, that the wishes of the patient for spiritual help and succour must be respected, and priests and clergymen will generally visit homes if they are told of the need. Such arrangements should only be made at the request of the patient, but it must be remembered that sometimes spiritual comfort is not sought because the patient is

denying the possibility of death; once death is accepted such aid may be suddenly requested. This does not necessarily reflect on the essential faith of the patient but is part of the process of coming to terms with death. The second reason concerns the provision of total care; it can be devastating to the nurse to find that following the death of a patient the rituals and customs of his religion have not been observed. For example, at the death of a Jew the body should not be touched and the Rabbi should be called. As was stressed in Chapter 4, in order to ensure that religious beliefs are respected the nurse herself must have some knowledge of the basic tenets of the main religions as well as knowing the beliefs and wishes of her particular patients, with a special emphasis on those who are terminally ill.

When death is accepted it is common for the patient to wish to settle his affairs and to put things in order for those who are left behind. Mrs Baker will undoubtedly be concerned about the future care of her children and the need for Sarah to be able to lead as normal a life as possible. If patients wish to talk in this way they should be encouraged to do so and not be fobbed off with, 'Don't worry yourself about it, we shall sort it out and care for everyone'. This is to take all responsibility away when in fact the reverse should be encouraged; encouragement towards the maintenance of present standards as opposed to the immediate encouragement of false hope. The assessment should include an estimate of the normal standards, and the nursing plan should attempt to maintain them. A home help may be one answer (although, as always, with the agreement of the patient) and in this case the home help would work under the directions of the patient. The standards of 'self' are important too; Mrs Baker is anxious to wash and dress herself carefully every day, probably to put up a good front for her children but perhaps simply because she has always been neat and tidy. The nurse might well observe that there are cosmetics and perfumes in the bedroom or bathroom that suggest the lady is particular about her appearance and tactful questions might reveal that she has her hair set once a week. If Mrs Baker is determined to keep herself looking as she did before illness intervened, for whatever reason, a voluntary group could be asked to take her to the hairdressers or to arrange for a hairdresser to visit the home. For men, daily shaving may be very important to self-esteem.

Fear of pain is common among those who are terminally ill, and no more so than when the diagnosis is known to be a cancer. The

work of Cicely Saunders[2] and the hospice movement has shown
that even severe pain can be controlled, especially if drug therapy is
combined with psychological stability. However, care in the hospice is continuous and can hardly be emulated in the home. It is
therefore necessary for the nurse to gain the fullest information
about drug therapy from the doctors, and to determine methods of
reviewing drug effectiveness from the beginning. In this way,
patient and nurse can discuss the fear of pain, and plan together to
meet changing needs. This aspect of care is mentioned under the
heading of 'assessment' because it is an essential aspect of caring for
the terminally ill and must be considered at all the stages of the
nursing process, from the beginning.

The family of a dying patient will experience similar emotions to
those of the dying person himself, including denial, anger, depression, and finally acceptance, but not necessarily at the same time as
the patient is experiencing these emotions. Again care must be on an
individual basis and the nurse will need to understand the dying
process and to accept that relatives may actually stay away from a
dying relative. This may not signify any lack of love, but merely that
the relative is denying the imminence of death. Assessment of the
family response should be based on the knowledge of the defence
mechanisms that may be used.

The acceptance of the death of a loved one is different from the
acceptance of one's own death. What actually is death, and what is
on the 'other side'? Where does the dead person go? These are
questions relatives may ask, and some may actually say that their
own fear of death makes the prospect of somebody dying in their
home—the home in which they must afterwards continue to
live—unwelcome, frightening and eerie. While the wellbeing of the
dying patient is important, so is the future wellbeing of those who
will be left behind and they will need support in their preparations.

Planning care

Assessment and planning are made difficult in caring for the terminally ill when patients and their family demonstrate contradictions
in need, and scorn caring activities or are even abusive in their
derision of them. Contradictions are common where there is denial
of terminal illness or where the patient wavers between acceptance
and renewed hope. The fact that defence mechanisms are being used
to excess must be the basis for the assessment of need and planning
of care, and not the contradictory messages themselves. Where

anger is turned upon the nurse, she may respond with a feeling of resentment or personal affront, rather than accepting the right and need of the individual to verbalise his inner feelings. Uncertainty about the therapeutic value of her relationship is bound to occur and the nurse herself may then be in need of support from colleagues who can listen and give objective support.

These two points highlight the difficulties that exist in formulating a nursing care plan for the terminally ill. The nurse may be confident of achieving a caring situation one day, only to find herself unable to communicate or contribute the next. Plans should not be changed rapidly however, as a greater knowledge and understanding of the dying process will make clear. What then should the nursing care plan include?

Physical care will include the maintenance of bodily functions. Constipation may cause unnecessary suffering; ill-fitting false teeth (a common occurrence as weight is lost) will cause mouth ulceration and feeding difficulties; pressure sores will also cause unnecessary suffering and should be prevented; and, finally, there is the need to control pain and assist in the maintenance of appearance.

Psychological care will not include unrealistic reassurance or encouragement. The amputee or the agoraphobic must indeed be encouraged to look on the 'sunny side', or 'round the corner', but with the dying such phrases are meaningless. Silence, presence and touch are more important. Being with the patient in silence is an important nursing contribution in itself, and the time available needs to be utilised appropriately. The accent in planning care for the dying must therefore be on flexibility; routines will be difficult to adhere to anyway because of the fluctuating and contradictory nature of dying.

Fear of solitude is common in those who expect death, and at the same time relatives and friends may deny the realities and stay away. Nurses may gain support at such times from the clergy, or from local self-help groups such as Dorothy House and the Marie Curie Foundation. The latter will also provide a night-nursing service for the terminally ill, and the Foundation's existence is invaluable. Liaison between all involved in the care plan is essential, and especially in the careful recording of drugs administered and any reaction to them. For example, if nausea and vomiting are significant side effects the drug will need to be changed, or its route of administration altered.

Terminal illness entails an increasing loss of function and

strength, and therefore an increasing degree of dependence. The nurse must plan for this, perhaps by bringing in a commode to be placed in the bedroom rather than allowing the patient to struggle to the toilet, or by setting up a 'sick room' downstairs so that the patient does not feel isolated when bed-bound nor the family tired out by constant running up and down stairs. If the nurse is to organise things in this way she will need to use all her skills in communicating her proposed plans to the patient in order to gain total agreement. Mrs Baker might well prefer to struggle with stairs and toilet, and put up with the tiredness, until such time as the children are all aware that their mother is dying. Or she might feel that the children must have the downstairs room in which to play and watch television while she has a period of solitude and quiet.

A state of increasing dependence in itself is often feared, and a feeling of demoralisation often develops as independence is lost. Here the expertise of the professional is often welcomed, because professionalism is accepted where the attentions of relatives would be embarrassing. This applies especially to intimate acts such as bodily washing and toileting. For example, someone like Mrs Baker may not wish to ask her daughter to empty commodes, clean her after toileting or wash her vulva. The nursing plan will take this into account if the reasons for the patient's requests are understood. If the emotional aspect is not recognised, the nurse could decide that the needs of the patient are simply for unskilled care, for anyone can empty commodes and assist with washing.

It is interesting to note that much of the literature about death and dying is concerned with the discovery and documentation of psychopathology or with the course that individual diseases and ageing processes will follow. There is very little written about the possibility of the dying patient facing death positively and actually gaining from the experience, and yet it is known that the patient's initial fear and denial of death will often disappear or decrease with the passage of time. The fact is that impending death can be coped with and nursing staff have a crucial role in building up a relationship of trust with the dying person, within which all fears—past and future—can be openly discussed.[3] Death is inevitable, and patients should be helped to prepare for it. This may involve assistance with making a will and nurses should seek the help of a solicitor if at all possible. (Chapter 22). Dying patients may also need to discuss their wishes to give personal items away to friends and relatives, and

their arrangements to ensure those left behind are cared for adequately.

Any nursing care plan will not end at the death, but will continue to provide support for relatives. Schoenberg *et al.*[4] have highlighted the phenomenon of 'anticipatory' grief, the growing sense of bereavement in relatives and friends who are anticipating the loss of a loved one. Whether it occurs before death or at the time of death, friends and family should be encouraged to express their grief—be it by crying, shouting or walking away. Nurses are no longer 'taught' to maintain composure on meeting death and if composure is not felt, emotion must be accepted. This can help relatives in expresssing their own grief, for when the professional in attendance makes no attempt to suppress emotions the role model is shown to be human.

The nurse who is planning the care of relatives could well follow guidelines concisely laid down by Schneidman[5]:

1. Total care of the patient needs to include contact with survivors-to-be.
2. Begin as soon as possible.
3. Remember that there will be less resistance in talking to a professional person, especially one who has no axe to grind and no pitch to make (e.g. nurse, doctor).
4. The role of negative emotions towards the deceased—anger, envy, guilt—needs to be explored, but not at the very beginning.
5. The professional plays the important role of reality tester—the quiet voice of reason.
6. Medical evaluation of the survivors is crucial. One should be alert for possible decline in physical health and in overall well-being.

Implementation and evaluation

It is probably fair to say that in caring for the terminally ill, the lines between the four stages of the nursing process are blurred. The very nature of dying requires that assessment is continuous, because changes in patient need and especially psychological need, are themselves continuous. Change requires re-assessment, which in turn will lead to further changes in the nursing care plan, and a constant need for re-evaluation.

Conclusion

The nurse working with a dying patient requires a great deal of support, including the availability of colleagues with whom her personal reaction to an individual death can be explored. Nurses have their own beliefs, experiences and feelings about death, which may limit their ability to support their patients and their families if, for example, they are denying death when the patient has accepted it. Nurses should be able to end a nurse-patient relationship if that relationship is no longer therapeutic, and here the support and understanding of colleagues is vital.

Trained community nurses are no longer subjected only to the 'cure training model' and are exposed to the subject of death during formal training. Death is not viewed as a nursing failure, but it remains for the patient a highly significant experience, and a uniquely individual one. Terminal care, as Eliopoulous[6] observes, 'requires a fine blend of sensitivity, insight and knowledge of the vast topic of death'. It is hoped that the bibliography will contribute towards this, together with the following list of resources and agencies which might be of help to the nurse in caring for the dying.

References

1. Kubler-Ross E. (1969). *On Death and Dying*. New York: Macmillan.
2. Saunders C. (1972). A therapeutic community—St Christopher's Hospice. In: *Psychosocial aspects of terminal care*. New York: Columbia University Press: pp. 3–15.
3. Earle A., Argondizzo N., Kutscher A. H., Goldberg I. K. (1976). *The Role of the Nurse in the Care of the Dying Patient and Bereaved*. New York: Columbia University Press.
4. Schoenberg B., Carr C., Peretz D., Kutscher A., Goldberg K. (1974). *Anticipatory Grief*. New York: Columbia University Press.
5. Shneidman E. S. (1976). *Death: Current Perspectives*. New York: Aronson Jason.
6. Eliopoulous C. (1980). *Geriatric Nursing*. London: Harper & Row.

Further Reading

Board of Inland Revenue. Leaflet: *Income Tax and Widows* (IR23).
Cartwright A., Hockey L., Anderson J. L. (1973). *Life Before Death*. London: Routledge and Kegan Paul.
Department of Health and Social Security. Leaflets:
  Death Grant (NI 49 and NI 196).
  Your Benefit as a Window (NP 35 for first 26 weeks; NP 36 after the first 26 weeks).

Epstein C. (1975). *Nursing the Dying Patient.* Virginia: Reston Publishing Co.
Jury D., Jury M. (1976). *Gramps.* New York: Grossman.
Kastenbaum R., Aisenberg R. (1972). *The Psychology of Death.* Berlin: Springer.
Lamerton R. (1977). Going deeper into care of the dying. *Nursing Mirror;* March 3: 64–65.
Marris P. (1958). *Widows and Their Families.* London: Routledge and Kegan Paul.
Parkes M. (1975). *Bereavement: Studies of Grief in Adult Life.* Harmondsworth:· Pelican.

Section IV

Policies for Care

> The district nurse is a generalist who must be prepared to cope
> with any condition in any setting and must have the profes-
> sional competence and awareness to identify when and where
> specialist help, of any form, is required . . . she must have the
> knowledge and ability to contact and acquire help in the best
> interests of her patients.
>
> Report of the Panel of Assessors on District Nursing. (1978)

Since information about the various services contributing to the
patient's health and welfare is often neglected in the basic nurse
training this section is devoted to an attempt to remedy that omis-
sion.

District nurses are often in close and confidential contact with
their patients. Sometimes they are the only people visiting the home
on a regular basis and are therefore most likely to know about the
unmet needs of the patient and his family. Helping the patient to
meet his wider needs is part of total patient care, since ill-health and
disability are generally caused by the interrelationship of many
factors. For this reason it is important that district nurses understand the work and the policies of other disciplines and how, and
from where, the patients may obtain help. Some patients. like John
Davis, will need a vast range of services, others, like Mrs Cray, will
need to be persuaded to use the services that are available, while a
number will be capable of organising any help they may need for
themselves. Each patient presents an individual pattern.

The history of the development of the various services for care is
complex and inconsistent. Although the Beveridge Report of 1942
hoped to produce an integrated and coherent plan for all the social
services, for the most part the different services, and the benefits

they each offer, have, like Topsy, 'just growed'. Each service stems from a different tradition. Some have their roots in the voluntary organisations, most have been subjected to change due to political or ideological considerations and all have been influenced, and continue to be influenced, by the vagaries of the finanacial situation.

Because of this complexity it is impossible to deal with each service in detail but, if the district nurse understands the organisation of the services, the principles which guide them and the main controlling legislation, the day to day details can be filled in from up to date guides and leaflets to which every district nurse should have access.

Some services are universal, that is to say, they arise from the assumption that the state has a responsibility to protect a minimum standard for all citizens in such areas as health, education and incomes. The philosophy behind universality was that, being the concern of all, and not merely the poor and the powerless, there would be pressure to keep standards high. On the other hand, the Beveridge concept of a minimum standard for all immediately raised problems, because firstly, flat-rate benefits linked to flat-rate contributions were necessarily low, secondly, what is subsistence level varies with households depending on their special needs and how they organise their budgets and thirdly, poverty is relative. The poverty line shifts with the expectations of society; not being able to afford the expenditure necessitated by custom, such as sending your grandchildren birthday cards, represents social deprivation. However, to raise the universal benefits to cover all exigencies would be immensely costly, and there has to be some element of selectivity to deal with special needs. It is this selectivity with its complicated variations from service to service that makes the benefits and their entitlement so confusing, and for this reason they are set out in Appendix I for easy reference.

Since finance is the main controlling factor in all services, and as its provision is a minefield of misconception, a chapter has been devoted to this. Not only is the Health Service the service that concerns the district nurse most, but also for historical reasons it belongs to a different tradition from the other services. It is, in fact, the joker in the pack, so for these reasons it merits a separate chapter. However, the other social services are even bigger spenders of public money than the National Health Service and it must not be forgotten that they can effect the health of the patient as

much, if not more, than the provisions of the Health Service.

Finally, because district nursing is about the provision of nursing care a chapter has been devoted to the development of nursing policies, both in England and the countries of the European Community, with particular reference to the effects that these changes of policy have had on district nursing in the past fifty years.

Chapter 17

Policies for Financing the Health and Social Services

Across the spectrum of the developed world social and health services are financed in a variety of ways. Each country structures and pays for its services according to its own needs and resources, and its philosophy towards social and health care. The method of finding money for such services depends on interrelated, but at times apparently arbitrary factors, so that countries with the same health needs may deliver and pay for their services in strikingly different ways. Countries influenced by the Catholic Reformation continued to emphasise the role of the Church and institutions in health care, while the Protestant countries stressed the importance of individual and family responsibility, and fostered the concept of domiciliary care, the family doctor and the parish nurse. Whether countries use more nurses and fewer doctors can often be traced to the historical position of women in particular countries. A high ratio of doctors in countries such as Italy tells us more about the position of women in Italy than it does about the present Italian health needs.

How much a country spends on its social services depends not only on its total wealth but also on the priority it gives to social and health needs. Obviously countries with a high *per capita* income can afford programmes undreamed of by poor agrarian societies, but whether spending is effective depends on the state of knowledge and technology, how the services are delivered and whether they are meeting the real needs of the population. High spending on health care does not necessarily produce lower mortality and morbidity rates. In this respect it is of little avail for developing countries like the oil states to buy expensive hospital technology when their real needs are those of an agrarian population for better sanitation and food distribution.

Because of their success in overcoming the hazards of poor sanitation and their control of infectious and parasitic diseases the

developed countries are in stage three of the demographic transition and have an ageing and slowly growing population (Fig. 2.1, page 12). The health and social problems of these countries are now complicated and obdurate and it is this fact above all others that accounts for their cost. The conquest of bacterial infection by controlling animal and human waste, and through immunisation programmes and antibiotic therapy, was comparatively cheap. There will be no second bonus.

With the proviso that the comparison of international statistics is fraught with difficulty, it will be seen from Fig. 17.1 that in 1977 health service expenditure in the United Kingdom as a proportion of the Gross National Product was less than most competitor countries. However, Fig. 17.2 shows that by using the yardstick of perinatal mortality England and Wales were well up in the league, and in fact have only recently been overtaken by France and Japan. Although the proportion of the GNP devoted to any service is important, other factors, which are often difficult to quantify, are equally so, and these include barriers to the use of the services or the failure to deliver them to those whose needs are the greatest.

In 1974 Robert Maxwell analysed the health care systems in the developed world and placed them on a spectrum with those like the United States which rely mainly on private enterprise on the right, and towards the left those like Britain whose services come mainly from taxation, with Russia, a fully collective society, at the extreme.[1] In spite of these variations, however, the survey showed that no matter what the political philosophy, all systems were relying more and more on public finance; all were facing the ineluctable problem of soaring medical costs, higher wages for health service workers and the fact that the main users of the service were the old, the disabled or the very young; in other words, groups least able to pay charges or insurance premiums. In the United Kingdom the number of people over the age of 75 years has risen by 63 per cent since 1951. In 1979 the amount spent in the hospital sector for each individual in that age group was £365 compared with the national average of £80.[2]

The British philosophy towards health care and the social services

Present health and social policies have their roots in the nineteenth century where the destitute were dealt with by the Poor Law and those above the pauper line, but in need and deserving, were often

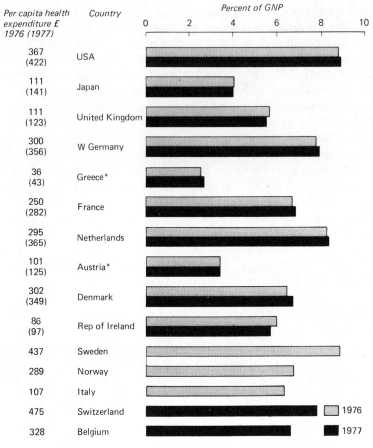

Fig. 17.1. International comparisons of health care expenditure expressed as a proportion of GNP and per head of population, 1976 and 1977. (By permission of HMSO).

relieved by one of the charities so much a feature of Victorian England. This fact is important because the Poor Law system might have been the foundation of the Welfare state, but unfortunately, as it became more repressive after 1834 so it became more unpopular, and the twentieth century was concerned with finding an alternative to the Poor Law rather than an extension of it.[3]

Two important breaks with the Poor Law at the beginning of the century were crucial to the subsequent development of the social services. The first was the *Old Age Pension Act* of 1908 which provided a small pension to the low paid over the age of 70 years on a non-contributory basis; the other was the *National Insurance Act* of 1911, which, on the contrary, worked on the insurance principle and covered low paid workers for unemployment benefit and medical treatment.

At the beginning of the second world war the government set up a Reconstruction Committee under the chairmanship of Sir William

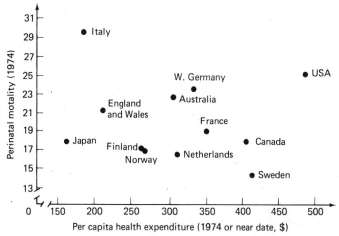

Fig. 17.2. Per capita health expenditure and perinatal mortality, 1974 (statistics provided by the Maxwell Survey quoted by the Royal Commission on the NHS).

Beveridge to prepare plans for the social services after the war. The Beveridge Report, issued in 1942 was the foundation of all post war social legislation and was built on the contributory scheme of 1911 to which various accretions had stuck like barnacles. There was a weekly contribution which provided for sickness, unemployment, old age, maternity, industrial injury and funeral benefits; both contributions and benefits were paid at a flat rate and it was envisaged that benefits would be sufficient to keep everyone above the subsistence level. But flat-rate contributions are hard on the low paid and therefore benefits had to be minimal. Beveridge, aware of this, argued that the scheme left scope for individual effort, thrift

and voluntary endeavour. The scheme legislated for a pluralistic society, allowed for a certain freedom of choice and left room for that other traditional arm, the charitable organisation.

Imaginative though the plan was it was soon in difficulty. The National Health Service interlocked with other social legislation, and budgets were prepared on the premise that once the backlog of illness was treated the nation would become healthier and demands for care would decrease. It was argued that the higher marriage-rate would mean that fewer people were living alone and it was this group who were the high users of the service. It was not foreseen that earlier marriage meant a higher divorce rate, and also, that there would soon be an increasing discrepancy between the life expectancy of the sexes. Furthermore, it was not understood that good health care does not reduce the demand for care, it increases it. People live longer to have more incidents of ill-health, and good care of itself raises expectations.

The financial problems of the health service were exacerbated by inflation, the change in the demographic profile (Fig. 2.1, page 12), and the great increase in medical knowledge and technology.

As it was impossible to increase the flat rate contributions steeply, the service was increasingly supplemented from general taxation. In 1948, to devote $3\frac{1}{2}$ per cent of the GNP to the Health Service was considered exorbitant, and in 1953 the Guillebaud Committee was set up 'to find ways of avoiding a rising charge on the exchequer'. After three years, when the cost had risen by some £100 million, the Committee was unable to offer any alternative method of financing the service. Twenty years later the Royal Commission came to much the same conclusion.

Financing the health and social service today

For half a century medical knowledge appears to have grown exponentially; more can be done for patients than there is money or manpower to achieve. Since not all needs can be met, choices must be made. But professional men and women pursue excellence and they do not like doing less than they know that they could if the resources were available, and this leads to conflict. Moreover, rationing the services and deciding who should receive organ transplants and who should be resuscitated usually falls on the professionals and this raises moral and ethical issues which create anxiety. On the other hand, if the Government intervenes with guidelines,

or consumer bodies offer advice, this is seen as 'interference with clinical freedom'.

The total budget for the National Health Service is now over £10 000 million, the steep rise in the last few years being mainly attributable to rises in wages and salaries (Fig. 17.3). After adjustment for inflation this is a *per capita* rise of over 267 per cent in 30 years. Nevertheless, in 1979 the slight drop to 5·5 per cent of the GNP created an outcry because the health service needs another

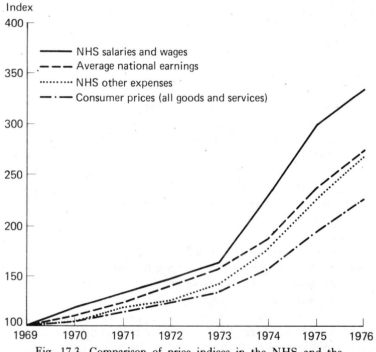

Fig. 17.3. Comparison of price indices in the NHS and the national economy: 1969 = 100. (By permission of HMSO).

one per cent increase on its total budget every year merely to maintain its existing services and cope with the increasing numbers of elderly.

As there is no prospect of the total wealth of the country increasing, the next question is how should the money be divided between the competing services? Because of the fall in the number of school children it has been possible to reduce the amount of taxation allocated to education, but all the big spenders in the social services

are in some way related to health. Health and welfare are intrinsi-
cally bound and although Social Security takes the biggest slice of
government spending, pensions in England are lower than those in
the leading European Economic Community countries. It makes
little sense to save the lives of pensioners in expensive Intensive
Care Units and return them to homes that they cannot afford to
heat. Housing is fourth in the spending league, but to take money
from that would mean more people suffering from ill health due to
substandard housing, and more people like Mrs Adams continuing
to cope with the inconvenience of an outside toilet. Even the smaller
budgets for services like libraries impinge on health. Man does not
live by bread alone.

Where the money comes from and where it goes

The 5·5 per cent of the GNP allocated to the National Health
Service now comes mainly from taxation. (Fig. 17.4). The contribution from the social security stamp has declined from 16 to 9·8 per
cent in the last 16 years although in the past it has been even lower
than at the present. The 2·2 per cent that comes from payments by
patients includes about 0·5 per cent from charges to private patients
in National Health Service beds. Another small source of revenue
comes from charges to insurance companies for treatment of road
traffic accidents.

The total revenue from all sources is divided by the Department
of Health and Social Security between the three main arms of the
service with approximately 15 per cent going to the personal social
services managed by Local Authorities, about another 15 per cent
to the family Practitioner Services to pay for practice expenses and
fees to doctors, while the lion's share of about 65 per cent is routed
to the Regional Health Authorities to pay for hospital and community health services, and of course since 1974, this has included the
salaries of district nurses. Similar arrangements exist for the countries of the United Kingdom with each reallocating money to the
appropriate authorities within the country. After deducting monies
earmarked for special Regional services the remainder is then allocated to the Health Authorities within the Region or country.

Health Authorities must spend their money within 'cash limits'
which means that their allocation cannot be supplemented even if
there are large salary awards or changes in VAT; anticipated rises
are allegedly accounted for in the original allocation. Apart from

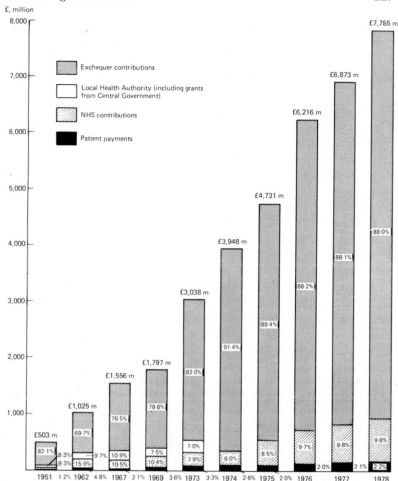

Fig. 17.4. National Health Service: sources of finance, United Kingdom. (By permission of HMSO).

keeping within their cash limits, Health Authorities have a duty to spend within the broad guidelines laid down by the Department.

Alternative ways of financing health care

Many people argue that other countries can spend more on their health services because they are financed by insurance schemes or direct charges to patients and that people are willing to pay more if

they see a relationship between what they are paying and what they are receiving.

This argument ignores several facts. Firstly, the high users of the health services are those least able to pay charges and it makes little difference whether they see a relationship between what they are paying and what they are receiving. In England over 60 per cent of all patients are exempted from prescription charges, while in Germany it is calculated that if health charges continue rising at the present rate, and the years of retirement continue to lengthen, by 1985 workers will actually need to pay insurance contributions equal to their salaries. Secondly, ill health strikes unevenly, and many of the long term sick could not have made provision for such an eventuality however provident they might have been. Thirdly, as already mentioned, high spending does not necessarily produce better community health. Such yardsticks as we possess indicate no clear correlation between these variables. At times, when England was one of the lowest spenders on health in the Western world, she had also one of the lowest infant mortality rates and one of the best life expectancies. The USA, the highest spender shown in Fig. 17.2 has, at present, almost the highest perinatal rate, while Japan, the lowest spender, has one of the lowest perinatal rates and, incidentally, one of the best life expectancies. Finally, there is the problem as to what is a 'right' charge for an item of medical service, and there is evidence that fees and charges rise rapidly for the well insured.

Paradoxically, one reason why the British system apparently gives value for money is that, in spite of the fact that administration is the scapegoat for all its alleged ills, it is in fact comparatively simple, and the Royal Commission on the Health Service (1979) found no reason to believe that it was over-administered.

By no means everyone welcomed the National Health Service, and since 1948 a number of alternative methods of financing the service have been suggested—particularly by the medical profession. These range from state lotteries to the encouragement of private medicine and complex insurance schemes, or direct charges to patients at the point of delivery. Since the cost of the Health Service is an emotive issue all governments have tried to contain the costs, and most have explored the possibility of some charges, but even with the most determined 'market' approach, charges will only yield a fraction of the total cost. The Royal Commission came to the conclusion that even if patients were charged £20 a week for their stay in hospital (at 1978 prices) it would make little difference to the

overall budget. Moreover, there is no concrete evidence to suggest that charges of themselves deter frivolous demands, and they might, as they did in the past, deter true needs. For example, would a charge of £5 for a visit to casualty be offset by a rise in long-term disability due to untreated wounds?

The strongest contender as an alternative system is that of a national, or semi-national, insurance scheme on an actuarial basis like motor insurance. However this is not as simple as it sounds; if the scheme were national and earnings related it would be indistiguishable from income tax and few people would see the relationship between the charge and the service provided. If, on the other hand, there were options for different premiums, like private insurance schemes at the moment, with the users reimbursed depending on their coverage, this would lead to higher administrative costs, hardship for the under-insured, a divisive service and different standards of care given to different patients, a prospect that most doctors and nurses find distasteful. Perhaps the most compelling argument against changing the system now is that most countries relying on such schemes are in difficulties and every European country is facing the fact that costs and claims are rising faster then either wages or the GNP.

Dividing the cake in the national health service

Since neither the GNP nor the proportion allocated to health care are likely to rise in the future, and there seems little hope of finding finance from elsewhere, we are left with the problem of making fairer and more efficient use of the £10 000 million we are currently spending. There are two main ways in which distribution might be changed: geographically and between the different branches of the service.

Geographically

Historically the health services have always been unevenly distributed. In the voluntary system where honorary doctors gave their services free to the hospitals, but made their money out of private patients, they tended to concentrate in London and the South-East where more private patients lived. This tendency was aggravated by the depression of the late 1920s when there was a southern drift of the population; but for climatic, occupational and socio-economic reasons the greatest health needs were in Wales and the North. In 1842, Edwin Chadwick (1800–90) noted that the labourer in Liverpool

had half the life expectancy of the labourer in the rural South; this discrepancy, although less marked, has continued. The North still has an infant mortality rate higher by five per thousand than the most favoured region, and one third more deaths among children under 14 years. However, to suggest that a redistribution of the health services would of itself change the position is to misunderstand the relationship of the curative health services to prevention. 'There are many reasons why chronic sickness or days lost from work are higher in the north than in the south; lack of provision of hospital beds is not one of them.'[4] In 1980 the working group chaired by Professor Sir Douglas Black reported concern about continuing inequalities in the health of the nation; the chances of pregnancy ending in a dead baby are twice as high for the wife of a manual worker as for the wife of a doctor, lawyer or university professor, and this discrepency, and others like it, have continued unchanged for the last fifty years. 'Sadly, the Government has refused to increase spending on the obstetric services even though such expenditure could be balanced by savings in other directions'.[5]

In 1976 the Resource Allocation Working Party (RAWP) produced formulae by which populations, weighted by the indicator of mortality experience, received more according to their need, the favoured areas marking time. When the Health Service budget was increasing, such plans, though crude, were acceptable, but in a period of retrenchment it means that the 'giving' areas actually suffer cuts and the receiving areas merely mark time. Now the rough justice of the RAWP formulae are questioned; poor health is due to more things than are controlled by the National Health Service.

Distribution of money between the branches of the service.

The acute general hospitals have always attracted more money; the interesting and the dramatic afforded prestige, and prestige brought in donations and medical students. On the other hand, the medical services that grew up under the shadow of the Poor Law were poorly provided and housed. This first budget in 1948 was allocated according to the current costs of the service at that time. The poor remained poor.

The reorganisation of 1974 did nothing to alter the allocation of resources, but the Family Practitioner Service remained outside the control of the Health Authorities as an open-ended service and as this service does not operate with cash limits it gets proportionately

more during a time of retrenchment. Although it is agreed that an increase in resources for primary care is desirable this is a haphazard method of redistribution and is doing nothing to encourage joint planning, a situation which may improve when District Health Authorities are established.

From time to time the Department issues guidelines about the need to move capital and revenue resources to the underprivileged branches of the service. However, distribution is bound to be slow because over 70 per cent of hospital costs go on salaries and wages and there is little that can be done about this in the short term. Moreover, because medical training is expensive it is axiomatic that all who train as doctors must be found posts, and the number of students qualifying has increased by one third in ten years. All consultant posts have a revenue consequence and most have a nursing manpower consequence so there is the added charge of nursing salaries. This is the fundamental reason why the transfer of resources to the community will be slow.

The future of the health services

Resources for health care are finite and must be used effectively, but obsession with cost-effectiveness can have dangers and the ethical considerations cannot be ignored. Can we, for example balance the 'cost-effect' to the community of so many more years of working life for a patient by giving him a transplant against the consequent diversion of money from, perhaps, such things as long-term care or preventive medicine? Practices may be grouped, streamlined and centralised; specialist services may be put on a more economical regional basis, but the money saved may be at the expense of what the patient values most, to be treated as an individual.

One way of employing resources more effectively, although in the long run it will not be cheaper, is by making the members of society aware of their personal responsibility for their own health. Much current ill-health is due to unwise habits and behaviour, which include the effects of alcohol, inappropriate (if expensive) diets, smoking, addiction to drugs, whether prescribed or otherwise, and the effects of air and water pollution by a society on the make. It makes little economic sense to push up tobacco sales in order to garner the tax and at the same time to spend millions on thoracic surgery, and, equally perversely, fail to use the media for health education because it is 'too expensive'. Nor does it seem

logical to budget in anticipation of road accidents and yet fail to enforce the wearing of seat belts. The district nurse, so often in a long and close relationship with her patients, is in a position to influence them both by example and advice, for although preventive medicine is primarily the role of the health visitor all members of the team have a part to play in health education.

References

1. Maxwell R. (1974). *Health Care, The Growing Dilemma*. McKinsey Survey.
2. The Office of Health Economics (1979). *Compendium of Health Statistics. The Cost of the National Health Service;* p. 1.
3. Fraser D. (1973). *The Evolution of the British Welfare State*. London: Macmillan; p. 50.
4. The Royal College of Nursing (1977). *Evidence to the Royal Commission on the National Health Service*. London: Royal College of Nursing; II, 8.
5. Smith T. (1981). The child-death cycle that could be broken. *The Times;* Jan. 27.

Further Reading

Brown R. G. S. (1978). *The Changing National Health Service*. London: Routledge and Kegan Paul.
Garner L. (1979). *The NHS—Your Money or Your Life*. Harmondsworth: Penguin Books.
Maxwell R. (1974). *Health Care: The Growing Dilemma*. London: McKinsey.

Chapter 18

The Development of the National Health Service

The hospital services of the nineteenth century developed along three main lines: the voluntary system with its roots in the charity hospitals; the provisions of the Poor Law, which eventually came under the aegis of local government and at the end of the century extended hospital services to non-paupers; and the mental hospitals, which were first under the Lunacy Commission, then in 1913, under the Board of Control.

There were also lines of health care in the community: some, like the Queen's District Nurses or the 'Lady Health Missioners', had their origins in voluntary societies; others, like the School Health Service, came into being because of legislation and were statutory. For the sake of convenience the statutory community services, and often their associated welfare services, were placed under the control of the Local Authority Public Health Department and the Medical Officer of Health.

The health services evolved piecemeal to meet changing needs, with the voluntary services often showing the way; but although this rich variety enabled adaptability and flexibility the services were confused, unevenly distributed and full of anomalies. More important, by the 1930s many health services were almost bankrupt and all the stratagems of 'popular' insurance schemes, charges to patients, national and local appeals and Flag Days were merely the rearranging of the deck chairs on the *Titanic*; the new possibilities of medicine and the expectations of patients were about to overwhelm the ship.

The structure of the national health service

In spite of the fact that plans for a comprehensive health service had been discussed since 1909, when the Beveridge proposals were put forward in 1942 the various vested interests could not agree, and the 1944 White Paper aroused deep passions and positive hostility from

the British Medical Association. In order to break the deadlock the Minister of Health, Aneurin Bevan, (1897–1960) in the new Atlee administration, produced a compromise solution which largely gave the services back to the people who had run them before and was particularly generous to the medical interest. *The National Health Service Act* 1948 took the services as they had developed so far and fixed them by legislation; it was, as it were, a snapshot of the services as they had evolved by 1946 (Fig. 18.1).

The structure exhibited many of the old historical divisions; the main change was that all types of hospitals were brought together within the Hospitals and Specialist Services division but even here some of the old dichotomies remained, with the mental hospitals having separate Management Committees and the teaching hospitals remaining outside the control of the Regional Hospital Boards. The service was tripartite, with each division funded from a different source. The administration of the hospitals was delegated to Regional Hospital Boards consisting of members appointed by the Minister; the Boards devolved responsibility to Hospital Management Committees, who were accountable for the day to day running of the hospitals in their group, but the teaching hospitals had separate Boards of Governors and were directly responsible to the Minister. The general practioners, who had been particularly vociferous in opposition to the service, managed to retain their independent status and had a contract *for* service, not *of* service, and were remunerated through Executive Councils by per capita payments and a complicated system of re-imbursement for practice expenses. The general practitioners retained their independence but the price they paid was their isolation from other branches of the service. The Local Authorities lost control of their municipal hospitals but retained responsibility for the Community Health Services which now included the domiciliary nursing services, preventive medicine and most of the personal social services. A divorce had been made between preventive and curative medicine and between the institution and the home, but at least the community health and the social services remained in wedded partnership in spite of matrimonial quarrels.

Criticism of the national health service—Green and White Papers

The National Health Service achieved its broad objective. A reasonable standard of health care became available to all citizens

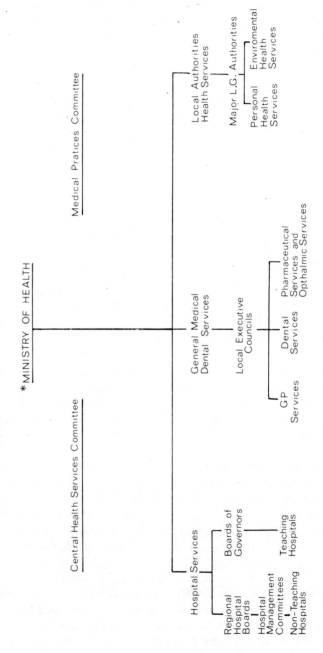

THE STRUCTURE OF THE NATIONAL HEALTH SERVICE

*MINISTRY OF HEALTH

Central Health Services Committee

Medical Pratices Committee

Hospital Services

Regional Hospital Boards
Hospital Management Committees
Non-Teaching Hospitals

Boards of Governors
Teaching Hospitals

General Medical Dental Services

Local Executive Councils

GP Services
Dental Services
Pharmaceutical Services and Opthalmic Services

Local Authorities Health Services

Major L.G. Authorities

Personal Health Services
Enviromental Health Services

*Became the Department of Health and Social Security in 1969.

Fig. 18.1. The structure of the NHS. (From McKeown, T. and Lowe, C. R., *An Introduction to Social Medicine.* Blackwell, 1966.)

whatever their financial position and when charges were made there were usually exemptions. Furthermore, as Chapter 17 has shown, by such crude measuring rods as we have, it gave value for money. Nevertheless there was much to criticise. Firstly, because the service had to be a compromise it inherited the old—and often outdated—priorities and it was primarily an 'ill-health service' with the prestige, money and manpower going to acute general medicine. Secondly, the services, including the ancillary services like dentistry, were geographically unevenly distributed and branches of health care like mental health and long-term care received proportionally far less than general medicine. Thirdly, because of their divisions the services were poorly co-ordinated and communication between the different parts was poor or non-existent, and in addition their complicated structure made them bewildering to the average citizen. As late as 1966 the survey *Feeling the Pulse*[1] showed that district nurses were often working in isolation and that general practitioners were ignorant of their nursing qualifications, frequently sending their patients to hospital for treatment that was well within the scope of the district nurse. Moreover, hospital staff, lacking understanding of the patient's home conditions and having little contact with the community health services, often sent patients like Mr Adams home to unsuitable conditions with no proper provision for further care. In fact the Dan Mason research study *Home from Hospital*[2] is full of such examples. Surveys like this and *Care in the Balance*,[3] brought home to the health professions that the barriers in the service were being paid for in terms of unnecessary suffering and it was these reports, as much as anything, that made people take a more urgent look at the need to unify the services.

Meanwhile, as professional conferences discussed 'unification', those working in the community health services embarked on experiments to make the delivery of care better co-ordinated and more effective. District nurses and health visitors in some areas were 'attached' to specially selected groups of general practitioners, and by 1963, these experiments provided an impetus for the *Committee on the Future Scope of General Practice*[4]. This committee, under the chairmanship of Dr Annis Gillie, found that many elderly patients needed a variety of services but they were often unaware that these services existed or of their entitlement to them—a finding of both *Home from Hospital* and *Care in the Balance*. To overcome these problems the committee recom-

mended that district nurses, health visitors, midwives and social workers should be attached to group medical practices to form a *Primary Care Team*. Within the next ten years 60 per cent of all health visitors and most district nurses were attached to group practices, and while there were losses as well as gains, most participants would agree that communication has improved even if in some cases the 'team' concept is more honoured in the breach than in the observance (Chapter 5).

The reform of the social services

While the Minister of Health, Kenneth Robinson, was preparing the first Green Paper on the Unification of the Health Services in 1968, the social workers were looking at their future. The personal social services, like the health services, had developed from voluntary organisations and the Poor Law; some were offshoots of other services like education, and some had come from the Public Assistance Committees of the 1930s. But poverty and ill health are linked as Edwin Chadwick showed in 1842[5] and the Black Committee demonstrated in 1980[6] and the health and social services frequently dealt with the same users. Therefore, when the Local Authorities, set up after the 1888 Act, took more responsibility for the personal social services they found it simple to group them under the Medical Officer of Health. However, there is no denying that the services were confused, with different Authorities trying different administrative patterns. By the 1960s the social workers themselves were anxious to improve their training and career structure; indeed, many of their problems were analogous with those of the nursing profession in the nineteenth century when they tried to establish themselves as a profession.

Because of these factors, and new attitudes towards social problems, in 1966 a committee was set up under the chairmanship of Sir Frederic Seebohm, 'to review the organisation and responsibilities of the Local Authority personal social services in England and Wales and to consider what changes are desirable to secure an effective family service'.

The report, which was published in 1968, concluded that the only solution to the present confusion was the establishment of an independent Social Services Department in each Local Authority under the control of a Director of Social Services. The report was welcomed by the social services, and in spite of warnings from the Central Health Services Advisory Committee about the need to

keep health and welfare integrated, the *Local Authority Social Services Act* came into force in May 1970.

The reform of the health service

Ever since a 'health service' was first considered in 1909 many people thought that the logical structure would be within the framework of local government, and the first plan for the National Health Service in 1944 was based on this concept, However, although this was a tidy solution it had become increasingly impractical. Firstly, the cost of the Health Service was now so great that it would destroy the delicate balance between the rates and the exchequer grant and, secondly, the medical profession thought such a plan would interfere with their clinical freedom and they would not co-operate with such a scheme. However, since health depends largely on other social services and factors outside medicine it is important that the administration of the health and social services be viewed as a whole and concurrently. Once the social services were placed firmly within local government the reform of the health services had to be linked with the reform of local government.

The Royal Commission on Local Government, set up in 1966, reported in 1969 and recommended that outside the Metropolitan areas there should be about 61 'Unitary' authorities, which it was thought, would be large enough to deal with the demands of the modern services and small enough to have a local identity. The Royal Commission's report (Redcliffe-Maud) was accepted in principle and new plans for a reformed health service were put out based on the Unitary authorities, that is to say a single tier health authority covering an area much the same as the now proposed 'single district' areas. In May 1970 the Labour administration fell from office.

The reorganisation of the health service

The incoming administration rejected the plans for a reformed health service and much of the report of the Royal Commission on Local Government, and prepared a new White Paper on Local Government reform which was in fact the basis of the *Local Government Act of 1972*. This Act provided for a two tier system with 44 County Councils covering the old traditional boundaries and six new ones like Avon and Teesside carved out of old counties. Below the County Council tier there was the District Council which was to be responsible for services like housing and slum clearance, refuse collection and amenities such as parks, although some services,

confusingly, involved both types of authority. The structure of the Local Authority service and the fact that the social services were now under the aegis of the new County Councils, determined the shape and structure of the reorganised health services. The Secretary of State for the Department of Health and Social Security consulted with the Brunel Institute of Organisation and Social Studies whose advice was reflected in the policy of consensus management with 'maximum decentralisation and delegation of decision making downwards matched by accountability upwards'.

The structure

In order to unify the services, which was the *raison d'être* of the exercise, the personal health services, including of course the district nurses, were brought under the control of Regional Health Authorities (which covered the same areas as the old Hospital Boards). Scotland, Wales and Northern Ireland had their own Health Departments and organised their services on similar lines except they had no 'regional' tier.

Below the Regions there were Area Health Authorities (Fig. 18.2) based on the 44 units of local government outside London. The Areas were intended to be co-terminous with the Local Authorities, with which they were to set up liaison committees, while the special needs of the teaching hospitals were met by designating certain areas as 'Teaching'. Because they were based on the old counties the Area Health Authorities were uneven in size; some were so large that they had to be divided into six districts, while others were 'single district areas'. The other outstanding anomaly was the fact that in England the Area Health Authorities were not given responsibility for the Family Practitioner Services and, although they allocated about 20 per cent of their budget to the Family Practitioner Services, the Authority had no control over how the money was spent.

The Primary Care Team

The independence of the practitioner services had consequences for the Primary Care Team as a whole. The doctor may himself employ a practice nurse and claim 70 per cent reimbursement from the Area Health Authority, which means that the practice nurse is accountable to the doctor and not to another nurse. On the other hand, district nurses, midwives and health visitors who were also attached were accountable to their nursing officer and had their contracts

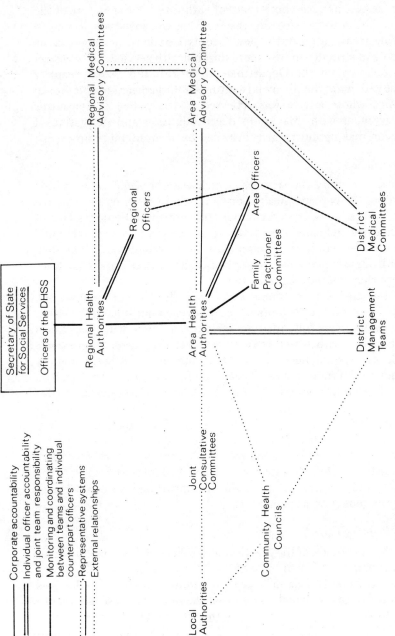

Fig. 18.2. Structure of the reorganised Health Service (from Management Arrangements for the Reorganised National Health Service, HMSO, 1972).

with the Area Health Authority. To complicate matters, social workers have their contracts with the Local Authority and are responsible to a Director of Social Services, whose area may not be the same as that of the Area Health Authority. This confusion of responsibility and accountability has legal and human consequences and may place the nurse in a dangerous position, a situation dealt with more fully in Chapter 22. Moreover, failure of communication within the team because members are accountable to officers in different places may have tragic consequences for patients and clients, and children have died because of poor inter-team communication.

Criticism of the reorganised health service

Although it was agreed that the health services must be unified and reorganised the proposals when they came met with much criticism and hardly any journal on health matters expressed approval. Firstly, the health services were divorced from the social services, and no papering over the cracks could disguise this; secondly, there was concern about the loss of Medical Officer of Health with his distinctive role; thirdly there were still anomalies—for example, the teaching hospitals were still set apart and the family health services were outside the main structure. Now this lack of co-ordination affected district nurses in a way that it had not done in 1948, for now most district nurses were attached to family practices.

The loudest complaints, however, were about the structure of the service. It was alleged that the number of tiers of management would delay decision making and would be expensive of resources. Moreover, it soon became clear that consensus management and worker participation without sensible discrimination would mean a vast increase in the number of committees, and one Authority reported having to consult with 26 committees before any decision could be taken. In 1976, the government having changed again, the Wilson administration appointed a Royal Commission, 'to consider in the interests of both the patients and those who work in the National Health Service the best use and management of the financial and manpower resources of the National Health Service'.

The Commission's report of 1979 made it clear that by no means all the problems of the National Health Service stemmed from reorganisation and that many were there before 1974. However, they pointed out that inasmuch as managerial problems arise from the structure of the service itself, these problems were due to the fact

that each 'tier' of management had a team of officers and each member of the team was responsible to the appointing Authority for the services in his or her control. This meant that an Authority with six Districts had to deal with seven teams and some 31 chief officers, but Area Officers were only advisory, and although they had a duty to 'monitor' they were not empowered to instruct if they did not like what they monitored. In this situation, matters that were once dealt with by the head of a department were now passed up and down the management chain.

The Commission agreed that the management arrangements of the service were cumbersome, but it recommended that the Regions should be retained and given more power and a positive financial role. Below the Region there should only be one management tier carrying operational responsibility for supplying services and co-operating with local government. The Commission advised that 'these Authorities should be formed from existing single District Areas and by merging Districts or by dividing Areas'. It was stressed that the new pattern should be flexible and should take into account geographical, historical and demographic considerations.

The Commission saw the Community Health Councils as having the two-fold task of representing the public to the Health Authority and of informing the public about the health services. The Councils had been more successful with the former task largely because they lacked resources and were not sufficiently involved by the Authorities, and of course, because they had been excluded from anything to do with the family practitioner services. The Commission recommended that the Community Health Councils should be strengthened.

Reorganising the reorganisation

In a repetition of the life cycle of confrontation politics—whatever their colour, the incoming administration in 1979 did not accept all the findings of the Royal Commission. However, it did agree that the criticisms about the structure were well-founded and issued a document called *Patients First* which was in fact about management structure rather than patients. The document stressed that another major upheaval of the services should be avoided and suggested that delegation of authority below the Regions should be to District Health Authorities which should be seen in terms of social geography and, outside London, should cater for populations

of about half a million people. The old multi-district areas are now being structured into new unitary Health Authorities of which there will be approximately 170. More power is to be given to individual hospitals and the Secretary of State has suggested that the titles of Matron and Hospital Secretary should be reinstated.

The 1981–2 Reorganisation leaves many criticisms untouched. It does not deal with the problems raised by consensus management and the need to differentiate between the subjects which merit worker participation and the consensus of the team, and those where management must manage. Nor does it deal with the divorce between health and welfare, and now there will be even less coterminosity because District Authorities will not match local government areas. There is a move to bring the Family Practitioner Service within the ambit of the District Authority although whether this will result in effective co-operation and co-ordination of health care plans remains to be seen. The Flowers Committee and the London Planning Consortium have now attempted to deal with the special problems of London and the demands made by so many teaching hospitals within so small a radius, where demands must either be rationalised and reduced, or they must be met. Whatever the pressure or vested interest they cannot be ignored.

Since health depends largely on services lying outside the National Health Service and beyond the scope of mechanistic medicine, the question remains as to how these services can be correlated when they are under different authorities and how they can be made responsive to the needs of the average citizen. Moreover, as the resources for the service are finite and are paid for out of taxation it seems reasonable that the consumer should have some say in the establishment of priorities. At present the choices are made mainly by professionals and clearly their opinion is of paramount importance, especially about the possibilities, or dangers, of a particular course of care. But in a service which is mainly about non-curable complaints, and where what is being provided by the service is mostly intervention and support, it appears sensible that the general public should have an opportunity to express a view on whether they want more home helps and meals on wheels or whether they wish to see more hospital beds and possibilities for transplant surgery. Mrs Cray might well prefer a ground floor flat to anything the Health Service can offer, an indoor toilet would be more beneficial to Mrs Adams than drugs for her arthritis, while cuts in school meals could devastate the Green family. The medical

profession decides who in society is 'ill', and as a corrollary, it makes decisions on how the money should be allocated to those labelled 'ill'. The time has come to modify this concept.[7]

References

1. Hockey L. (1966). *Feeling the Pulse*. London: Queen's Institute of District Nursing.
2. Skeet M. (1974). *Home from Hospital*. 4th ed. London: Macmillan Journals.
3. Hockey L. (1968). *Care in the Balance*. London: Queen's Institute of District Nursing.
4. *The Future Scope of General Practice* (Gillie Report) (1963). London: HMSO.
5. Chadwick E. (1842 reprinted 1965). *The Sanitary Conditions of the Labouring Population of Great Britain*. London: Longman.
6. Social Services Committee. (Black Report). London: HMSO.
7. Kennedy I. (1981). *Unmasking Medicine*. London: Allen & Unwin.

Further Reading

Bruce M. (1968). *The Coming of the Welfare State*. 4th ed. London: Batsford.
Fraser D. (1973). *The Evolution of the Welfare State*. London: Macmillan.
Owen D. (1976). *In Sickness and in Health*. London: Quartet Books.

Chapter 19

The Social Services

Social services may be statutory or voluntary; they may deal with personal services such as social security or with non-personal services like education, housing and employment. Many of our present statutory services have their origins in voluntary action as with district nursing itself and most of the child care services. Often they were formed in response to a special need; for example a Royal Commission in 1861 found that the majority of school leavers could not read a newpaper and the report led to the idea of cheap elementary education, and in 1885 the Commission on Housing gave rise to the revolutionary idea of 'council houses'. The solutions were usually pragmatic, unco-ordinated and were in fact often merely attempts by society to accept some responsibility for the industrial revolution and for what Professor Titmuss later described as 'socially generated dis-service and socially caused dis-welfare'[1].

After the *Local Government Act* of 1888 the new authorities assumed responsibility for some of these services with varying degrees of accountability to central government, with each authority adopting its own pattern. At first these services were concerned with the administration of the Poor Law through Boards of Guardians, but soon other duties became statutory such as the setting up of Local Education Authorities after the *Education Act* 1902 (Fig. 19.1). On the other hand, some duties were merely permissive; after 1850 municipal councils were allowed to provide public libraries and by the end of the century civic pride and new wealth had produced a rash of museums, galleries, parks and those other cultural facilities that were so much the hallmark of the late Victorian city. Generally speaking, by the end of the century the sanitation and personal health services were grouped in the Public Health Department under the Medical Officer of Health who was the most important officer in the sanitary movement. However, many health services were in fact outside his control and these included the new style 'hospitals' that had been built under the Poor Law after 1867. Meanwhile the social and welfare services

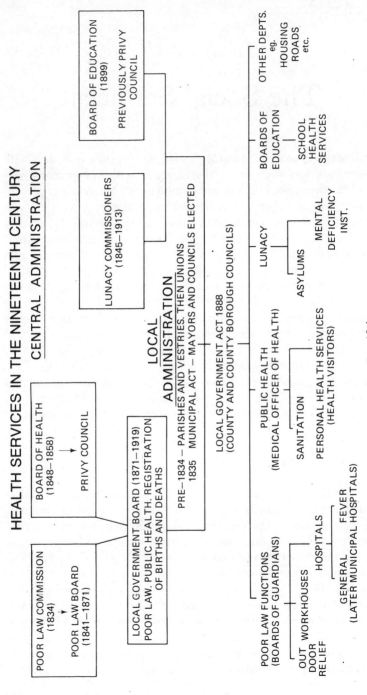

HEALTH SERVICES IN THE NINETEENTH CENTURY

CENTRAL ADMINISTRATION

POOR LAW COMMISSION (1834) → POOR LAW BOARD (1841–1871)

BOARD OF HEALTH (1848–1858) → PRIVY COUNCIL

LUNACY COMMISSIONERS (1845–1913)

BOARD OF EDUCATION (1899) PREVIOUSLY PRIVY COUNCIL

LOCAL GOVERNMENT BOARD (1871–1919) POOR LAW. PUBLIC HEALTH. REGISTRATION OF BIRTHS AND DEATHS

LOCAL ADMINISTRATION

PRE–1834 – PARISHES AND VESTRIES. THEN UNIONS
1835 MUNICIPAL ACT – MAYORS AND COUNCILS ELECTED

LOCAL GOVERNMENT ACT 1888 (COUNTY AND COUNTY BOROUGH COUNCILS)

POOR LAW FUNCTIONS (BOARDS OF GUARDIANS)
OUT DOOR RELIEF
WORKHOUSES
HOSPITALS
GENERAL (LATER MUNICIPAL HOSPITALS)
FEVER

PUBLIC HEALTH (MEDICAL OFFICER OF HEALTH)
SANITATION
PERSONAL HEALTH SERVICES (HEALTH VISITORS)

LUNACY
ASYLUMS
MENTAL DEFICIENCY INST.

BOARDS OF EDUCATION
SCHOOL HEALTH SERVICES

OTHER DEPTS. eg. HOUSING ROADS etc.

Fig. 19.1.

developed ad hoc and were spread through all the departments of the local authority.

All social and welfare services impinge on health and, with the possible exception of Mr Evans—provided he returns to his old job—all the cases in Chapter 1 will require a number of different services. However, it is probably the personal social services with whom the district nurse will have the most contact.

The personal social services

In the past, social work was usually associated with philanthropic and charitable organisations, although some welfare work was done by officials of local government departments. For example, the School Board attendance officer often found hardship in the homes he visitied—perhaps children were not attending school because they had no shoes; the housing departments began to employ welfare officers, and perhaps best known of all was the relieving officer who assessed people for 'Parish relief'. However, both the state and the voluntary system operated within the economic philosophy of *laissez-faire* and differentiated between the 'deserving' and the 'undeserving' poor, justifying their intervention with the former on the grounds that if people could be 'got back on their feet' they would return to work, which helped the market economy. Morally, of course, the work ethic was all important.

Since the Second World War, attitudes have changed because of the greater understanding of social problems and their causes, and as a reaction to the massive misery caused by inter-war unemployment. Nearly a quarter of the population on the dole made a mockery of the concept of the 'work ethic'. After the Beveridge Report in 1942 there were new ideas about what was meant by a 'welfare state' and with a change of emphasis from utilitarianism (Chapter 22) to humanitarianism it was regarded as reasonable that the state should intervene to ward off the worst effects of stress in all classes.

For these reasons, and others, the social services changed their ideas about the organization of communal services to meet social needs, but while the social services were fragmented through different departments there was little chance of developing these ideas, nor of improving the training of social workers themselves. Discussion of this problem led to the setting up of the committee under the chairmanship of Sir Frederic Seebohm which reported in 1968 and, although not all the philosophy of the report was put into

practice, this was the basis for the *Local Authority Social Services Act* 1970. The Act set up a Social Services Department which carved out an empire from other departments; home helps, services for the disabled and mentally handicapped were taken from health departments; other services, such as the responsibility for children in care, from the Children's Department, and other social responsibilities were hived off from education and housing. The original concept was for a community service for groups of 50 000 to 100 000 people, but the *Local Government Act* 1972 made this impossible because most of the county areas were too large. In order to overcome the problem *Social Service Departments* have been set up in each of the metropolitan and non-metropolitan counties and in the 33 London boroughs: they therefore often cover areas unequal in size, and also areas that have no matching Health Authorities, and this is a matter that will not be put right even when the Health Authorities are based on the smaller 'Districts'.

The Social Services, many of which have their roots in voluntary organisations, are trying to establish a fully professional service; they cover a wide range of problems which often involve the whole family and its environment, and for this reason they try to offer a 'family orientated service'. However, although the training of social workers is now comprehensive and generic, certain aspects of the work can be divided into different skills which for convenience can be grouped into: services for children, the physically handicapped, the mentally handicapped, the elderly and services dealing specifically with income need.

Services for children

In 1946 the *Care of Children Committee* (the Curtis Report) recommended the setting up of Children's Departments under the aegis of the Home Office and the appointment of Children's Officers who, incidentally, took over some tasks from the health visitor and unwittingly hastened the divorce between health and welfare. Although the new Children's Department tended to concentrate on what had already happened it did eventually lead to a more preventive approach, and in 1963 the *Children and Young Persons Act* required authorities to take steps to diminish the need to take children into care. Since then there have been a number of experiments including the idea of cash payments to relative or friends, or for payments for someone to live in with the children. Although this

was hailed as a new idea it was in fact a device often used by the Overseers of the Poor in the eighteenth century.

Children may come into care either through a court order or because the authority is fulfilling its duty under the *Children Act 1975*. Court cases usually arise from matrimonial, wardship or criminal proceedings, and in matrimonial cases where it seems that neither parent should be given custody, the child, or children, may be committed to the care of the Local Authority. Court cases may also arise from offences committed by children, and although children under the age of ten cannot be charged they may be taken into care. Apart from court cases, children may come into care because they have been abandoned or because for some reason the parents or guardians are incapable of providing for the child. It must, however, be emphasised that a Local Authority has no power to keep a child against the wishes of the parents although it does have a duty to ensure, as far as possible, that the child will have proper care. Only on rare occasions, after stringent conditions have been fulfilled, will an Authority overrule the wishes of the parents.

In this area come the problems arising from suspected non-accidental injury to children. The battering of children is not new and literature is full of reference to it, but recent reports such as that of the National Society for the Prevention of Cruelty to Children[2] must come as a shock to a society that is both affluent and better educated than previous generations. Identifying children at risk is difficult but the latest surveys show that the families at greatest risk are those where the parents are young and immature and lack the ability to respond to the needs of a demanding child. In nearly half the cases of child abuse marital discord is a factor, and the lower income groups (particularly when unemployed) are heavily represented. In 1974 the Department of Health and Social Security issued a memorandum on the subject,[3] and all Authorities have been urged to set up Area Review Committees whose local policies should be known to district nurses.

Services for the physically handicapped

Because of increased longevity the number of handicapped people in the community is increasing. In 1944 the *Enducation Act* laid down that handicapped children should receive appropriate education and the *Disabled Persons (Employment) Act* provided for a Disabled Persons Register, the appointment of Disablement Resettlement Officers and for the setting up of Industrial Rehabilitation Units,

work which was eventually extended by the *Chronically Sick and Disabled Persons Act* of 1970, the provisions of which are all important to someone like John Davis.

The aim of all work with disabled persons is to assist them to independence within their limitations, help them to come to terms with their disability and to give help and support to their families. Disabled persons are defined as 'those who are blind, deaf or dumb, or who are substantially and permanently handicapped by illness, congential deformity or old age'. Local Authorities have a duty to make known to such persons the services they offer. The needs of the severely disabled like John Davis are complicated and require the co-ordination of many services which in his case have already included the health and housing services and the Social Services Department and may well soon involve others. For some patients the employment services will be vital and for others the educational services may be important.

It is useful to remember that the Open University has a special service for handicapped persons, has made a study of meeting their particular educational needs, and manages to cope with the severely disabled in Summer Schools.

Services for the mentally ill and the mentally handicapped

The services for the mentally handicapped have passed through many vicissitudes with needs and attitudes changing.[4] Some mental illness has declined, particularly that which was the sequela of acute infections, but there is evidence, difficult to measure, that anxiety and depression are less well tolerated than they were formerly. Furthermore, in a technical society with a rigid notion of the 'rate for the job' it is more difficult to find work for, or to fit in, the mentally handicapped. The electronic age favours the quick and slick.

Although about five million people a year consult their doctors about mental health problems, few are admitted to hospitals and even then their stay is likely to be short, which of course means that all problems have to be dealt with in the community. Before the *Social Services Act* of 1970 the psychiatric social workers, who worked from the department of the Medical Officer of Health, often had a close relationship with the local mental hospital, the psychiatrists, the qualified mental nurses and, if they existed, the community psychiatric nurses. Now the psychiatric social worker has disappeared and this, together with the divorce between the

hospitals and the local authorities occasioned by the 1974 reorganisation of the health services, means that there is a lack of co-
ordination in the services dealing with mental ill-health.

In particular there has been disquiet about the co-operation of
the services dealing with mental handicap. The Social Services are
responsible for mentally handicapped persons in the community, if
they are in hospital or residential care the Health Service is responsible, while under the *Education Act* of 1975 the Education Department has a duty to provide suitable education. In order to try and
resolve some of the problems a *Committee on residential care for the
mentally handicapped* was set up under the chairmanship of Mrs
Peggy Jay. The committee came to the conclusion that a new caring
profession should be created with all workers trained in a course
designed to qualify students for a Certificate of Social Service. This
suggestion has not found much favour with the nursing profession
although to some extent it was similiar to the long term solution
proposed by the Committee on Nursing in 1970 (The Briggs
Report). However, whatever its merits or demerits, the proposal is
likely to founder in the foreseeable future because of the lack of
money to pay the extra 60 000 staff it would require.

Services for the elderly

There are now some 16 per cent of the population past the age of
retirement compared with 6 per cent in 1911 and the percentage in
the higher age groups is increasing. It is the over 85s, of which Mr
Adams is a typical representative, who will make the greatest
demands on the Health Service (Fig. 19.2). Fortunately the problem is partly offset by the fact that the younger retirement groups
are fitter, more independent, have greater expectations of continued activity, and with better pensions and facilities, they are able
to continue to play a role in the community. Indeed they themselves
often make a significant contribution to the voluntary services. On
the other hand, this very independence and the tendency to move to
'retirement areas' often cuts them off from the younger generation.
Moreover, smaller families and smaller houses, the mobility of
much employment, and the fact that daughters and daughters-in-
law often work outside the home, all militate against older people
living with their children even if they wished to do so, which they
usually do not. All these factors make family support in times of
crisis that much more difficult.

Ageing is a variable process; Mrs Cray at 68 has aged early

whereas Mrs Adams seems to have coped into her 80s, but the document *A Happier Old Age*[5] points out that the proportion of people who are bedfast and housebound rises steeply with age, with mental infirmity becoming an increasing problem. The Almshouse, that legacy of the Elizabethan Poor Law, was the traditional way of dealing with the unsupported 'aged infirm', and in 1960 there were still 37 000 old people in Part III Accommodation in old

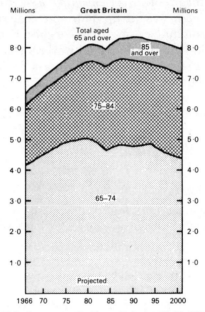

FIG. 19.2. Elderly persons in Great Britain, 1966–2001. (By permission of HMSO).

converted Poor Law institutions, and in some cases 'conversion' was more apparent than real. Since then, with a greater understanding of the needs of old people, and the fact that residential care is becoming increasingly expensive, there has been a reversal of policy and there is more emphasis on keeping the elderly mobile and at home, which of course has enormous implications for district nursing.

When it is clear that an infirm person can no longer cope alone it

is always worth finding out if any particular service is available to them; for example, do they belong to any particular Church or denomination, for most have homes from old people and some of the old Dissenting groups like the Quakers offer a number of services. It is worth finding out whether patients have served in the armed services and if they belong to the British Legion, or whether they are members of a professional organisation or occupational group or trade union which offers facilities. Most people have a touchstone somewhere. In dealing with elderly nurses, help may be from the Counselling, Help & Advice Together (CHAT) of the Rcn which has a directory of funds and trusts. The more usual services offered by Local Authorities and voluntary societies are listed in Appendix 1 and 2.

Services dealing with poverty

At the end of the nineteenth century Charles Booth (1840–1916) pointed out that for most people income and need followed a cyclic pattern. Young couples with no children were comparatively well-off but when children arrived and the wife stopped working the needs rose and the income fell. When the children were grown up and working (probably at the age of 13 years) there was another period of comparative ease, only to be followed by hard times again when the bread-winner stopped working because of age. Basically, the provision of benefits in the twentieth century has aimed at restoring income at least to subsistence level during the troughs of childbearing, sickness, unemployment and old age.

Different countries and ideologies have met these needs in different ways. In France, when the birth rate fell sharply, generous child allowances were introduced; in England when it was feared that the unfit school children would not be suitable as recruits to the army, there was the provision of a school health service and school meals. In both countries, be it noted, welfare provisions were related to the defence needs of the country.

In England, for historical reasons, we have dealt with the main needs of Booth's cycle through a pragmatic variety of contributory and non-contributory benefits. Contributory benefits are as of right, that is to say they are universal and paid to all people who qualify regardless of income or class, although it must be stressed that payments do not derive from actuarial calculations and are supplemented from taxation. On the other hand, non-contributory payments are usually, though not always, subject to a means test;

that is, they are selective and paid to those whose needs are the greatest. Usually these are families whose total income is below the offical 'subsistence' level. This level varies with inflation and the district nurse should have some idea of the current rate. Benefits can be complicated and may take the form of cash or kind, such as school milk, clothing grants, and rebates on rent or rates. (*See* Appendix 3).

Other statutory services

Apart from the personal social services, the work of the district nurse may be affected by the operation of other statutory services, including education, employment, housing and a range of legal services.

The education service

At the end of the nineteenth century, England was at least 60 years behind her neighbours in the field of general education, and to try to remedy this Parliament created a Board of Education followed by the great *Education Act* of 1902 which made elementary education to the age of 14 years compulsory. The Fisher Act of 1918 empowered Authorities to raise the school leaving age and also made provision for more medical services and the greater care of defective children. However, the main educational services of today stem from the *Education Act* of 1944 introduced by R. A. Butler as part of the overall Beveridge report. All fees for maintained schools were abolished, the system of primary, secondary modern and grammar schools established, and provisions for dental and other services strengthened. In the past twenty years there has been a continuing move towards the comprehensive system and in 1972 the school leaving age was raised to 16 years.

The school health service

This service is of particular concern to district nurses because patients are often concerned about the health of their children, or, as in the case of Mrs Baker, the health of the parents reacts on the children, and for this reason the school nurse must be seen as part of the primary care team.

The school health services have their origins in the revelations of the *Committee on Physical Deterioration* of 1904 which showed that 40 per cent of Army recruits were physically unfit—and the Army's standards were hardly high. In 1907 the *Education (Administrative Provisions) Act* required Authorities to provide for the medical

inspection of children, thus making the Board of Education a health authority, and in spite of protests from the British Medical Association, the services were extended to give treatment for minor ailments. At the same time, Authorities were empowered to provide school meals and milk, a move that provoked much protest and outraged letters to *The Times*. After the *Notification of Births Acts* of 1907 and 1915 more Authorities began to employ health visitors and to attach them to the Medical Officer of Health, consequently they often assumed responsibility for the health of school children. Some Authorities, however, especially in the large towns, preferred to employ specially recruited school nurses and, if necessary, to give them an in-service training.

After the setting up of the National Health Service it was questioned whether the school medical service was still necessary, since now children had the right to free medical treatment. The debate, which was not unrelated to the desire to cut costs, meant that the position of the school nurse was not clarified and the service took on the mantle of Cinderella. But hopes that the service would be redundant soon faded. Children now stayed at school longer, they matured earlier, they had psychological and emotional problems about examination pressure and competition which were unknown in earlier years. Old problems like malnutrition have largely disappeared, although they may still be met in immigrant groups, but their place has been taken by the complicated problems arising from an affluent society such as obesity, smoking, drinking and drug taking, to say nothing of the fact that in 1978 there were 4600 pregnancies in girls under 16 of which 3000 ended in abortion.[6]

Today the school health service tries to fulfil three main aims: to be a health education service, an occupational health service, and to provide liaison with other services. Since 1974 the school health services have been the responsibility of the National Health Service, with each Health Authority having a Child Health Nursing Officer who is responsible for co-ordinating all the health services for children, a function which will fall to the District Health Authorities when they are set up.

In 1976 the *Court Committee*[7] recommended that there should be an integrated Child Health Service, with each group medical practice having one doctor with paediatric training and a similiarly qualified health visitor who would oversee other child visitors and school nurses. The committee also recommended that each school should have its own nominated doctor and nurse, trained in educa-

tional medicine, who would act as general mentors to the children. The report has not been implemented, partly because it goes against the philosophy of the primary care team where workers are 'all purpose', and also because of cost and because health workers have already undergone enough upheaval. Nevertheless, the report is a salutory reminder that child health care in England is now falling behind other Western countries and there is no room for complacency.

Special schools. Every Authority has a duty to provide education for the different categories of handicapped children; as far as possible children are taught in normal schools and referrals are made after discussions with those responsible for the school health service and the head teacher. In some cases where either the numbers are few or the home conditions are poor it will be necessary to send children to a boarding school; Alison Green is fortunate in that she is able to go to her special school daily since it is important that she stays with her family.

Nursery schools. Although these have existed since the Education Act 1944 they have always been in short supply and in 1967 the Plowden Committee recommended that children in deprived areas should be given better than average schooling to compensate for their social and environmental deprivation. For this reason there has been a tendency to concentrate such schools in deprived areas, but for families relying on the mother as the bread-winner, or even partial bread-winner, the lack of nursery schools can mean real difficulty and can lead to unsatisfactory child minding.

Housing services

The *Housing Acts* of 1885 and 1890 allowed Local Authorities to provide working class houses, but as this was seen as interference with the market system with a vengeance, little was done, and the provision of cheap houses came mainly from charitable trusts like Peabody or Guinness. The First World War saw the beginning of rent control, and although in the inter-war period there was some council house building it was often of poor quality and design, but as the country recovered from the economic slump there was a burst of suburban building, and owner occupation spread down the social scale.

During the Second World War a Ministry of Town and Country Planning was created with the hope of avoiding the mistakes of the

past unplanned development, but the overall shortage was so great that the aim was only partially met. Since then much attention has been paid to the way in which cities grow. Originally the city centre was the high point of prestige but in the late nineteenth century it became increasingly fashionable to move away from the scene of work.

Different classes, however, have different abilities to compete with one another in terms of housing and of transport, and those with no cash tend to get trapped in areas of high density living. The once desirable becomes undesirable; working men move to the next zone with white collar workers moving further away. Cities, therefore, develop in concentric circles with the ripples spreading outward. It will be noticed that Mr Fisher commutes from a dormitory town to the city. Post-war speculation, assisted by convenient bomb damage, has tended to concentrate on office blocks and luxury flats in the centre of cities and now it is the outer ring of the centre, once so fashionable, that has become the twilight zone. Because of planning blight these areas tend to be poorly served with health and education services and for this reason they become even less desirable. The three generations of the Green family are likely to be trapped for some time.

Post-war planning emphasised the need to tie housing schemes in with road networks and to avoid the evils of ribbon development. People like Mrs Cray were rehoused in tower blocks which, it was thought, would break down barriers and give social cohesion. What was not foreseen was the high maintenance costs and the invitation to vandalism, and these flats have been particularly unpopular with mothers of young children and with elderly people, and since the partial collapse of Ronan Point in 1968 few authorities have continued with this type of building. Recently there has been a move to rehabilitate old buildings but unfortunately, not before whole neighbourhood communities have been obliterated beyond recall.

The pattern of housing

The Department of Housing is responsible for housing policy but the actual administration is devolved onto Local Authorities, with functions divided between the County Councils and the Districts. Basically there are four types of housing: owner-occupied, Local Authority, voluntary housing associations and privated rented accommodation. In the last 25 years owner-occupation has doubled but Local Authorities still supply one third of the total stock. Local

Authority housing is usually allocated on a points system and it is estimated that there are over a million people like the Greens waiting for a council house.

Rights of tenants

Most tenancies are protected by the *Rent Act,* but rents are not now controlled; instead they are fixed by the Rent Officer who works within a Local Authority area, but who is not a servant of that Authority and who is in fact employed by the central government. Objections to rents will be heard by the Rent Assessment Committee where the appellant can be represented by a solicitor or some other authorised person if he so wishes.

Since housing conditions may well affect the health of the occupants the district nurse should know something of the many improvement, repair and special grants for which householders and landlords may apply to bring a house up to a reasonable standard. Sometimes the nurse may find a patient suffering hardship, or even being in danger of injury, because of disrepair; in such cases the Local Authority may issue an order requiring that the repairs be done and the danger removed. The Authority also has the power to act in the case of deficient sanitation and to recover the costs later and, similiarly, they can take steps to insure that property, and sometimes people, are cleansed of vermin and that rats and mice are eradicated.

The employment services

These services are most important to the district nurse when she is dealing with disabled people and in this respect they are discussed elsewhere. It is important to remember, however, that the Department of Employment has directly employed Nursing Officers who give help and advice on nursing matters.

Voluntary organisations

Probably half the population of Victorian England was poor. The lowest tenth, the 'perishing classes' found relief from the Poor Law; for those who managed to keep above the pauper line but who were distressed because of illness, accident, unemployment or some other disaster, there was a wide range of charities.

Victorian charity was a response to the growing disparity between rich and poor in an increasingly affluent society, and was largely prompted by the Christian belief in good works, and the

notion that it is 'more blessed to give than to receive'. The Victorians firmly believed that the personal connection was more valuable than the cold hand of the state. There was also a growing concern about law and order; the powerless, impoverished masses were a focal point for criminal activity and political agitation. Finally, there was the evangelical point of view; as General Booth of the Salvation Army put it 'you can't save a man's soul when he is hungry'.

In 1861 there were 640 charities in London alone, and to bring some order to the chaos of overlapping and competition the Charity Organisation Society was formed. Some of these charities were the forerunners of later statutory services such as the National Society for the Prevention of Cruelty to Children, which pioneered much of the Child Life Protection legislation, or St Dunstan's which demonstrated the need for the services to the blind.

Many branches of social work have a similiar lineage. However, after the Second World War as the statutory services took over more and more of the social services and as social workers put their work on a client basis, the role of the voluntary societies began to look ambigious. In this atmosphere the voluntary societies tended to experiment and to pioneer new forms of service, (for example, the after care of prisoners, hostels for unmarried mothers, support for drug addicts) while, at the same time, supplementing the statutory services with such things as meals-on-wheels. However, the Seebohm Committee, while fully accepting the need for a professional service, saw the voluntary societies, not as a secondary source, but as a positive force for 'developing citizen participation in revealing new needs and shortcomings'.

In recent years there has been a burgeoning of voluntary societies, many of which receive government subsidies. The expectation of help with social needs, like expectations for health care, rises faster than professional manpower and official resource can keep pace, and social workers, like professional health workers, need to rationalise their skills and promote community self-help.

There are about 77 000 organisations registered with the Charity Commission of which over 10 000 were formed between 1960 and 1970—a figure which gives the lie to the idea that modern society is lost to self help and voluntary endeavour. Furthermore, it must be remembered that the needs for social help are much more complicated than in previous generations. At the beginning of this century anyone of reasonable intelligence could comprehend the services to

which they were entitled—which were pretty few. Now, with the best will in the world, this is manifestly untrue. Who, for example, understands exactly who is entitled to a rate rebate?

However, the great rise has been in the number of self-help groups, particularly where sufferers of a disease or disability, such as ileostomy patients, spastics or alcoholics, form a group to help one another; the afflicted have an empathy with the afflicted and often form not only a society for mutual aid but also a pressure group. Mr Fisher, John Davis and Alison's parents can all be helped by such groups.

The greatest difference between the Victorian charity and the present day voluntary organisations is not the current emphasis on 'self-help', (the Victorians tutored by Samuel Smiles (1812–1904) were strong on that), but the fact that Victorian society saw charity as an *alternative* to state aid whereas today it is a supplement and a spur to state welfare. But perhaps, more significantly, voluntary organisations are supported by all classes of society instead of merely being seen as a duty of the rich towards the poor; the builder's wife may well be delivering meals to the retired judge who is housebound because of his arthritis and arteriosclerosis, money does not buy service and the days of housekeepers are over.

Professor Ralph Dahrendorf in the Reith lectures of 1975 suggested that there was an urgent need for society to get away from the work ethic that has been so much the basis of the Protestant capitalistic society, where 'work' is seen as something that a person is paid to do for so many hours a day, then at a certain age is 'put out to grass to the world of non-work'.[8] He went on to point out that there a need to adopt a more flexible notion about work and retirement, and to ask why, provided that in our affluent society we have enough for reasonable subsistence, the early retired or the redundant cannot undertake some useful work according to their various abilities without being penalised or accused of undercutting? This might well prove more interesting and rewarding than participating in those 'retirement hobbies' which are sometimes merely filling in time.

References

1. Titmuss R. (1968). *Commitment to Welfare*. London: Allen & Unwin.
2. National Society for the Prevention of Cruelty to Children (1979). *Annual Report*.
   Also (1976) *Child Victims of Physical Abuse*.

3. Department of Health and Social Security (1974). *Memorandum on Non-accidental Injury to Children.* London: HMSO.
4. Baly M. E. (1980). *Nursing and Social Change.* 2nd ed. William Heinemann Medical Books; Chapter 7 and 20.
5. Department of Health and Social Security (1978). *A Happier Old Age—a discussion document.* London: HMSO.
6. Davies S. (1980). What every child should know. *The Times;* Feb. 21. (Comment on the report of the Joint Working Party (1979) *Pregnant at School and Schoolgirl Mothers.*)
7. *The Future of the Child Health Services* (Court Report) (1976). London: HMSO.
8. Dahrendorf R. (1976). *The New Liberty.* London: BBC Publications.

Further Reading

Family Welfare Association (1980). *Guide to the Social Services.* London: Family Welfare Association.
Townsend P. (1979). *Poverty in the United Kingdom.* Harmondsworth: Penguin.
Townsend P. (1965). *The Poor and the Poorest.* London: Bell.

Chapter 20

Policies for Nursing

Until the nineteenth century nursing tasks had been carried out by a variety of people ranging from aristocratic ladies and devoted Augustinian nuns to village nurses, medical students and paid attendants. No one asked 'what was the proper task of the nurse'; people were cared for by the person on hand and care varied according to the changing mores, the knowledge available and the expectations of the community. By no means all care was bad, indeed some of it was devoted beyond praise, and nursing care often gave more comfort than the medical treatment of the time. However, Miss Nightingale was right when she pointed out that nursing, even if devoted, was for the most part untrained. In spite of the general belief that 'every woman makes a good nurse', Miss Nightingale insisted that 'the elements of what constitutes good nursing are as little understood for the sick as for the well'.[1] When she said that she used 'the word nursing for want of a better' Miss Nightingale clearly meant that nursing should apply to something more than 'the application of poultices and the administration of medicines', and her concept embraced a whole range of social and environmental factors that cause ill health and which the nurse must be trained to prevent, or advise and treat when prevention has failed. The cryptic comment that 'the causes of the enormous child mortality are perfectly well known . . . the remedies are just as well known and among them is not the establishment of a Child's Hospital',[2] shows that she considered an understanding of the causes of illness to be essential to nurse training;—it was for this reason that nurses needed to be educated.

The Nightingale reforms

In spite of the opposition from doctors who believed that 'nurses were in the position of housemaids and needed only the simplest instruction',[3] the Nightingale School opened at St Thomas's Hospital in July 1860 with carefully selected pupils of 'good education and moral standing' doing a year's training. The pupils were

supernumerary to the work force but the training and supervision were rigorous. In 1866, in order to augment the strained Nightingale Fund, pupils were admitted in two ways; ordinary pupils who did a two year training and who received maintenance and £10 a year, and the 'lady probationers' who paid for their training and did a year's course. Miss Nightingale herself did not like the division, and stressed that all must do the same course with the same supervision, but the Fund needed the money and the 'ladies' who were inevitably better educated and the fastest learners, were valuable in pioneering the Nightingale system.

The policy was that the new nurses, once trained, should take positions as superintendents in hospitals elsewhere and, in nursing matters, make the position of matron or 'nurse superintendent', supreme. To do this they had to wrest power from the doctors, chaplains and hospital administrators, and while there were some casualties the new matrons, duly backed by Miss Nightingale herself, usually triumphed and apostolic succession was assured. This had an important effect on the administration of the voluntary hospitals which became tripartite, with the matron having direct access to the Board of Governors. When this access was lost, after the inception of the National Health Service, nurses reacted sharply and the restoration of this administrative right was one of the main reasons for the setting up of the *Committee on Senior Nursing Structure* in 1966.

However, although the new Nightingale system offered educated women as escape from what Miss Nightingale called 'busy idleness' at a time when there were few other opportunities, by the end of the century out of the 63 000 or so paid nurses, it is doubtful if even 10 000 had been trained in the reformed system. Nevertheless, the idea that nurses needed to be selected and trained had taken root, and thanks to the efforts of the *Workhouse Reform Movement* and of people like John Stuart Mill and Miss Nightingale herself, after the passing of the *Metropolitan Poor Act* of 1867 and the building of new infirmaries for the pauper sick, the Poor Law authorities themselves began to employ paid nurses and, after 1873, some also introduced their own training schemes. In 1881 a Royal Commission recommended the general accessibility to these hospitals, and by 1891 the citizens of London had the right to use the hospitals for infectious fevers that were being erected by the *Metropolitan Asylums Board*.

As time went by these too began to train nurses for 'fever nursing'

which, owing to the new knowledge of bacteria that was accumulating, was an art in itself. But generally speaking, the hospitals administered by the Boards of Guardians, even if the patients were no longer all paupers, attracted fewer candidates for nurse training, and the standard of selection was less rigorous than in the voluntary system. Thus began the great divide between nurses trained in the voluntary hospitals and those in the municipal system.

Apart from nurses trained in the voluntary and Poor Law systems, in general and later in specialist hospitals, there were nurses specially trained for nursing in the community (Chapter 21) although, as with their colleagues in hospital, for many years the untrained outnumbered the trained.

Miss Nightingale never ceased writing and talking about the need for the prevention of illness by health education, and she realised that the 'health missioners' attached to the various visiting societies also needed a definite training. The great 'sanitary movement' which followed the publication of the report of Edwin Chadwick and the Health of Towns Commission in 1845 had produced a spate of sanitary societies, and some, like the Salford Ladies Health Society, actually employed women to visit and instruct mothers in domestic hygiene. Miss Nightingale's contribution to this movement was that she designed a training scheme for such visitors 'who were not nurses' but who would form a back up service to the new trained district nurses. Her plan for a course of lectures in 1890 classed as technical education, is important because it established the idea of health visitor training within general education and also the fact that hospital training was not a necessary prerequisite for such work. Health visitors, who had a variety of backgrounds, including medicine, continued on this basis with Bedford College and the Battersea Polytechnic offering training schemes by 1907.

The campaign for state registration

The rise of a large middle-class in the nineteenth century produced an increased demand for services of all kinds which led to the growth of 'professional' occupations, and, as each tried to enhance its status by examinations and diplomas, so there was a demand for 'registration' and the denial of practice to the unregistered. Doctors had been registered since the Medical Act of 1858 and it was not long before the new style matrons were clamouring for registration for nurses. However, there were difficulties, not least of which was the problem of defining the limits of nursing practice. It is compara-

tively easy to say what is the law—and therefore what is the lawyer's province—but it is less easy to define nursing care. Furthermore, was it to be a two or even a three year training, what standards were to be set, and did the mere length of training guarantee safe practice? If the standards were high then what about the livelihood of all the others who practiced nursing? Above all, there were Miss Nightingale's wise reflections on the nature of nursing which, as she pointed out, needed not only the acquistion of knowledge but had another aspect, the vocational, which could not be tested by an examination. The nurse has 'to nurse living bodies and spirits'.[4]

Undaunted by the difficulties, the registrationists led by Mrs Bedford Fenwick, the erstwhile matron of St Bartholomew's Hospital, founded a variety of organisations to further the policy of registration for nurses, the best known of which was the *Royal British Nurses' Association*. The movement was to some extent associated with the suffragette campaign which at the beginning of the twentieth century was at its height. Nursing, except in the mental hospitals, was almost entirely feminine and, not without reason, attributed its difficulties in advancing as a profession to the general position of women in society. Partly because of the association with the militant wing of the suffragette movement, but mainly because of dissension in the profession itself and the conflicting advice given to the Committee on Registration (1904), the early Registration Bill of 1908 came to nothing, and soon the general expectation of war obscured its claim on the attention of the government.

Nursing organisations and their policies

The Royal British Nurses' Association, the National Council of Nurses and the Matrons' Council all had as their main aim the registration of nurses, a three year training and a high registration fee. These early associations tended to be exclusive and there was much dual membership. On the other hand, at the beginning of the century the rapidly growing Trade Union movement was expanding into hospitals, especially in the county asylums and the Poor Law hospitals. The Trade Union movement was essentially male dominated and linked to the new 'Labour' party; if women were recruited at all they either had their own under-funded association or a separate, and often powerless, section. Most nurses remained unorganised.

The First World War highlighted the lack of organisation in

nursing and the fact that there were no national criteria to judge what was meant by 'a trained nurse'. To overcome some of these problems the leaders of the Joint War Organisation of the British Red Cross and the Order of St John put forward the idea of a new *College of Nursing,* unattached to any political movement and not associated with either the registrationists or the suffragettes, with a constitution in line with the other professional 'Royal Colleges' and with power in the hands of the members themselves.

The policy of the College of Nursing, which was set up in April 1916, was to promote the better education of nurses and uniformity of the curriculum; to recognize 'approved' schools of nursing and to maintain its own register of persons who had certificates from such schools; and generally to pursue such objectives as 'would advance the art and science of nursing'. By the end of the war the College had about 15 000 members and as it increased in strength it too pursued the cause of registration but in a somewhat more accommodating manner.

When the new Ministry of Health was set up in 1919 it was clear that some form of registration would have to come, not to protect or enhance the status of the nursing profession as the early campaigners had intended, but to protect the public from the vast numbers of women who had had nursing experience in the war and called themselves 'trained'. Many thought that the College of Nursing would be the registering body, but the Royal British Nurses' Association was still campaiging for its own rigid Bill and in the internecine warfare that followed, the exasperated Ministry eventually set up its own statutory body, *The General Nursing Councils* under the *Nurses' Registration Act* of 1919 which allowed for a separate Council for Scotland and another for Ireland (to be the Northern Ireland Council after 1922). Thus, the profession lost the right to control its own basic education.

The General Nursing Council was controlled by the Ministry who also had the responsibility for the oversight of the health services. Before the war because impoverished hospitals had been quick to see the advantages of biddable, educated probationers, and because of the lack of opportunity for a career for women elsewhere, there seemed a never ending stream of devoted young women coming forward to nurse. As about one third of these recruits left fairly quickly the main labour force of many hospitals had come to be made up of probationers, a fact that would have made Miss Nightingale turn in her grave.

The Ministry of Health was in no position to help the finances of either the voluntary hospitals or the municipal system and therefore it could do no more than accept the status quo; the new Council was designed to accommodate nurse training *as it was at that time.* Accordingly, the Council recognised most hospitals giving a training and divided the Register into five, and later, six parts. There was a part for nurses trained in general hospitals and, because they had a different training, a part for male nurses; then there were also supplementary parts for the nursing of fevers, children, mental diseases, and finally, a part for the care of mental defectives.

This fragmentation of the basic training was against the educational policy of the College of Nursing who had been looking at developments in America and who favioured a 'comprehensive training' with specialisation to follow as in medicine. However, this was an issue on which the profession has always been split. Miss Lückes, the matron of the London Hospital, giving evidence to the Select Committee on Registration in 1904 had argued that it was 'a waste to train all for everything'.[5] The mental nurses saw little advantage in would-be psychiatric nurses doing a training in a general hospital and the health visitors have always been sceptical about the value of a spell in an acute general hospital as the foundation to a career in health education.

The new Nursing Council brought some order, eventually only approving schemes that met its standards, and set up machinery for removing the names of unsuitable practioners, but because it fixed with legislation a training and education that ought to be evolving to meet new needs, its contribution to the advancement of the art and science of nursing was hardly revolutionary.

The inter war years

Policies for nursing remained pragmatic and disparate. The different branches had come from different traditions; not only was the Register divided into six parts, there was also that other division between those trained in the voluntary and the municipal systems where not only the social status of the patients, but often their diseases, and certainly the structure of the administration, were different. A 'trained nurse' compassed a much wider range than say, a trained doctor or solicitor. Furthermore, mental nursing had come from the county asylums, first under the Lunacy Commission then under the Board of Control and mental nurses had taken examinations under the aegis of the *Medico- Psychological Associa-*

tion since 1891 and many regarded its certificate as of more value than that offered by the General Nursing Council. Also, mental nurses tended to organise through trade unions so there was practically no point of contact between general and mental nursing.

Midwives had always been a separate profession. Miss Nightingale had tried to found a school of Midwives at King's College Hospital but it had closed because of puerperal sepsis; nevertheless the College of Midwives was formed in 1881 and was influential in getting the *Midwives Act* of 1902 passed which set up the *Central Midwives Board* as an independent examining body with the College of Midwives responsible for the post-certificate courses.

Health visitors, as already pointed out, were originally not necessarily nurses but often had another qualification such as a female sanitary inspector or medical practioner, and usually did a special course such as the one organised by Bedford College. As time went by, with more emphasis on maternity and child welfare, nurses tended to predominate and particularly nurses with more than one certificate.[6] In 1925 health visitor training became the responsibility of the Ministry of Health and more full time courses were set up in technical and other colleges, including the College of Nursing, with the Royal Sanitary Institute becoming the examining body. In 1946 all health visitors were required to be state registered nurses and to hold the first part of the certificate of the Central Midwives Board, and finally, in 1962, the Royal Sanitary Institute handed over to the *Council for the Training of Health Visitors*.

Apart from the *Queen's Institute for District Nurses*, dealt with more fully in Chapter 21, which was another training and examining body, the Royal College of Nursing as it became after 1928, was offering its own certificates for post-basic courses which in 1932 included the Certificate of Industrial Nursing (later called Occupational Health Nursing) and a Ward Sisters' Certificate. At the same time the sister tutors were usually qualified through a Diploma of the London University and later registered as 'tutors' with the General Nursing Council, while the Diploma in Nursing of the London and Leeds Universities offered registered nurses a more demanding course in the basic sciences and the philosophy relating to nursing. To complicate matters even further there were a number of 'national certificates' which might be taken before or after training in such fields as orthopaedics, ophthalmics and tuberculosis (later thoracic nursing) or in tropical diseases.

Policies for nursing since the establishment of the national health service

Unlike the First World War, the 1939–45 war did not attract large numbers of nursing recruits and in 1946 30 000 beds had to be closed because of the nursing shortage. The government tried to make good the deficit by any means and these included short, 'crash' courses for ex-service auxiliaries, not re-introducing the educational entry test and the introduction of a variety of cadet schemes, often without safeguards, and relying on the work of 15-year-olds. The results of these measures were to affect nursing for the next twenty years.

Meanwhile the nursing profession itself was looking for ways to meet the new demands on nursing, and partly as the result of the Horder Report the *Nurses Act* of 1943 was passed which established a Roll for 'assistant nurses' with the General Nursing Council. However, the new grade was not universally welcomed and for a long time only marginally affected the shortage. In the early years assistant nurses (later known as enrolled nurses) were confined to work in the long stay hospitals but eventually they were accepted as a valuable component of the nursing team in all hospitals, including the mental hospitals in 1967 and also in the district nursing service.

The new demands of the National Health Service highlighted two main problems for nursing. Firstly the need to change the system of training and education to meet the new health needs and expectations of patients, and to meet the aspirations of nurses themselves, and secondly to improve the economic status that nurses had inherited largely as the result of being a woman's profession. The two problems were related and were, to some extent, a vicious circle.

Nursing education

There were three major reports on nurse training within the first eighteen years, The Nursing Reconstruction Committee (Horder), The Working Party on the Recruitment and Training of Nurses (Wood), and A Reform of Nursing Education (Platt), all of which, if accepted, would have placed more emphasis on community nursing.[7] It is now a matter of history that these reports, although widely debated, failed to bring about the necessary legislation to bring about a change in the status of the student nurse and the

educational programme. Finally, in 1970, as the result of pressure from the profession itself which was brought to a head by a fall in recruitment due to low pay and dissatisfaction with the standards of training, the government set up *The Committee on Nursing* under the chairmanship of Professor Asa Briggs (later Lord Briggs). The recommendations of this committee were important for district nurses because it was the first committee to plan for nursing within an integrated health service, and the first to offer a plan based on the total health needs of the community rather than the service needs of hospitals.

The Committee's recommendations in 1972 were generally well received although the various training councils were unable to agree on the structure of the new council and this subsequently raised problems for district nursing (Chapter 21). The Committee saw nursing education as a continuum in much the same way as had earlier committees, but whereas the Platt and Horder reports had thought that the range of people attracted to nursing was so wide that it was necessary to have two basic courses, the Committee on Nursing recommended a single portal of entry. The Committee's plan was that all students should take five modules in a foundation course which would lead to a Certificate in Nursing, but contrary to the advice given by the Royal College of Nursing and other professional bodies, the learner was to remain a Health Service employee. Some students would stop there but others would take modules in greater depth leading to registration, with the student free to build in a variety of patterns. Finally, the Certificate of Higher Education would replace the various special trainings and the separate examination bodies and there would be further links with universities. This last certificate would take the place of the various post-basic nursing certificates including the present certificate for district nursing.

Although the recommendations were accepted in principle it was not until April 1979 that the *Nurses, Midwives and Health Visitors Act* reached the statute book with the new Central Council and the boards for the separate countries being set up in 1981. This Central Council will eventually take over all the functions of the General Nursing Council but it is likely to be some time before it is ready to introduce a new and integrated system of basic education. When it does so it will have to take into account two factors that were not apparent in 1970; first, the impact of the Labour Laws, especially the *Employment Protection Act,* on contracts for 'apprentice'

labour, and second, the far reaching effects of the Nursing Directives of the European Economic Community.

Nurse management

Apart from education and pay the other great concern of the nursing profession after the setting up of the Health Service was the structure of nursing administration, and related to it, the career structure. The old style did not fit the tripartite structure of the hospital service nor yet the new pattern for the Local Authority services. The Committee on Senior Nursing Structure under the chairmanship of Sir Brian Salmon (1966) attempted to rationalise and simplify the position by proposing three bands of administration, top, middle and first line, with only two grades in each. Unfortunately in some cases the report was hastily implemented and without sufficient preparation, and some of the fundamental philosophy was often ignored. Nevertheless, the implementation did restore the nursing voice to the decision making levels, and, contrary to popular myth, it actually reduced the ratio of nursing administrative posts to ward posts.

A similar report was introduced for the community nursing services under the chairmanship of Mr E. Mayston and was important for district nurses because it merged the three arms of community nursing, midwifery, 'home nursing' and health visiting. The report recommended that the structure should be based on geography and not on function, and that at the top, the policy making level, a Chief Nursing Officer should be appointed to co-ordinate the nursing services and to provide a single line of communication on nursing matters to the Medical Officer of Health. In middle management only one grade was recommended, which equated with the Senior Nursing Officer in the Salmon structure. However, when dealing with first line management there was a fundamental difference between the community and the hospital services; nurses in the community had an additional training and functioned as independent practitioners, and it was difficult to make a valid comparison because the community nurse had to organise her own priorities and work load without other nursing support. The committee considered therefore, that all grades in the community services should receive management training.

The implementation of the Mayston report was overshadowed by the reorganisation of the health services (Chapter 18) but the fact that there was a clear 'line' structure for services that were inte-

grated made it comparatively easy to dovetail with the hospital services. But for the Salmon and Mayston reports, the reorganisation of the health services would have proved even more traumatic for nursing than was the case.

The European Community regulations

These regulations are now important to nursing. Article 57 of the Treaty of Rome requires the mutual recognition of diplomas and qualifying certificates and the co-ordination of conditions of practice. The original intention was to give different nationals the same legal rights, but the first directives went beyond this and drew a distinction between the legal position and the need for 'certain minimum standards' as a basis of recognition. This led to a long and involved debate but fortunately a Permanent Committee of Nurses was set up which negotiated on behalf of nurses. The Directives issued by the Commission are only concerned with broad parameters regarding the quantitive aspects and they point out that emphasis should be on the quality of training. Each country has to have a 'competent authority' responsible for implementing the directives which in the case of Britain is the General Nursing Council until it is replaced by the Central Council for Nurses, Midwives and Health Visitors.

The Nursing Directives

The requirements are broad and flexible: all nursing recruits must have ten years general education, and the quantitive requirements are that the training should be 4600 hours or three years, although it is recognised that mere duration is meaningless and it is likely that in the future training will be measured in terms of hours. However, it seems clear that only the registration of course of the Committee on Nursing would be acceptable, but the main problem arises in ensuring that students of nursing have theoretical knowledge and experience in the seven areas laid down by the directive, which include: general and specialist medicine, general and specialist surgery, child care and paediatrics, maternity care, mental health and psychiatry, care of the old and geriatrics, and home nursing. Although these can be accommodated in the proposed 'modular' system, if they are to be anything but perfunctory then there is little chance of the student giving much service to the wards and this must raise the question as to whether she should be on the pay-roll and counted as 'ward staff'.

These Directives are of course important for district nurses since *all* students must now have experience and teaching in home nursing and this can only reasonably be done on a one to one basis. It will be time consuming and it implies that all district nurses must be able to teach students, which requires a different skill from that exercised when teaching patients. There are at present 56 000 students in training.

Conclusion

Policies for nursing have undergone a change in the last thirty years. In many ways the wheel has gone full circle because having cured the 'curable' and prevented, or intervened with, much that is now preventable, we are left with the inescapable fact that we must all age and eventually die, and before we leave this world what we are most likely to need is care. Therefore, more and more the nurse must take on the role of the prescriber and organiser of care, and administrative support services and nursing education must now be directed to this end. For six of the cases described at the beginning of this book medicine can now do little, but good nursing care can still do much; for two at least the best hope is that good care will see the patients 'comfortably out of this world' and it will support and comfort the relatives, and other carers, to the end and beyond.

References

1. Nightingale F. (1859. Facsimile ed. 1970). *Notes on Nursing.* London: Duckworth; 16
2. Ibid; 17
3. Woodham Smith C. (1950). *Florence Nightingale.* London: Constable; 345
4. Ibid; 571
5. *The Select Committee on the Registration of Nurse* (1904). London: HMSO; 15
6. Ministry of Health (1919). *The Training of Health Visitors* (Circulars 4 M and C W). London: HMSO.
7. Baly M. E. (1980). *Nursing and Social Change.* 2nd Ed. London: William Heinemann Medical Books; Chapters 14 and 23.

Further Reading

Baly, M. E. (1980). *Nursing and Social Change,* 2nd Ed. London: William Heinemann Medical Books.

Section V

The Professional District Nurse

A district nurse, competent to undertake duties in the community, will be held individually accountable for the professional standards of her own performance and must understand the legal and professional implications of caring for patients in their own homes.

Panel of Assessors for District Nurse Training, 1978.

In their evidence to the Briggs Co-ordinating Committee the Panel of Assessors stressed the fact that the district nurse has unsupervised access to the homes of people who are ill, frail and at risk, and that there was therefore a need for a high standard of professional conduct and practice to safeguard both the patient and the nurse.

Although this need is common to all nursing, because the district nurse works alone, and is isolated from her medical and nursing colleagues, questions about professional responsibility, accountability and ethical considerations have an even greater urgency.

This urgency is now exacerbated by the fact that the nurse may be dealing with patients with a wide variety of religious beliefs, or none at all, and that advances in medical knowledge and technology have produced ethical problems undreamed by earlier generations. For these reasons, and because in the past there has been much confusion about the professional responsibility of the nurse, and in the present there is much concern about her extended role, two chapters have been devoted to the basic questions that must guide and influence nursing practice, and to the way district nursing itself developed as a profession.

Chapter 21

The Development of District Nursing

Although it is commonplace to think of professional nursing beginning with the Nightingale reforms of 1860, from time immemorial men and women with a vocation have cared for the sick in their own homes. Some like the Vincentian sisters in the seventeenth century, belonged to orders that gave a training and had rules about bedside care that few would quarrel with today. Moreover, there have been periods when nurses attending patients in their own homes were trained in extended duties such as lancing, blood letting and later, vaccination. The performance of such tasks largely depended on who was on hand to do them.

Nursing in the community in the nineteenth century

The old Poor Law Committees usually employed parish nurses to care for their pauper sick in their own homes and, even after the Amendment Act of 1834 (the New Poor Law) it was often found to be cheaper to care for the poor sick at home rather than put them in the workhouse. The standard of care offered to paupers varied widely—as did the nursing duties which at times embraced everything from administering dangerous drugs and applying leeches to minding the baby. However, by the standards of the times, and the general expectations for care, by no means all parish nursing was bad and records suggest that many earned their patients' gratitude.

The pauper sick were cared for by the employed 'Parish' nurses and doctors while the non-pauper 'poor sick' were often cared for by one of the many charities or visiting societies. In the middle of the nineteenth century efforts were made by charities to employ a more elevated cadre of women with some training in nursing, a notable experiment being that of Mrs Elizabeth Fry who, in 1840, founded a Nursing Institution in Devonshire Square, London. Although the scheme was inspired by the Deaconness movement of Kaiserswerth it was not particularly successful because the objectives were

muddled and the nurses lacked systematic training; indeed it was this confusion of spiritual proselytising with physical nursing that made Miss Nightingale vow that she would rather found a 'highly paid profession of nursing than a religious order'.

In 1859, William Rathbone, a wealthy shipowner in Liverpool, employed Mrs Robinson from St Thomas's Hospital to nurse his wife in the final stages of her consumption; Mrs Robinson so impressed her employer—a proof if one were needed that not all nursing before 1860 was bad—that he retained her to look after the 'poor sick' in the surrounding area. William Rathbone was of Quaker stock and came from a family with radical political views and a history of philanthropy, and he realised that good nursing not only alleviated suffering but it prevented pauperism by restoring the bread-winner to work; a nice example of charity going hand in hand with nineteenth century utilitarianism. Since Mrs Robinson could do little on her own Rathbone consulted Miss Nightingale who was just starting her school of nursing at St Thomas's hospital, about the possibility of supplying *trained* nurses to look after the sick in their own homes. Miss Nightingale gave the matter much consideration and eventually suggested that the Liverpool Infirmary be persuaded to train its own nurses for hospital work and home nursing in a joint training scheme. The Liverpool Infirmary co-operated—no doubt spurred on by the fact that Mr Rathbone promised a new training school built at his own expense, and the first 'trained' nurses were allocated to the districts of Liverpool in 1863.

The Liverpool scheme is important because it was the model for other provincial schemes and was at times at odds with the views and objectives of the later Queen's Institute of District Nursing. Each 'district' was run by a Ladies Voluntary Committee which was responsible for collecting money and dispensing welfare and each Committee had a Lady Superintendent who was not a nurse but who supervised the work of nurses. Such superintendence was contrary to Miss Nightingale's dictum that 'only those who have undergone the training should rise to the position of Superintendent.' This is the heart of the conflict about 'amateur' and 'professional' that dominated so much of the correspondence about district nursing in the later part of the nineteenth century.

In 1868 Mr Rathbone became a Member of Parliament for Liverpool, and as he then spent much time in London he was soon involved in a venture of the Order of St John of Jerusalem to

promote district nursing in London. Miss Nightingale was again consulted and although she was now out of London managing the complicated affairs of the Nightingale family and their two houses she found time to write *Suggestions for Improving the Nursing Service for the Sick Poor.* These suggestions formed the basis of *The Metropolitan Nursing Association* which was founded in 1874 with Miss Florence Lees, one of Miss Nightingale's ablest pupils, as superintendent. Disciplined and well-educated, Miss Lees shared Miss Nightingale's view that 'district nursing should be a profession for educated women rather than a craft for the lower orders',[1] which was contrary to the opinion held by the ladies of Liverpool.

It is clear from the content of the lectures given by Miss Lees that she herself was adept at a number of skilled techniques, which is no doubt why the doctors of the day were not enthusiastic about the idea of the new style district nursing as 'an occupation for educated ladies'. The doctors argued that the new nurses would take the bread out of their mouths, but it must be remembered that many of the sick poor could not afford a doctor and for many poor families the district nurse *was* the substitute doctor; well might Miss Nightingale say 'the district nurse would carry more responsibility than her hospital colleague because there would be no doctor to call on.'

The candidates for The Metropolitan Association were carefully selected and spent nine months training in the Home in Bloomsbury followed by a year's training in a hospital operating the reformed nurse training system and, finally, a further six months studying district nursing. Apart from the theoretical knowledge required, the standard of conduct and ethics was strict. Nurses were not to interfere with the religious beliefs of the patients or influence them in any way, which of course was the antitheses to the philosophy of Mrs Fry's Institute and the Raynard Bible Nurses. Furthermore, nurses must be prepared to do everything necessary to put even the most degraded dwellings in 'nursing order', and on no account were they to accept gifts. An interesting injunction was that a patient's hair should never be cut off unless it was hopelessly infected since it was better to take any trouble rather than lessen the patient's self-respect. A maxim that might stand at the heart of the Nursing Process.[2]

Queen Victoria's Jubilee Institute for Nurses

In 1887 after much diplomacy and counter-diplomacy the greater part of the Women's Jubilee Offering of £70 000 to Queen Victoria

was given for an extension of district nursing schemes and this
provided for the foundation of the Queen Victoria Jubilee Institute
for Nurses. A provisional committee was set up with Miss Lees,
now Mrs Dacre Craven, one of its moving spirits. A niece of Mr
Rathbone, Rosalind Paget, who had trained as a nurse at the
London Hospital was appointed as the first Superintendent and,
with the help of Mrs Dacre Craven, advocated a system of training
on the lines suggested by Miss Nightingale and practiced by the
Metropolitan Nursing Association. The new nursing force was
organised in County Associations and the distinctive uniform and
the badge worn as a pendant were approved by the Queen herself
who spoke of 'my nurses'. By 1896 there were 539 Queen's Nurses
who appear to have been carefully selected and groomed for leadership but they were a small minority and for the most part district
nursing was done by untrained or partly trained nurses, supplied by
religious organisations or the various 'Nursing Associations' that
had sprung up in different parts of the country, of which the
Liverpool Association was a prime example. Apart from these,
there were of course 'village nurses' who simply hired themselves
out for gain.

Eventually, some of the Associations, if they came up to the
standard required by the Queen's Jubilee Institute, affiliated to that
body. As in the hospital world, there was a wide divergence of
opinion as to whether actual nursing needed educated women and
much ink was spilt on the need, or otherwise, for examinations,
with the Liverpool Lady Superintendents definitely against such an
idea. However, much of this controversy must be related to the
wider issue of the clamour for the emancipation of women and the
suffragette movement and the problem of women's labour in a
society gradually becoming more egalitarian.

After the *Midwives Act* of 1902 the Institute required its midwives to be certificated with the Central Midwives Board and
gradually the Queen's Institute began to supervise the 'village
nurses' and select suitable candidates for a full training. Inevitably
it was the Queen's nurses who raised the standard and who—like
the Nightingale nurses in hospitals—became the model for emula-
tion, albeit not without much parochial, and often unseemly,
infighting between the different Associations.

In 1919 State Registration at last became a reality and although
the register was divided into parts and the standard was not high it
was now at least possible to differentiate between the trained and

the untrained. Registration with the new General Nursing Council now became a prerequisite for starting district nurse training for which the Queen's Institute retained the responsibility. In 1928 the charter was revised and the name changed to The Queen's Institute of District Nursing. Throughout the inter-war period a large proportion of district nurses were trained and employed through the agency of the Queen's Institute, although in 1936 the *Midwives Act*, in an effort to improve maternity care, required all Local Authorities to employ salaried midwives, and this some did by employing directly through their Public Health department. Each authority was a law unto itself but there was a tendency for rural authorities in particular to use Queen's nurses for combined duties, nurses who were often triply trained and who did much to enhance the image of the district nurse.

Like so many other voluntary societies the Queen's Institute pioneered the way for a statutory service, for in 1948 the National Health Service Act required what the Act described as 'home nurses' to be provided by all Authorities. A working party set up in 1955 to consider the training required for such nurses noted that out of the 9203 district nurses then in employment less than half were Queen's trained, and because of the increased demand for such nurses it was decided that other arrangements should be made for their training. In 1959 a Panel of Assessors was set up to advise the Ministry of Health, which reduced the length of training from six months to four. The District Nursing Advisory Committee took over the organisation of training as an interim measure, but although the granting of a National Certificate had the effect of increasing the number of nurses with a 'certificate' it was a retrograde step because the district nurses now had no independent educational body and the emphasis was on numbers rather than preparation to meet the future health needs of the community. In 1968 the Queen's Institute finally surrendered its training responsibility.

District nurses, having lost the prestige once offered by being 'Queen's nurses' with a distinctive uniform and the affection it attracted, now felt their position as the Cinderella of the primary care team, more acutely because since 1962 their colleagues in the team, the health visitors, had had an independent Council for Training and Education of Health Visitors which provided a longer, more heuristic and prestigious educational programme. The Committee on Nursing (Briggs) which reported in 1972

recommended that nurse training should be seen as a continuum and that more emphasis should be placed on community care, and the district nurses looked to the implementation of the Committee's recommendations to put their anomaly right. However, because the training bodies that were to be replaced by a Council for Nurses, Midwives and Health Visitors were fearful that the new training to be offered for their specialty would be lower than they had already achieved, they demanded, and eventually received a separate committee within the proposed new structure. This left the district nurses in the same anomalous position, and still a far cry from the days of the superior standard of education demanded by Dame Rosalind Paget which had made them the envy of the nursing world. In 1979 the Panel of Assessors was reconstituted and enlarged its membership which, together with the professional organisations and district nurses themselves, lobbied in a manner worthy of Florence Lees. By dint of determination district nurses now have their own committee and premises under the aegis of the Central Council for Nurses, Midwives and Health Visitors, and a new curriculum has been approved. In 1981 this training will be mandatory before anyone can use the title and practice as a district nurse.

District nursing as a profession

Much of the debate about district nursing at the end of the nineteenth century turned on the question of whether or not it could be regarded as a profession. Discussion centred on the fact that the district nurse was required to do many non-nursing tasks and was involved in social questions beyond her competence. Therefore, the argument ran, district nurses should be honest working women but be supervised by Lady Superintendents who could deal with the social and welfare problems. Usually these superintendents were from a class much involved in charitable work and they were, as Mary Stocks points out in all fairness, 'not only well educated but experienced in social work'.[3]

Miss Nightingale and Miss Lees had other ideas. Miss Nightingale always insisted that a nurse must be educated because she had to be what she called 'a sanitary missioner' and teach people. This wider concept required educated women and a system in which nurses were accountable to a trained nurse for nursing matters. Paradoxically, the Nightingale experiment proved its worth as medicine became more scientific, and the younger doctors soon

found that the educated nurse—originally trained to organise and give care—was a valuable assistant in the new technical medicine, and could be trusted to do much of the measuring and recording. It is therefore slightly ironic that nursing was hailed as becoming a profession at a time, when in hospitals at least, it became to a large extent, an adjunct to another profession. In this respect the district nurse, concerned with giving care and unsupported by doctors, had a greater claim to be considered as an independent professional.

It was this coincidence of the rise of the Nurse Superintendent, to whom the nurse was supposed to be responsible for nursing matters, and the use of the nurse as the doctor's assistant, to whom she was responsible for clinical matters, that led to confusion about her professional responsibility and her accountability. Not only were the public and administration often misled, but nurses themselves had a muddled perception of their own role.

The hallmarks of a profession

Many writers have tried to describe the distinguishing marks of a profession but setting aside Plato's immortal phrase, 'the pursuit of excellence', perhaps the most succinct is that given by Sir Harold Himsworth because he manages to reduce to two main hallmarks most of the characteristics given by other writers.[4] These are set out more fully in *The Professional Ethic* especially written for nurses by Norah Mackenzie.[5]

Sir Harold argues that for a profession to exist at all there has to be a 'social contract' between society and the professional body. Society has a special need, and in order that this need can be met it allows the professional person 'the status, authority and privilege necessary for him to discharge his duty,' and it tacitly agrees to this person being above the law in certain respects. For example, the doctor and nurse are allowed to handle dangerous drugs and to do certain things to patients that in other circumstances would be an offence, lawyers are allowed to possess incriminating information and not be made to disclose it. In return for these privileges society requires that the professional person has a special competence and skill to meet the needs that brought the profession into being. If doctors can order their patients to take dangerous drugs or make incisions into their bodies, then society wants a positive assurance that the training and skill is of the best. Therefore, the first hallmark of a profession is that it embodies a *competence and skill that is more than ordinary*. This skill must always be improving, and for this

reason requires the continual prosecution of research which is the essential criterion of professional endeavour.

However, it is not just 'competence' that distinguishes the professional person, and the second hallmark relates to the fact that professions deal with people and there is a special relationship between the practitioner and his client. As knowledge advances and science becomes more esoteric so medicine (and other professions) become less intelligible to the man in the street, and with every step towards more specialisation he becomes more vulnerable. How then can the patient or the client be sure that his professional adviser will act for his particular good? Of course he cannot be sure, but the bridge across this doubt is trust, and for this reason the professional person 'must act always so as to increase trust'. This is the reason why professions not only have registers of qualified practitioners, but why they also remove the name of anyone who is deemed not to be a fit and proper person. What constitutes improper conduct may vary from profession to profession, but the outstanding reason is always the betrayal of the special trust; in the case of doctors and nurses it is the misuse of drugs and the abuse of a relationship with a patient, whereas in law and accountancy it is the misuse of information or the client's money. Any conduct, however, on duty or off, which destroys trust in the profession may be cause for disciplinary action. Therefore, the second hallmark of a profession is that it adheres to a *standard of conduct and a code of ethics more exacting than that expected of the public in general*. It is for this reason that taking industrial action that inflicts harm on one's patients cannot be reconciled with professional status. Harm destroys trust and without trust the professions are helpless.

Is nursing a profession?

It is generally agreed that Miss Nightingale's aim to raise nursing to the status of a profession was realised inasmuch as nurses were trained and had 'competence and skill'. Later, the General Nursing Council ensured that no one could practice as a 'nurse' who was not, by the Council's standard, a safe practitioner. In 1921 the Council set up a Disciplinary and Penal Committee to deal with those nurses whose conduct, on or off duty, had in some ways destroyed trust. Broadly speaking Sir Harold's two main hallmarks were met, but there were large areas of doubt.

Firstly, while many nurses did possess a high degree of competence, the standard for registration was not high and it might only

be in one branch of nursing. The reason was that, because of the squabbles within the profession in 1919, nursing allowed the control of its basic education and training to pass to the Ministry of Health who was also responsible for the staffing levels. An important hallmark of a profession was surrendered—that it controls its own educational programme. On the credit side the profession did keep control of its post-basic education and although this was consistently higher it was to some extent dictated by the level of the foundation course.

In addition, the nursing profession did not possess a 'body of knowledge extended by united effort'. Much nursing, including district nursing, was concerned with how things were done and not why they were done, and a great deal of nursing practice was based on folklore rather than scientific findings. The position is now changing; the demographic profile and the changed health needs set out in Section I are placing a fresh emphasis on nursing care. Medicine can do little for Mr Adams, but planned nursing and co-operation with other agencies can do much, and thanks to this realisation there are nurses who, by virtue of research, practice, education and experience are extending the body of knowledge about nursing practice. For example, sheer longevity, if nothing else, highlights the importance of a scientific approach to the care of pressure areas.

There has also been confusion about professional responsibility, as was mentioned earlier. Not only have nurses not had a clear perception of their own responsibility, but the confusion has been confounded by other and conflicting ideas about their role including those of the doctors and of official administration.[6] If the nurse is merely an assistant to someone else 'who takes responsibility' then there is little obligation to provide further training, refresher courses, libraries, journals, text books and all the other essentials for professional growth. Failure to meet the true needs of a profession means that eventually, cut off from the necessary tools, we become the way we are perceived.

Remaining a safe practitioner

If district nurses are to fulfil the first hallmark of a profession, 'to possess skill and competence above the average extended by united effort and continual reseach', then certain obligations are laid upon them. This implies a pooling of knowledge and experience which can only be achieved by meetings and conferences at various levels,

or by the written word. One thing is certain, in a time of rapid professional change, excellence cannot be pursued in isolation. In this respect group practice offers an opportunity for interchange of knowledge, experience, opinion and new developments as reported in professional journals, and although there has not been much favour for the Court Committee's idea of a 'designated specialist paediatric nurse and doctor', nevertheless, members of the team will have different interests which can be used as a source of sapiential authority on an informal basis. Apart from this, each member of the team has a duty to participate in meetings, designed to advance the practice of his or her particular branch of health care, held outside the practice locality. If people do not do this the ideas of the team will become conservative and inbred.

The pursuit of excellence can only be carried out by regarding qualification as a first step in continuing education. There must be a commitment to regular professional reading through journals, and every practitioner should possess his or her basic reference books. Also, as will be seen from Chapter 22, ignorance of new knowledge is no excuse in law if a patient has suffered avoidable harm. The aphorism, 'half that you teach your students today will be out of date in five years; the trouble is you do not know which half', must now be speeded up, and even recently qualified nurses can no longer rely on how they did it in training.

The philosophy behind the Committee on Nursing was that nursing education should be seen as a continuum, with a progression towards specialist qualification for those who have the ability and motivation. Even then, however, some abilities will not be fully developed, and it is important that district nurses who have the motivation and ability to do so take opportunities for further study, not necessarily because it 'will make them better nurses' but because it makes life richer and more satisfying.

The Diploma in Nursing with its emphasis on the wider issues appeals to a number of nurses working in the community, and having an additional training they then have a start over their hospital colleagues. For others with specialist interests, such as geriatric nursing, there are opportunities through the Joint Board of Clinical Nursing Studies. Others, after years of vocational training, may feel cut off from the main stream of general education and may wish to broaden their horizons through general diploma or degree courses, and in this respect the Open University offers a number of courses related to community care.

Nursing as a research based profession

One of the most cogent reasons for denying that nursing has a professional status is that its practice is based on tradition modified by trial and error and not on scientific understanding. Some have argued that nursing is primarily a practical matter and to such arcane and pretentious flights nurses should not aspire. But, if nursing has been defined as 'assisting the patient, sick or well, in the performance of those activities contributing to health or its recovery that he would perform unaided had he the necessary strength, will and knowledge'—if this is the case, then it follows that the nurse must understand what is involved, and the interpersonal relationships that occur when she assists with these activities. Practice must be based on proper understanding and the results of professional action must be seen and evaluated.

In the past nursing has not had that group of research workers that are the usual concomitant of a profession, and research has not been the basis of the foundation training nor yet of post basic education. However, in the last decade or so strides have been made; nurse research officers have been appointed to the Department of Health, to the General Nursing Council (now the Central Council) to the Royal College of Nursing, the Queen's Institute and to Health Authorities. A number of universities involved in nursing education supervise research into nursing practice and train nurse researchers, while the Royal College of Nursing has a Research Society and there are a number of opportunities for research appreciation.

For district nursing to become research based there is a need for some district nurses with special aptitude to be trained as research workers and to identify nursing problems on the district that are either specially obdurate, or are now changing and in need of further study. Although comparatively few will be so trained and not all research yields valuable results, all professional nurses should be aware of the main tenets of the research approach and the different types of methodology, and all should be able to read a research report with understanding. Moreover, they should know and act on such research as has been validated, such as the Norton Pressure Scale, and they should continually question their own practices. It is the duty of every district nurse to those she trains not to hand on blind obedience to standard practice, but to advocate a questioning of what we do, why we do it, and even, whether it needs to be done at all.

Research should not be seen as a thing apart but should inform all practice, for this reason the authors of this book decided against a separate chapter on research, and also, because, like Miss Nightingale's 'handicraft of nursing', it cannot be taught in a manual.

References

1. Stocks M. (1960). *A Hundred Years of District Nursing*. London: George Allen and Unwin; p. 44.
2. Dacre Craven F. (1889). *A Guide to District Nurses and Home Nursing*. London: Macmillian & Co London (quoted by Stocks, 1960[1]).
3. Stocks M. (1960). *op. cit.;* p. 30.
4. Himsworth H. (1953). Change and permanence in education for medicine. *The Lancet*, Oct. 17; p. 789.
5. Mackenzie N. (1971). *The Professional Ethic*. London: English University Press.
6. Anderson E. R. (1973). *The Role of the Nurse*. London: Royal College of Nursing; Research Project Series 2, Number 1.

Further Reading

Baly M. E. (1980). *Nursing and Social Change*. 2nd ed. London: William Heinemann Medical Books; Chapter 24, Appendix 8.
Hockey L., Macleod Clark J. (1979). *Research for Nursing*. Aylesbury. H. M. and M.
Mackenzie N. (1971). *The Professional Ethic*. London: English University Press.
Stocks M. (1960). *A Hundred Years of District Nursing*. London: Allen and Unwin.

Chapter 22

Ethical and Legal Considerations

When Stephen Undershaft in Shaw's *Major Barbara* told his father that he had the qualifications for becoming a politican because he 'knew the difference between right and wrong', his father regarded this as a joke because, as he said, it was a subject that had always puzzled philosophers and baffled lawyers. We by no means always know 'what things we ought to do' as recent debates on medical ethics demonstrate all too clearly.

Nurses, if they claim to be professional people, cannot stand aside from ethical issues; indeed being closest to the patients they should be their advocates. Apart from a duty to speak up in public debate or in the professional press about the use of scarce resources or questions of an abuse, for example, the failure to get proper consent for a transplant, nurses are confronted with their own ethical problems for which the answer is by no means always clear.

The professional ethic

The fact that professions lay down ethical codes is indicative of how important the subject is to professional people. The International Council of Nurses issues its own code but this is only a general statement endorsing the fact that 'nurses believe in the essential freedoms and the preservation of human life', and 'that their actions will be unrestricted by considerations of nationality, race, colour, politics or social status'.[1] This is little help to nurses in specific situations; what, for example, is meant by 'essential freedoms', equality before the law or equality of opportunity, including opportunity for health care? Does 'life' include the embryo from conception and 'life on the machine'? As the Rcn discussion document on ethics points out 'Codes are never a substitute for individual moral integrity'.[2] But if we are left relying on individual integrity what guides can practitioners find to help them make the right decisions in controversial matters?

Some people will say that there is no dilemma, and that their own religious beliefs or personal philosophy provide all the answers. Stephen Undershaft belonged to that group. But religious creeds are usually in archaic language, and in a time of rapid change even the most devout and learned can draw different conclusions from the same basic teaching, as the terrible conflict at the time of the Reformation serves to testify. Moreover, although religious teaching lays down guidance about living it is usually couched in general terms or through parables and can be interpreted equivocally. Nor have the great moral philosophers been more explicit, but at least they have shown the questions that ought to be asked. This is the value of including some moral philosophy in all professional education.

Nearly two and a half thousand years ago Socrates (469–399 BC) asked the abiding question, 'How ought men to live'? and tried to find the answer through dialectical logic, working out by question and answer, what contributes to virtue and what makes a good citizen. Socratic teaching was written down by his disciple Plato (427–348 BC) who fused it with his own philosophy and the concept of the 'idea' or 'ideal', the eternally existing pattern of which individual things are but imperfect copies. Plato held that right behaviour stemmed from a proper balance of the elements within us and that correct harmony led to goodness; therefore, balanced actions were just actions, that is to say, they were disinterested actions, and hence, the figure of Justice is often depicted holding a pair of scales. The Socratic tradition emphasised that if man was wicked it was due to his ignorance, therefore virtue must be pursued through the pursuit of knowledge. Aristotle, (348–322 BC) whose ethics were the lodestar of mediaeval philosophy, stressed that good could only be achieved through contemplation and the rational principle, which is why his works on politics and ethics were closely related. Stephen Undershaft, brought up in the nineteenth century Public School classical tradition, thought the same. The Greek system of thought dovetailed with the Christian ethic with which it was largely in tune, and this fusion gave the moral philosophy which governed western civilisation until the coming of modern science. Even after that it was commonplace to describe subsequent philosophy as a 'footnote to Plato'.

A new attempt at laying down principles of behaviour came in the eighteenth century with the philosophers of the so called 'Enlightenment' who challenged the idea of an innate conscience and whose

work gave rise to the principle of 'the greatest good for the greatest number' and Bentham's idea of 'utilitarianism' which was the underlying force of so much nineteenth century legislation.

The greatest influence on modern moral philosophy, however, has undoubtedly been Immanuel Kant (1724–1804) who maintained that 'goodness' was not an inborn characteristic and that 'good feelings' such as sympathy could lead to wrong actions. For Kant a human action is only morally good when it is done for the sake of 'duty', that is to say it is done for a disinterested reason; Kant places much emphasis on the right motivation. To find a governing principle Kant posited two imperatives, the second of which is generally known as the 'categorical imperative' and states *'Act only on that maxim through which, at the same time you can will it, will become a universal law'*, sometimes rendered as 'am I willing that everyone should act the way I am acting now'. Although much Kantian philosophy is difficult and convoluted, nevertheless Kant does provide a useful working guide in dealing with patients and colleagues. It is always well worth questioning our motivation. Kant, like Plato, is explicit about the danger of inflicting harm for our own ends, which of course would include harming patients to achieve a salary award, but he offers no golden key about the problem of disinterested harm to avert a greater harm. For example, are war, civil disobedience or revolution ever justified?

Philosophers such as Bertrand Russell have looked at 'the right action' in terms of contemporary values and mores; others have tried to rethink moral philosophy in terms of current problems, for example, overpopulation and finite resources. Still others, especially since the first explosion of the nuclear bomb, have been concerned whether in fact all knowledge *is* good and whether truth *should* be followed wherever it leads, even if it leads to genetic engineering and to the abyss.

Meantime, as life becomes increasingly complex the practical problems for the district nurse multiply. Records on the computer and the ever-increasing size of the 'team' change the old concept of confidentiality; there are new questions about the 'pill' and who should be on it; and the possibility of prolonging life artificially raise terrible dilemmas about 'saving life at all cost'.

Some ethical problems for nurses

Confidentiality

In recent years a number of inquiries, particularly into the deaths of

children in care, have highlighted the strain that the commitment to
confidentiality can place on the professional worker. Nurses have,
quite rightly, taken from the doctors that part of the Hippocratic
Oath which says 'whatever I see of the lives of men which ought not
to be spoken of abroad, I will not divulge, deeming that on such
matters we should be silent.' But what should a nurse do if she
suspects that a child, or an old or disabled person, is being cruelly
treated and abused? Such suspicions can place the nurse in a
difficult position, and she has to weigh up whether the danger is
immediate and whether reporting her suspicions would risk having
the door closed against all workers and thus making the last state
worse than the first.

The district nurse is less likely to come across child abuse than
her health visitor colleague but she may well suspect abuse or gross
neglect of an old person, and the guidelines laid down by the
Department of Health dealing with suspected child abuse could be
adapted. In the case of an emergency, if the person in question is
already apparently injured, there should be prompt consultation
with the doctor and possibly the social worker with a view to getting
the patient removed to hospital for an assessment. However, if
suspicions are not strong enough to warrant this the nurse should
discuss the case with the family doctor and at least one senior
colleague, or a colleague in a different profession. The risks should
be weighed and a case conference called. Senior nursing staff should
ensure that nurses know what to do when faced with such a
dilemma. In the end the nurse herself must decide when to seek
advice and her judgement will be based on her knowledge and
experience, and on how well she made that initial assessment. For
example, an inexperienced nurse may well have overestimated the
ability of a family to cope when faced with the burden of giving
continual care to someone like John Davis, and have given the
family more responsibility than they can stand. Sometimes we hear
what we want to hear and all to often we listen to what people are
saying rather than grasp what they are trying to tell us.

However, in the event of a tragedy such as a patient being injured,
or even killed, by relatives, it must be remembered that no-one
involved is above the law. Professional workers have been severely
criticised in court for failing to report suspicions about neglect, and
it was of little avail when they told the judge that they were 'trying to
establish a client/worker relationship based on confidence.'

There may be cases where a nurse is subpoenaed; if so she must

appear in court and give evidence on oath, and to refuse to do so is contempt of court. If a nurse is called as a witness she should take care to confine her answers to factual, truthful statements and never allow herself to be drawn into giving an opinion. This is something which must be left to the 'expert witness'. If the nurse feels uneasy about the prospect of cross-examination she should get advice from her organisation. Fortunately, in actual practice conflicts concerning confidentiality and the requirements of the law are comparatively rare, but there have been cases where doctors have been prepared to be prosecuted rather than betray a confidence and journalists have gone to prison rather than reveal their sources. Each professional must judge for himself whether a principle is at stake, act accordingly and be prepared to take the consequences.

There may be other problems concerning confidentiality. Sometimes the nurse through her own perspicacity learns something that the patient wishes to be secret, or the patient or relatives, in a moment of stress, may reveal something and then beg the nurse to say nothing. Such confidences must be respected and are best forgotten and certainly not recorded. However, if it impinges on the health of the patient, then the nurse should try to get the patient to accept help voluntarily. Such situations can be delicate and time-consuming; they may involve such problems as wife-battering, an unwanted pregnancy, fear of violence due to mental disorder or alcoholism, or suspicions of drug addiction. On these occasions the nurse must give such lonely support as she can until those concerned are ready to accept help; but there may be rare occasions when the matter seems so serious that in the interest of the greater good, and perhaps the safety of other people, confidence has to be broken. This is a big decision, but if it has to be taken the person concerned should be warned that in their own interests and possibly someone else's, another person must be consulted; this of course could very well in the first instance be the doctor or the social worker. Never act behind the patient's back. Once the step has been taken, provided it is done honestly, the patient may well be relieved that the decision to act has been taken from them. In fact this is something the nurse needs to be quick at discerning: the occasion when 'Don't tell anyone' means 'Please help me'.

Saving patients from themselves

It has been pointed out in Chapter 13 that an order for compulsory

removal will only be made in exceptional circumstances, but nurses sometimes come across people who are elderly, confused and apparently unable to cope with their hygiene and nutritional needs, but who refuse help and are determined 'to keep their independence'. This is a great problem and likely to get worse, since it is expected that by 1985 the age group over 75 years will have increased in numbers by 20 per cent. Because of the discrepancy between male and female life expectancies many of these will be women living alone, and as they get older, some will be eccentric and some confused. But who is to say that they should not be allowed to finish their lives among the unwashed dishes if they are determined to do so? 'Is life a boon?' asked W. S. Gilbert in *The Yeomen of the Guard,* but not everyone worries about staying alive until July when 'perchance they might have died in June'. If we start coercing those we regard as unfit to live alone, what criteria do we use, and who will watch the watchers?

No one can be forced to accept help against their will but the district nurse who may have been the friend of the family for a long time is often in a good position to give advice early and to apply gentle persuasion when things begin to go astray, and she may be able to ease patients into the idea that sheltered accommodation is not necessarily the end of all independence. The secret lies in getting people to make the decision before they become confused, but this is advice more easily given than taken.

Suspicions of criminal activities

Sometimes it comes to the nurse's notice that a family she is visiting is engaged on some illegal activity and she may wonder if she has a duty to the law. It is not the job of the nurse to play policeman; if those plants in the front garden could possibly be cannabis, so be it; or if she becomes aware that Mr Evans is conducting a rewarding side-line while off sick, that is not her concern. However, as in the case of confidence, there may be rare occasions when she has to consider the greater good. Not many district nurses are going to stumble on a cache of home made bombs, but there may be other instances such as the much discussed dilemma about the patient who arrives at surgery with an apparent bullet wound of the shoulder after the news of a bank robbery. There can be no rules in such cases, except that a patient's confidence should only be betrayed if some greater issue is at stake and this calls for personal judgement,

wisdom and, above all, the ability to see a situation from several perspectives.

Terminal care and the wishes of the patient

The Victorians accepted death and talked about it, largely because theirs was, at least superficially, a religious society, but also because, with a high death rate and a high birth rate, both were frequent occurences. Now, in a secular society and with death a less frequent visitor, it has tended to become a taboo subject, and this failure to be able to talk about death is at the root of some of the current problems concerning the wishes of the patients themselves, and their adviser's ideas about what is best for them. However, it must be remembered that a person is not obliged to accept medical treatment, even if refusal may result in an earlier death, and there is no legal, moral or ethical obligation to use drugs, or apply treatments if they can at best be described as prolonging the process or distress of dying.

The nurse may well be troubled about patients dying alone with perhaps only intermittent care, but sad though this is, and however much it is an indictment of modern society, is it worse than being moved into hospital for the last few days of life? Although hospices like St Christopher's have provided centres of excellence and research and have to a large extent revolutionised the medical care of the dying, it is now important that, as far as is humanly possible, these principles be applied in the domiciliary setting. Of the cases outlined at the beginning of this book three are 'terminal' in the sense that they will not recover, and for two at least death is not far away. It is hoped that they will both be able to die at home, with dignity and as free from pain as possible, and that 'their nurse' will support them to the last.

Research ethics

The problem is now so pressing that most research centres have 'Ethical Committees'. The Rcn discussion document on ethics says that although 'the initiation of clinical research is usually a medical responsibility nurses have the right and duty to express opinions about the effect of such procedures on the patients under their care.' Miss Norton has suggested paraphrasing Miss Nightingale with 'it is the first duty of the researcher to do the patient no harm.' To which wise counsel it should be added, that if avoidable harm occurs the patient may seek legal redress through the law of

damages. Advising district nurses to be research-minded is not an invitation to rush into unsupervised studies which may do more harm than good; researchers must be trained and there must be sound reasons for the study. It must be remembered that patients have a right to withdraw and any duress put on a vulnerable group such as the old or the mentally handicapped is an abuse of professional power and can only bring research, and the profession itself, into disrepute. Whatever the purpose of a research study, it must be designed in such a way that the dignity of those participating is protected.

Communications about colleagues

In the hierarchical structure of a hospital there are exact procedures for staff appraisal and counselling but this is less easy within the primary care team, for to a large extent the members are independent practitioners. Difficulties may arise when colleagues know that a member of the team is failing in a way that is not obvious to the nursing officer. Failure may be due to domestic anxiety, poor health or incipient mental ill-health; it is no kindness to cover up until something does happen. Tragedies have occured this way. Probably the best person to take action is the colleague who is nearest at work, maybe the one with whom the nurse in question works in harness, or in the case of an enrolled nurse, the district nurse who supervises. Sometimes a sympathetic approach is enough to persuade the nurse to become amenable to help, but occasionally, particularly in the case of mental illness, the nurse is obdurate. At this stage someone has a moral duty to take action. However, if such action is contemplated the nurse in question should be told, because it is as important to be honest when dealing with colleagues as it is when dealing with patients or clients.

When making a report about a colleague there are several points to be borne in mind. A report (or reference) if it is true is not actionable, nor is it actionable if it is made in good faith and without malice to the person properly entitled to receive such a report. Privilege is lost however, if information is passed on to a person or persons not entitled to recieve it, and in the case of a district nurse this would include members of the team to whom she was not accountable. Finally, when dealing with a sick colleague it must be remembered that no approach can be made to her medical adviser without her express permission, and of course, no doctor would disclose information without the consent of his patient.

The records of patients

The practical considerations have been dealt with in earlier chapters but there may be ethical and legal implications. The fact that the care plan should be left in the patient's house is an indication that the plan must be factual and truthful. Other records must be kept in safe custody and should only be shown to persons entitled to see them. However, in this respect, there has recently been much disquiet about the increasing number of people who do have access to the patient's records, and with the district nurse taking a larger teaching role, this is becoming as true in the community as in the hospital. Everyone who has access to the patient's notes must be made aware of their obligation to safeguard confidentiality.

It is also important that patient's records are kept in a safe place and never lost; claims for damages may be brought at a later date, for example, a claim about the delayed effect of a drug, of which Thalidomide is the prime example. For this reason, if for no other, it is important that records are accurate, legible and intelligible.

The records to be kept when administering controlled drugs are laid down by the *Misuse of Drugs Act* 1971 and should be adhered to, but most Authorities have their own rules to ensure that prescribing and recording habits are uniform. Although patients' records are confidential they are not the property of the practitioner and they must be disclosed to the proper authority if asked, the prospect of which is a further warning that they should never include unsubstantiated opinion.

The district nurse and the law

Confusion about accountability and professional responsibility may lead to lack of clarity about legal responsibility. When professionals were self-employed the situation was obvious; the doctor who was negligent or the architect who designed a house that fell down were clearly liable for damages. However, when professionals are employed by someone else, probably the State, the situation is less obvious, nevertheless the principle remains: professional practitioners are responsible for their own professional acts. A district nurse is a member of a primary care team and is employed by a Health Authority, and is personally responsible for the treatment she carries out and for the drugs she administers even though these were ordered by another professional; she is also responsible for delegating tasks to a proper person. If the patient, his property or

his reputation suffer avoidable harm then the nurse in question may be liable to pay damages.

The duty of care—patients' rights

The nurse has a 'duty of care' for any patient with whom she deals and that patient has a right to expect that no avoidable harm will be done to him or his property, and 'harm' in this respect can include psychological factors such as anxiety caused by lack of, or even wrong, information. If the patient, or someone acting for him, feels that harm has resulted due to negligence there may be an action for damages and the action is likely to be brought against the person, persons, or corporate body against whom the claim is the most likely to succeed. However, even if the claim is initially brought against the Health Authority it must be remembered that the negligent person is also liable 'and indemnity may be claimed against that person'.

What constitutes negligence, and what harm, will be a matter for the law courts, and much will depend on the circumstances. If a nurse gives 1·0 mg of a well-known drug when the standard dose is 0·1 mg, even though the doctor himself misplaced the decimal point or did not make it clear, the nurse is negligent because a competent nurse should have queried the dose. The law expects a nurse to use initiative. If on the other hand, it was some esoteric drug and the wrong dose was ordered and given the nurse could not reasonably be regarded as negligent. If harm results during the giving of treatment, a claim for damages would be unlikely to succeed if proper precautions had been taken and the treatment was given in a proper manner, and provided that the patient had given consent, understood the implications, and was the proper subject for the treatment or procedure in question. It must be remembered that 'avoidable harm' includes damage to property, and the district nurse is in a much more vulnerable position than her hospital colleagues in this respect. What about all that clutter in Mr Adam's room all too easily knocked over, or the antique table at Mr Fisher's side all too easily marked? If the nurse causes damage patients may quite rightly expect to be compensated, and if they don't it is still an embarrassment.

Finally, patients may sue not only because of physical harm but because of damage to their reputation. For this reason it is important that suspicions about cruelty, neglect or criminal activity are only made to the proper person through the correct channels. It is

quite right to discuss fears that an old person is being underfed with the doctor, who would probably, in fact appreciate being informed, but it may bring an action if it is discussed with the neighbours.

There are a number of points for the district nurse to remember if a claim is brought and she herself is likely to be involved. Firstly, even if the claim is against the Authority she should seek advice from the professional, or other organisation, that manages her indemnity insurance cover. The claim may involve several members of the team who have different interests and whose evidence may conflict, and the unadvised lose out against the well-advised—there are always many versions of the same story. Secondly, the Authority may settle out of court but subsequently conduct an 'unofficial' inquiry and apportion blame, or it may be concerned in defending its management role, by contending that it employed the right staff in the right place and the equipment was adequate and properly maintained. On the other hand the nurse's defence might well be (and often is) that there were not enough qualified staff, or that the right equipment was not available. The managerial line of defence is not necessarily the same as that of the individual.

Apart from expecting that the nurse who has a duty to care will not be negligent, the patient also has the right to refuse treatment, and to touch someone without their consent is an assault. This may lead to a difficult situation with an obstinate, but ill and perhaps confused patient, who is refusing treatment or refusing to take prescribed drugs. If all persuasion by the nurse and relatives fails the patient must be left; no-one can be forced to receive treatment he does not want.

The nurse's rights in relation to patients

Although the nurse may not coerce a patient, likewise he may not assault her—unless of course she has forced an entrance against his wishes. If a nurse is assaulted by a patient she should withdraw as quickly as possible and a first sensible step would seem to be a discussion with the team as a whole. Maybe another member of the team would be more acceptable, or the patient may calm down, but if the patient continues to behave in a violent way to all comers then the team are quite within their rights to withdraw their services; indeed it would be folly to do otherwise. If a nurse is actually injured by a patient she should report the matter immediately and if

she suffers real harm the matter should be taken up with the Criminal Injuries Board.

Futhermore, the nurse is entitled to expect that the premises she enters will be safe, and although the health and safety regulations do not extend to private houses, owners and occupiers are required to keep their property safe under the *Occupiers' Liability Act* 1957. With the obvious proviso that the nurse herself must take reasonable care, if she is injured due to faulty property, say a faulty floor board or broken steps, she may well have a claim for compensation.

The National Insurance (Industrial Injuries) Act 1946.

District nurses, who are often without trained assistance, may sustain injury to themselves when they are actually giving care; and this particularly applies to lifting patients. As far as possible nurses should avoid situations where they may either injure themselves or the patient. If the patient is injured he may have a claim against the nurse, if the nurse is injured she should report it immediately and sign the accident book and if she is off sick she should make sure that a claim for industrial injury is lodged; this is payable no matter where the blame lies. Establishing the fact of 'industrial injury' is important, partly because injury benefit is higher than sickness benefit but, more importantly, if the disability goes on there will be a right to disablement benefit. If there is a delayed disability and the claim has not been established it is very difficult to do so retropectively. Claims under the National Insurance Act are as of right and have nothing to do with claims for compensation.

Wills and gifts

The district nurse may become the long-standing friend of the family, but she should be wary of being drawn into too close a relationship, particularly in pecuniary matters. Nurses are sometimes asked to witness a patient's will but if so she would do him a service if she made sure all was in legal order; the two witnesses must witness the signature and sign in the presence of one another. On the whole it is better not to be involved in such transactions and some Authorities have rules about this. The receiving or refusing of gifts can be a delicate matter, but any acceptance other than for the most trivial can be fraught with danger if the relatives are jealous, and large gifts, whether given or willed, may be challenged and regarded by the law as 'given under undue influence'. On the other hand, to refuse the memento from the grateful patient or relatives,

or the garden produce from the proud husband, may appear churlish, and nurses must use their discretion about small gifts and be guided by good manners and commonsense.

The duties and the position of the nurse

The qualified nurse is expected to be a safe practitioner within the limits of her training, but questions often arise about what are called 'grey areas'. The subject has been made unduly complicated by nurses being confused by 'certificates of authorisation' when in fact basic rules cover most problems.

The nurse should not undertake tasks outside her contract of employment. She should not, for example, agree with a doctor to do an immunisation clinic—however tempting the blandishments—unless the employing Authority agrees; the doctor cannot assume responsiblity for her and he does not employ her. If there is a professional accident while the nurse is doing a task outside her terms of contract, then in the eyes of the law she is doubly vulnerable, and the employing Authority would certainly be under no obligation to help with her defence. However this is not to say that nursing duties cannot or should not be extended, but if they are, there are certain precautions to be observed. The Royal College of Nursing and the British Medical association have issued a leaflet with which all nurses should be familiar, *The Duties and Position of the Nurse*[3].

The main points—as they concern district nurses—can be summarized as follows:

1 A technique outside the scope of routine nursing should only be assigned to a nurse after consideration of the circumstances and with the agreement of those concerned. The nurse assigned to such a task should receive proper training and supervision and be satisfied that she is competent to undertake the new duty.

2 There should be machinery for consultation between the nursing officers and the Family Practitioner Committees.

3 When agreement has been reached and it has been agreed that a nurse, or a group of nurses, should be deployed on duties normally considered outside the scope of routine nursing it should be reported to the employing authority and duly minuted.

4 Although Memorandum RHB 49/128 makes it clear that

Health Authorities are expected to undertake the defence of a nurse in proceedings against her, if the nurse has acted outside her authority such cases are to be referred to the Department of Health, but this does not absolve the nurse from personal liability for her own actions and there is no guarantee that the damages would be paid by the Department.

5   Because of the implications all nurses are urged to belong to a professional organization *providing individual legal cover.*

If these rules are followed nurses have little to fear about extended duties, bearing in mind that they must be safe practitioners at all times and that these tasks must not be delegated to untrained persons.

However, it is not the performance of procedures 'outside the scope of routine nursing' that necessarily worries the district nurse, but the whole concept of 'prescribing care' and using initiative in planning a regime of care that is not task-orientated. Moreover, the primary assessment can sometimes look perilously near 'diagnosis', but once again the same principles apply. The nurse must be a safe practitioner, inasmuch as her assessment must be based on sound knowledge and a physiological and psychological understanding of the patient's condition, and the care inititated should be that which a competent qualified nurse could be expected to prescribe. No one can expect more. Assessments are not infallible and patients may subsequently develop, or already have, an undiagnosed condition, that means that the care plan was wrong. This of course is not negligence. What must be borne in mind however, is that if a wrong treatment, drug or dose is given because the nurse *herself* is out of date, for example, through confusion over the metric system, this will be no excuse at law. The professional nurse has a duty to be, and to remain, a safe practitioner. Conversely, Health Authorities and senior nurses have a duty to see that opportunities are provided for up dating and refresher courses; this is particularly important for nurses returning to district nursing after a break in service.

The district nurse and the labour laws[4]

These laws, which are becoming increasingly complicated and frequently amended, apply to the district nurse as they do to any other citizen. Those most likely to affect her include:

The Contract of Employment Act 1972. This Act required that all employees, within 13 weeks of starting employment, be given a statement containing information about their rate (or scale) of remuneration, the frequency of payment, the terms and conditions of service—including the period of notice to be served—and the details of the grievance procedure. Apart from the 'contract of employment', professional workers can reasonably expect a job description and job specification, which should include the lines of accountability and the chain of command.

The Employment Protection Act 1975. This Act extended the previous legislation about unfair dismissal and enabled new tribunals to award the reinstatement of a dismissed worker; it reduced to 26 weeks the period of completed employment necessary before the worker could complain of unfair dismissal, and was more explicit about trade union rights and the time off allowed for union activities and other worker entitlements. Although this Act may be amended the principles governing dismissal, and other matters affecting nurses, are likely to remain. Any nurse who feels she has been unfairly dismissed or had her contract broken in any way should get in touch with her appropriate organisation. For the purposes of all Industrial Relations laws 'trade union' includes those organisations who have applied successfully to the Certification Officer and have been certified as 'independent unions'. These include organisations like the Royal College of Nursing, the Royal College of Midwives and the BMA.

Health and Safety at Work etc Act 1975. Although this Act does not apply to private houses, it does to clinics and old people's homes, and other public places where the nurse may work. It therefore behoves nurses to understand the main principles of the Act. These include ensuring that the working environment is safe and that equipment is in good order, that employees have adequate training and instruction, that entrances and exits are safe and there is a written-up policy on safety. The reason for the Act was that the incidence of accidents at work was unacceptably high, and the new legislation was designed to provide greater worker participation and awareness. Although there could be a danger of over-reaction, and 'safety' is not an end in itself, nevertheless district nurses should set a good example and make sure that the premises in which they work are as safe as possible, lest it be said that the cobbler's children are the worst shod.

Nurses and industrial action

Whether withdrawal of labour by the caring team can be justified must be a matter for individual conscience. However, there are certain legal points to be borne in mind and a number of practical considerations.

Technically withdrawal of labour constitutes a breach of contract and can be a reason for dismissal. Although the Employment Protection Act lays down safeguards concerning such a breach in the pursuance of *bona fide* trade union activity much would depend on the particular circumstances and the attitude of the employing authority, but certainly an unofficial walk out that left patients without cover might well be tested as a case for 'fair dismissal'. In addition, if a patient, or patients, suffered harm as a result of the withdrawal of labour they might well have a claim for damages. So far such a case has not arisen, but if it did there is no reason to suppose that if it were valid it would not be upheld.

Perhaps more important than the legal issues are the practical considerations. For withdrawal of labour to be effective in persuading the Government to offer more money, withdrawal must be widespread and inflicting harm and hardship. But deliberately inflicted harm is something most nurses could not contemplate, nor could they visualise the 'picketing' of volunteers that would be necessary to make a strike effective. To argue that labour can be withdrawn without affecting the patients is dangerous. It implies that the absent nurses would not be missed by the patients, or that they were doing non-nursing tasks, or that they were overstaffed in the first place. Although it is possible to visualise a situation in which there is a moral duty to make a protest, the caring professions, for better or for worse, must find other means than the withdrawal of labour to put pressure on authorities. A study of wage economics reveals that public sector wages and salaries are affected by a number of factors of which industrial action has seldom been one.[5]

Although it is not always obvious, the profession's best ally is the esteem of the public. During a period when nurses salaries were being held back because of a wage freeze, while industrial unions got large increases, *The New Statesman* carried a head-line 'District Nurses or Dockers?' and went on to say that no group of people were held in higher esteem than district nurses. The voters agreed with the *The New Statesman* and showed their disapproval of the

government's policy at the ballot box, and what was then a good salary award was achieved for nurses. But this unique esteem does not come because the district nurses are simply safe practitioners coming to families in time of trouble, but because 'they act always so as to increase trust.'

References

1. International Council of Nurses (1965). *Code of Ethics*. Geneva.
2. Royal College of Nursing (1976). *A Code of professional Conduct—a discussion document*. London: Rcn Publications.
3. Royal College of Nursing (1970). *The Duties and Position of the Nurse*. London: Rcn Publications.
4. Baly M. E. (1980). *Nursing and Social Change*. 2nd ed. London: William Heinemann Medical Books; p. 472.
5. Baly M. E. (1980). *Op. cit;* Chapter 26, p. 326.

Further Reading

Baly M. E. (1975). *Professional Responsibility in the Community Health Services*. Aylesbury: H M and M.
Martin A. (1978). *Watchdog for the Record*. London: Rcn Publications.
Moore G. E. (1976). *Ethics*. Oxford: Oxford University Press.
Royal College of Nursing (1980). *Guidelines on Confidentiality in Nursing*. London: Rcn Publications.

Appendices

Appendix 1

Guide to Health and Social Services

This appendix is divided into three sections:

A Health services, provided by Area Health Authorities (from 1982 provided by District Health Authorities) and by Family Practitioner Committees.

B Social services provided by Local Authority social services departments.

C Social services provided by other agencies.

A. HEALTH SERVICES

Service	Type of service provided	Notes
1. *Hospital services*	Inpatient care	Access via referral by GP
	Outpatient consultation	Referral by GP; GP can also arrange domiciliary visit by consultant
	Accident and emergency services	Self-referral to casualty departments. Some hospitals operate limited service for minor casualties only, with medical cover provided by GPs
	Maternity services—antenatal supervision, inpatient care, postnatal follow-up	Run in close conjunction with community midwifery and GP service; organisation varies greatly from district to district

Service	Type of service provided	Notes
2. Hospital-based specialist services	Diagnostic investigations	As requested by consultant or GP; for hospital inpatients and outpatients and for GP patients
	Physiotherapy	For inpatients and outpatients referred by consultant
	Occupational therapy	For inpatients and outpatients referred by consultant; limited community service provided through local authority social services
	Social work	Hospital-based social workers are employed by local authority social services
	Convalescence	Arranged by hospital social worker; infrequently available
	Infertility and genetic counselling	Access via referral by GP or family planning clinic
	Abortion	Access via referral by GP. Private clinics also available—access via referral by GP or voluntary organisation
	Treatment of sexually transmitted diseases (special clinic)	Self-referral welcomed; referral by GP not necessary

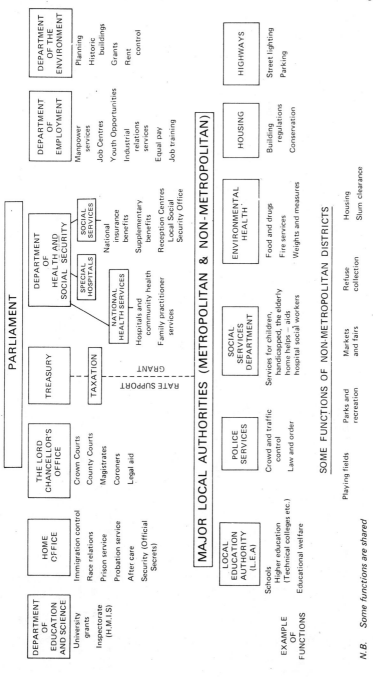

MAJOR LOCAL AUTHORITIES (METROPOLITAN & NON-METROPOLITAN)

SOME FUNCTIONS OF NON-METROPOLITAN DISTRICTS

FIG. 1.

N.B. *Some functions are shared*

Service	Type of service provided	Notes
3. *Transport to and from hospital*	Ambulance service	Sometimes run on an agency basis eg London Ambulance Service. Can be ordered only by GP or hospital except: i) for any accident (999 call) ii) for sudden illness outside the home (999 call) iii) maternity cases: by advance arrangement
	Hospital car service	Private cars driven by volunteer owners paid a mileage allowance. Can be ordered only by hospital
	Volunteer transport service	Run by many local voluntary organisations. Arrangements vary
	Expenses for travelling to and from hospital and for visiting	Patients on low incomes or supplementary benefit may be eligible. Usually arranged by hospital social worker. See leaflet H 11 available from local social security offices or hospital social worker
4. *Community health services* a) Health visiting	Advice about the care of young children, expectant and nursing mothers, the elderly, and others as referred or self-referred, by home visits and in clinics. Individual and group health education	Visits *all* families following notification of birth. Access by self-referral, or referral by any health or social agency. Usually attached to general practice (see Chapter 5)
b) Home nursing	Nursing care of the sick in their own homes and in health centres and surgeries	Access normally via referral by GP. Usually attached to general practice (see Chapter 5)

c) Domiciliary midwifery	Home delivery now rare but antenatal and postnatal care, including health education, provided in conjunction with GP	Sometimes attached to general practice, or some other form of liaison scheme. Considerable variety of schemes for early discharge following hospital delivery
d) Child health clinics	Health visiting advice. Developmental assessment including specific screening eg vision, hearing. Immunisation (see below). Welfare foods (see below)	Held in health centres, GP surgeries, health authority clinics, and sometimes premises such as church halls hired by the health authority
e) Immunisation	Primary immunisation for all children under 5 years against diphtheria, whooping cough, tetanus, polio, and measles. Other immunisation (eg TB) as necessary. Programme for older children (eg rubella) administered via school health service (see below)	May be given, usually by district nurse, at child health clinic or at GP's surgery. Other immunisations, i.e. for adults, come within family practitioner service (GP)
f) Welfare foods	Vitamin drops/tablets (A, D, C) for expectant and nursing mothers and children under 5 years. Subsidised baby milks	Available at antenatal and child health clinics
	Free milk	See Financial Benefits page
g) Family planning service	Advice on all methods of contraception including sterilization and free contraceptive supplies. Some special clinics for psychosexual problems and for young people. Domiciliary service available in some areas	Advice also available for women patients only, through GP services

Service	Type of service provided	Notes
h) Health education	Health education department acts as resource centre for advice and materials for all health service staff involved in health education. Also special programmes, and service to schools	
i) School health service	Medical examination	Usually at school entry and at age 12 or 13. Undertaken by school nurse or health visitor at the school, with follow-up home visits if necessary
	Health surveillance, including screening for head lice, foot defects, vision and hearing. Immunisation. Specialist facilities such as speech therapy and child guidance. Dental examination and treatment	
	Additional services in special schools for handicapped children	Also available through family practitioner dental service
j) Priority dental service	Dental care for expectant and nursing mothers and children under 5 years	Usually organised in conjunction with school dental service
k) Chiropody	Provided for elderly people in clinics or on a domiciliary basis; sometimes available for handicapped people and expectant and nursing mothers	Provided directly by health authority or by voluntary organisations such as British Red Cross Society, sometimes on an agency basis. Service very sparse in some areas

Service	Type of service provided	Notes
1) Loan of equipment	Equipment necessary for nursing people at home such as commodes, hoists, incontinence pads, etc.	May be provided directly by the health authority or by voluntary organisations such as British Red Cross Society on an agency basis. Level of provision varies from area to area
5. *Environmental health services*	Investigation and control of outbreaks of infectious disease. Maintenance of controls on food hygiene	Run by local authority environmental health department with advice and medical staff provided by the health authority

B. PERSONAL SOCIAL SERVICES

Service	Type of service provided	Notes
1. *Services for families and children*		
a) Day care	Provision of day nurseries; Registration and regulation of private day nurseries and playgroups; Registration and supervision of childminders	Any person who 'cares for one or more children under the age of 5, to whom they are not related, in their own home for a period of two hours or more in a day and for reward' must notify and be registered by the local authority and meet whatever conditions are required (e.g. limit on the number of children) as a condition of registration. Some authorities have training programmes for child minders
b) Residential care	Children's homes (residential nurseries, community homes which were formerly called approved schools, hostels for teenagers)	
	Foster care	Foster care now greatly preferred to institutional care. Foster parents are normally paid an allowance to cover cost of maintaining child; some authorities have salaried foster parents for handicapped or disturbed children

Service	Type of service provided	Notes
	Registration and supervision of privately arranged foster care	
c) Supervision of children in care	Residential or foster care, or supervision by social worker while child continues to live at home	Children may come 'into care' either as a result of a court order—e.g. when a child has committed a criminal offence or is 'exposed to moral danger' or 'beyond parental control, or if he is being ill treated or neglected—or voluntarily at the request of parents
d) Preventive services	Casework and counselling by social workers. Other services vary from area to area, e.g. adventure playgrounds, cash grants. Prevention of non-accidental injury to children; Area Review Committees developed jointly with health authorities	Developed since the 1963 Children and Young Persons Act Detailed procedures and guidelines vary from area to area but must conform to central guidelines laid down by DHSS
2. *Services for handicapped and disabled*		
a) Social work service	Casework, counselling, and advice on obtaining services and benefits	Responsibilities laid down by 1948 National Assistance Act greatly extended by the Chronically Sick & Disabled Persons Act 1970. The local authority is required to maintain a register of disabled people.

b) Home helps	Basic housework, but often includes 'extras' such as shopping, collecting prescriptions, etc.	Charges based on means test. Persons receiving supplementary benefit usually pay nothing. Number of hours service available to each client limited by restrictions on service
c) Meals on wheels	A hot meal delivered to the home, usually two or three times per week	Usually run by a voluntary organisation (e.g. WRVS) on an agency basis. Small charge
d) Occupational therapy	Mainly concerned with 'activities of daily living'; assesses the need for aids and adaptations to the home	
e) Provision of aids and adaptations to the home	e.g. replacement of steps by ramps, lift, downstairs toilet	Available for privately owned and council-owned property
f) Provision of telephone	All or part of the cost of installation and rental but not the cost of calls	Eligibility very restricted
g) Day centres and social clubs	Premises often used as base for other services, e.g. luncheon club facilities	Service varies greatly from area to area, considerable involvement of voluntary organisations
h) Transport facilities	Minibus or private car service, often run by voluntary organisations. Special car parking arrangements	NHS provision of 'tricycles' replaced by mobility allowance and provisions to assist in buying own cars
i) Holidays and outings	Usually provided by voluntary organisations but paid for by local authority	Provided by several voluntary organisations, sometimes alongside other services (e.g. British Diabetic Association) sometimes as the main purpose of the organisation

Service	Type of service provided	Notes
j) Residential services of various kinds	SS department may co-operate with housing department in allocation of council-owned property. Residential homes and hostels of various kinds	Severe shortage of suitable accommodation Also provided by voluntary organisations, e.g. Leonard Cheshire Foundation
k) Special services for blind people	Free radio, reduced rate television licence, books and periodicals in Braille or Moon, guide dogs—these services are often administered through Social Services Departments but not provided directly by them	Separate registration system for 'blind' and 'partially sighted' which, unlike registration as disabled, is medically assessed. Often includes elderly people whose sight is failing through age

3. Services for the mentally disordered

All services described in previous section may also be available for the mentally disordered. In addition the NHS Act 1977 gives powers to provide additional specialist services:	Special day centres, sheltered workshops, hostels	

4. Services for the elderly

Many of the services previously described are	i) To provide meals and recreation in the home and elsewhere	

available for the elderly but in addition a DHSS circular (19/71) lists the services which local authorities are empowered to provide specially for the elderly as follows:

ii) To inform the elderly of services available to them and to identify elderly people in need of services

iii) To provide facilities or assistance in travelling to and from their homes for the purpose of participating in services provided

iv) To assist in finding suitable households for boarding elderly persons

v) To provide visiting and advisory services and social work support

vi) To provide practical assistance in the home including assistance in carrying out adaptations or providing additional facilities to secure greater safety, comfort or convenience

vii) To contribute to the cost of employing a warden or welfare function in warden-assisted housing schemes

viii) To provide warden services for occupiers of private housing

Residential accommodation

Old people's homes

Originally provided under Part III of the 1948 National Assistance Act hence often referred to as 'Part III accommodation. Charges on a means tested basis.

Privately-owned old people's homes are registered with the local authority.

Service	Type of service provided	Notes
	Sheltered (warden assisted) accommodation usually flats or bed-sitting rooms	Provided in association with local authority housing department
5. Services for other groups		
e.g. vagrants, alcoholics, battered women	Residential services—hostels of various kinds, with or without social workers support	Services vary greatly from area to area. Special schemes in city areas funded by the Urban Aid Programme
	Day services—clubs and day centres of various kinds	

C. SOCIAL SERVICES PROVIDED BY OTHER AGENCIES

Service	Agency	Type of service provided
a) Housing	Local Authority Housing Department (non-metropolitan district councils & GLC)	1) Demolition of old housing, building new housing, improvement, management and repair of existing local authority housing 2) Assistance to private house owners—improvement schemes and mortgages 3) Responsibility for dealing with homelessness transferred from social services departments under the Housing (Homeless Persons) Act 1977
b) Education	Local Authority Education Department	1) Pre-school education—nursery schools 2) Primary and secondary education 3) Further and higher education—Polytechnics and Colleges of Further and Higher education administered by local authorities, Universities by University Grants Committee In addition to the schools and colleges themselves, the following services are also provided: i) school health service (provided by the NHS, see page 256) ii) special schools for handicapped children iii) social work (education welfare service)

Service	Agency	Type of service provided
		iv) school meals and milk v) financial grants for fares, maintenance and clothing vi) careers advice vii) youth and community service (youth clubs) viii) grants and awards for further and higher education
c) Employment services	Manpower Services Commission	Job centres Rehabilitation and resettlement service for disabled people (disabled resettlement officer) Training Opportunities Scheme (TOPS), Youth Opportunities Programme, Careers Service
d) Legal services	Legal Aid Scheme	Free legal advice from solicitors who choose to participate in the scheme; subject to means test Further information available from citizens advice bureaux
e) Probation and aftercare	Home Office	Supervision of people placed 'on probation' by the courts Prison welfare—social work support for prisoners' families After care of ex-prisoners

Service	Type of service provided	Notes
6. *Family practitioner services* a) Medical (general practitioner)	Primary medical care as defined in Chapter 5. GP is contracted to provide services 24 hrs a day and 7 days a week and is responsible for arrangements to cover his absence Some GPs provide special services, e.g. obstetrics, family planning Emergency treatment is available to anyone	*See Chapter 5* Individuals register with GP of their choice; GP also has the right to accept or not accept a particular patient A patient who cannot find a GP willing to accept him/her will be allocated to a GP by the FPC. List of local GPs is available from Post Office or Family Practitioner Committee
b) Dental services	Dental examination. Dental treatment. Supply of dentures. Preventive measures (e.g. fluoride treatment) not usually available as NHS but may be available privately	Lists of local dentists are available from Family Practitioner Committee. Patients do not register with a dentist as with a GP. Some dentists give only limited NHS services. Examinations free of charge but charges up to specified maximum payable for treatment except for: i) children under 16 years, ii) children over 16 years attending full-time school, iii) expectant and nursing mothers (i.e. within 1 year of delivery) iv) persons in receipt of FIS or SB, v) other persons with low income. See leaflet NHS 4
c) Ophthalmic services	Ophthalmic opticians can examine and test eyes, prescribe spectacles and supply them. Dispensing opticians can only supply spectacles prescribed elsewhere. Ophthalmic medical practitioners can examine and test	Initial eye test no longer depends on referral by GP. Examination and eye tests are free for under fives, but there is a charge for spectacles except for under fives, schoolchildren and people with low incomes (see

Service	Type of service provided	Notes
	eyes and prescribe glasses but do not supply them. More complicated eye disorders are treated by the hospital services	leaflet F1 available from opticians). This exemption covers only the cheapest NHS frames; more expensive NHS frames and privately manufactured frames have to be paid for and if chosen frames do not fit NHS lenses the lenses have to be paid for as well
d) Pharmaceutical services	Supply of drugs, dressings and appliances prescribed by GP, by hospital outpatient department, or by a dentist	Each item is charged for, except for patients in the following groups: i) children under 16 yrs ii) men over 65 years and women over 60 years iii) expectant and nursing mothers (i.e. within one year of birth) iv) people suffering from certain specified conditions v) people receiving SB or FIS vi) war pensioners for treatment of their accepted war disabilities vii) people with low incomes Non-exempt persons who need frequent prescriptions can buy a 'season ticket'. See leaflet M11

Appendix 2

Guide to Voluntary Organisations

There are thousands of voluntary organisations and this Appendix lists only a few of those most relevant to district nursing. Directories which give more information include:

Darnbrough, A., Kinrade, D. (1979). 2nd edn. *Directory for the Disabled.* Cambridge: Woodhead–Faulkener.

Family Welfare Association (published annually). *Guide to the Social Services.* London: FWA.

Sayer, K. (1979). *The Kings Fund Directory of Organisations for Patients and Disabled People.* London: King Edward's Hospital Fund for London.

Willmott, P. (1978). 4th edn. *Consumer's Guide to the British Social Services.* Harmondsworth: Penguin.

It is important for nurses working in the community to find out at local level which organisations operate in their area and what services they provide. Information about local services can be obtained from the following sources: public library; town hall or council offices; citizens advice bureau; community health council.

The main types of voluntary organisations are:

1. *Large nationally organised societies* which provide a wide range of services, sometimes acting as the agent of the Local Authority or the Health Authority to provide services such as meals on wheels, or transport services which the statutory authorities have a duty or the power to provide, e.g. British Red Cross Society, Citizens Advice Bureaux, Salvation Army, St. John Ambulance Brigade, Women's Royal Voluntary Service. These organisations have local branches whose address and telephone number will be found in the local telephone directory.

2. *Charities which provide financial help* for certain groups in need, or for research, e.g. National Society for Cancer Relief, Lady Hoare Trust for Physically Disabled Children.

3. *Education and pressure groups* set up to promote understanding and stimulate government action to deal with a particular problem, e.g. National Association for the Welfare of Children in Hospital, Association for Improvements in the Maternity Services.

4. *Self-help groups* made up of people who suffer from a particular disability, and their relatives. Some of these groups have local branches as well as national offices. The range of services provided varies from area to area, but at national level most of these organisations provide useful information services and act as pressure groups like those in group (3), e.g. Alcoholics Anomymous, Mastectomy Association.

5. *Local 'good neighbour' schemes* run by local churches, local women's organisations etc., which meet particular local needs such as home visiting, transport services, night-sitting, etc. Information about these organisations must be sought at local level from the sources listed above.

The organisations listed below are grouped, somewhat arbitrarily, under nine headings defined by 'client group'. This list is by no means comprehensive but the main organisations in each group can usually provide information about other organisations concerned with the same client group.

The Blind

Royal National Institute for the Blind, 224 Great Portland St, London W1N 6AA.

There are many organisations which provide specialist services for the blind and many 'special interest' groups covering a variety of recreational activities. Several are listed in the Kings Fund Directory mentioned above.

The Deaf

Royal National Institute for the Deaf, 105 Gower St, London WC1E 6AH.

British Assoc. for the Hard of Hearing, 16 Park St, Windsor, Berks. SL4 1LU.

Both of these are organisations who provide specialist advice and information about other organisations, and there are many 'special interest' organisations for deaf people.

Mental Handicap, Mental Illness, Behavioural Problems

Mind (National Assoc. for mental Health), 22 Harley St, London W1N 3ED.

National Society for Mentally Handicapped Children, Pembridge Hall, 17 Pembridge Square, London W2 4EP.

These are major national organisations providing a range of services and information, but they also have local branches which provide services and information locally.

Specialist organisations of particular relevance to district nurses include:

Al-Anon Family Groups, 61 Gt. Dover St, London SE1 4YE.

Alcoholics Anonymous, PO Box 514, 11 Redcliffe Gardens, London SW10 9BG (for local branches see local telephone directory).

Depressives Associated, 19 Merleys Way, Wimborne Minster, Dorset BH21 1QN.

Open Door Association, c/o. 447 Pensby Rd, Heswall, Merseyside L61 9PQ (agoraphobia sufferers).

Phobics Society, 4 Cheltenham Rd, Charlton-cum-Hardy, Manchester M21 1QN.

Samaritans, 17 Uxbridge Road, Slough, Bucks (over 100 local branches—see local telephone directory).

Schizophrenia Association, Tyrtwr, Llanfair Hall, Caernarvon, Gwynedd LL55 1TT.

Physically Disabled and Handicapped (General)

Association of Disabled Professionals, The Stables, 73 Pound Rd, Banstead, Surrey SM7 2HU.

British Sports Association for the Disabled, Stoke Mandeville Stadium, Harvey Road, Aylesbury, Bucks.

Disabled Living Foundation, 346 Kensington High St, London W14 8NS.

Disablement Income Group, Attlee House, Toynbee Hall, 28 Commercial St, London E1 6LR.

Disability Alliance, 5 Netherhall Gardens, London NW3 5RN.

Holidays for the Disabled, Ridgehanger Lake, Liss, Hants.

Motability, State House, High Holborn, London WC1R 4SX.

PHAB (Physically Handicapped and Able Bodied), 42 Devonshire St, London W1N 1LN.

Royal Association for Disability and Rehabilitation (RADAR), 25 Mortimer St, London W1N 8AB. (Formerly Central Council for the Disabled).

SPOD (Committee on Sexual Problems of the Disabled), 49 Victoria St, London SW1.

Wheelchair Action, 2 Merthyr Terrace, Barnes, London SW13.

Specific Disorders

Association for Spina Bifida and Hydrocephalus, Tavistock House North, Tavistock Square, London, WC1M 9HJ.

Back Pain Association, Grundy House, Teddington, Middx. TW11 8TD.

British Diabetic Association, 10 Queen Anne St, London W1M 0BD.

British Epilepsy Association, Crowthorne House, Bigshotte, New Wokingham Road, Wokingham, Berks. RG11 3AY.

British Migraine Association, Evergreen, Ottermead Lane, Ottershaw, Chertsey, Surrey KT16 0HJ.

British Rheumatism and Arthritis Association, 6 Grosvenor Crescent, London SW1X 7ER.

Cancer After-care and Rehabilitation Society (CARE), Lodge Cottage, Church Lane, Timsbury, Bath BA3 1LF.

Chest, Heart and Stroke Association, Tavistock House North, Tavistock Square, London WC1 9JE.

Coeliac Society, PO Box 181, London NW2 2QY.

Colostomy Welfare Group, 38-9 Eccleston Square, London SW1V 1PB.

CRACK (the young arm of the Multiple Sclerosis Society), 286 Munster Road, Fulham, London SW6 6BE.

Cystic Fibrosis Research Trust, 5 Blyth Road, Bromley, Kent BR1 3RS.

Haemophilia Society, PO Box 9, 16 Trinity St, London SE1.

Ileostomy Association, 1st floor, 23 Winchester Road, Basingstoke, Hants.

Invalids At Home Trust, 23 Farm Avenue, London NW2.

Leukaemia Society, 45 Craigmoor Avenue, Queens Park, Bournemouth.

Marie Curie Memorial Foundation, 124 Sloane St, London SW1X 9BP.

Mastectomy Association, 1 Colworth Road, Croydon, Surrey CR0 7AD.

Multiple Sclerosis Society, 286 Munster Rd, London SW6 6BE.

Muscular Dystrophy Group, Nattrass House, 35 Macaulay Rd, London SW4 0QP.

National Ankylosing Spondylitis Society, 4 Beaconsfield Rd, Clifton, Bristol BS8 2TS.

National Society for Cancer Relief, 30 Dorset Square, London NW1 6QL.

Parkinsons Disease Society, 81 Queens Road, London SW19 8NR.

Renal Society, Oak Cottage, Wises Lane, Borden, Sitting-bourne, Kent.

Spastics Society, 12 Park Crescent, London W1N 4EQ.

Spinal Injuries Association, 5 Crowndale Road, London NW1 1TU.

Urinary Conduit Association, 36 York Road, Denton, Man-chester.

Wireless for the Bedridden Society, Inc., 81b Corbets Tey Road, Upminster, Essex RM14 2AJ.

Children

BREAK (Davison Morley Trust), 20 Hooks Hill Road, Shering-ham, Norfolk NR26 8NL (holidays and short-stay emergency care).

Invalid Children's Aid Association, 126 Buckingham Palace Rd, London SW1 9SB.

Lady Hoare Trust for Physically Disabled Children, 7 North Street, Midhurst, West Sussex GU29 9DJ.

National Association for the Welfare of Children in Hospital, 7 Exton Street, London SE1.

National Society for the Prevention of Cruelty to Children, 1 Riding House Street, London W1.

Voluntary Council for Handicapped Children, c/o. National Children's Bureau, 8 Wakley Street, London ER1V 7QE.

(*Note*: all the societies dealing with specific disorders provide information, advice, and support for parents).

Marriage and Family Problems

Brook Advisory Centres, 233 Tottenham Court Road, London W1A 9AE.

Family Planning Association, Margaret Pyke House, 27-35 Mortimer St, London W1N 7RJ.

Gingerbread (The Association for One Parent Families), 35 Wellington Street, London WC2.

National Council for the Divorced and Separated, 13 High Street, Little Shelford, Cambridge CB2 5ES.

National Marriage Guidance Council, Harbert Gray College, Little Church Street, Rugby, Warwicks. (*Note*: there are specialist organisations for Jews and for Catholics with marital problems).

National Women's Aid Federation, 374 Grays Inn Rd, London WC1.

One Parent Families (formerly National Council for the Unmarried Mother and her Child),s225 Kentish Town Road, London NW5 2LX.

Pregnancy Advisory Service, 40 Margaret Street, London W1N 7FB.

Elderly People

Age Concern England, Bernard Sunley House, 60 Pitcairn Road, Mitcham, Surrey CR4 3LL (formerly National Old People's Welfare Council).

Elderly Invalids Fund, 10 Fleet Street, London EC4Y 1BB.

Help the Aged, 32 Dover Street, London W1A 2AP.

There are also many locally based voluntary organisations which provide a variety of benefits and services for elderly people; information can be obtained from the local branch of Age Concern, whose address and telephone number will be found in the local telephone directory.

Bereavement

Compassionate Friends, 50 Woodways, Watford, Herts WD1 4NW. (Bereaved parents).

Cruse: National Organisation for Widows and their Children, Cruse House, 126 Sheen Road, Richmond, Surrey. (Widows, Widowers and their Children).

Appendix 3

Guide to Social Security and Other Financial Benefits

The system of financial support provided by the state to individuals in need is highly complex. The government department which is responsible for the main benefits, i.e. social security benefits, is the DHSS, operating through local DHSS offices. Some financial benefits are administered through other departments, e.g. tax allowances through the Inland Revenue Department.

This appendix should be used only as a general guide; leaflets about each benefit, including details of who is eligible and how to apply, can be obtained from local DHSS offices, or from the DHSS Information Division, Leaflets Unit, Block 4, Government Buildings, Honeypot Lane, Stanmore, Middlesex HA7 1AY. A full list of leaflets is given in *Catalogue of Social Security Leaflets* (N I 146). The level of benefit is adjusted each year and so actual amounts are not included here.

The main groups of benefit as listed in this Appendix are:

A National Insurance benefits, payable to people who have paid National Insurance contributions and related to the type and level of contributions paid.

B Non-contributory benefits available to specified groups of people having a particular need, e.g. the severely disabled.

C Supplementary Benefits administered through local DHSS Offices for the Supplementary Benefits Commission.

D Other benefits.

A. NATIONAL INSURANCE BENEFITS (Contributory)

Benefit	Information leaflet	Who is eligible	Notes
1. Sickness benefit	NI 16	Paid for 28 weeks during certificated incapacity for work. Contribution conditions (Class 1 and Class 2 only) apply	Non-taxable. Reduced after 8 weeks in hospital (leaflet NI 9)
2. Invalidity pension	NI 16A	Paid after 28 weeks when sickness benefit ends if illness or disability continues	Non-taxable, except where paid with retirement pension. New state pension scheme started April 1978 divides pension into 2 parts: i) basic pension ii) additional pension related to earnings. See also Non-Contributory Invalidity Pension, page 338
3. Invalidity allowance	NI 16A	Supplement to invalidity benefit paid where person is chronically sick and at least five years below pension age; three rates according to age of onset	Non-taxable
4. Unemployment benefit	NI 12	Weekly benefit paid for up to one year if contribution conditions are satisfied	Not payable for up to 6 weeks where person has left his job voluntarily or been dismissed for misconduct

5. Maternity benefits	NI 17A		
a) maternity grant		Lump sum grant paid on mother's own or her husband's NI contributions	From 1982 will be paid to all irrespective of contribution record
b) maternity allowance		Weekly benefit payable from 11 weeks before EDD to 6 weeks after birth. Payable on mother's full NI contributions only	Amount reduced if contribution conditions not fully met
6. Death grant	NI 49	Lump sum payable on the death of a contributor or his/her spouse or dependent child	Amount varies with age of the person—lower for a child
7. Widows benefits	NI 13	Paid on the deceased husband's contribution record	All widows benefits are taxable
a) widow's allowance		Paid weekly for the first 6 months only	
b) widowed mother's allowance		Payable from end of 6 month period of widow's allowance; additional amount for each child	
c) widow's pension		Payable after widow's allowance ends to widows aged over 40 years at time of bereavement	Rate depends on widow's age at bereavement or when widowed mother's allowance ceases. New state pensions scheme started April 1978 divides pensions into 2 parts: i) basic pension ii) additional pension related to earnings

Benefit	Information leaflet	Who is eligible	Notes
8. Child's special allowance	NI 93	Payable to mother on the death of her former husband if the marriage has been dissolved and the former husband contributed to the cost of the children	Not taxable
9. Retirement pension	NI 15 NI 15A NI 15B NI 92 NI 105 NI 184 NP 32	Payable to men at 65 years and women at 60 years, provided they satisfy the contributions and have retired from work. Payable for men at 70 and women at 65 even if still working	Married woman can receive pension on husband's contributions when he retires, or on her own contributions at age 60. Amount of pension is increased if retirement is deferred. Extra payment to pensioners aged over 80 years. Subject to earnings limit, and amount reduced according to amount earned. Non-contributory pension paid to pensioners over 80 years New state pension scheme began April 1978 divided pension into two parts: i) basic pension ii) additional pension related to earnings Reduced after 8 weeks in hospital

Benefit	Information leaflet	Who is eligible	Notes
10. Industrial injuries benefits a) industrial injuries benefit b) industrial disablement benefit c) industrial death benefit	NI 2 NI 5	Paid where employee is unable to work because of accident at work or prescribed industrial disease, or dies as result of it. Almost everyone working for an employer is covered by the 'special element' in NI contributions; no other contribution conditions	Analagous to basic NI benefits but paid at a higher rate. Disablement must be medically assessed. Special supplements available: i) special hardship allowance ii) constant attendance allowance iii) exceptionally severe disablement allowance iv) hospital treatment allowance v) unemployability supplement

B. NON-CONTRIBUTORY BENEFITS (Special Groups)

Benefit	Information leaflet	Who is eligible	Notes
1. Child benefit	CH 1	Weekly benefit for each child up to 16 years (or 19 years if in full-time education) payable to whoever is responsible for the child (usually the mother)	Not taxable Basic amount is increased for one-parent families
2. Guardian's allowance	NI 14	Paid to person taking care of orphan child	Not taxable
3. Family income supplement	FIS 1	Families, including single parents, with at least one child where the head of the family is in full time work and where gross family income is below a prescribed level	The amount paid is equal to half the difference between the actual income and the prescribed level Eligibility for FIS automatically entitles families to certain other means tested benefits and exemption from NHS charges

Benefit	Information leaflet	Who is eligible	Notes
4. Non-contributory invalidity pension	NI 210	Payable to people of working age who have been unable to work for six months and who do not meet the contribution conditions for NI sickness benefit or invalidity pension	Not taxable. Rate reduced if other benefits are payable. Reduced after 8 weeks in hospital
	NI 214	Married women claimants must be able to show inability to perform household duties	
5. Attendance allowance	NI 205	Payable to adults and children over 2 years who are severely disabled either physically or mentally	Not payable until condition has existed for 6 months
a) higher rate		Person requires frequent attention or continual supervision by day and by night	Withdrawn after 4 weeks in hospital
b) lower rate		Person requires frequent attention or continual supervision by day or by night	
6. Invalid care allowance	NI 212	Payable to persons of working age who cannot work because of caring for a severely disabled relative. Married women are not generally eligible	Limited definition of 'severely disabled', 'relative', 'not gainfully employed', and 'regularly and substantially engaged in caring'. Withdrawn 12 weeks after own admission to hospital or when attendance allowance is withdrawn

Benefit	Information leaflet	Who is eligible	Notes
7. Mobility allowance	NI 211	Payable to persons aged 5-65 years who are unable to walk because of physical or mental disablement. Inability to walk must persist for three months from date of claim.	Taxable but recipients are exempt from paying road tax on their vehicles
8. War pensions a) war disablement pension b) war widows and dependants pension	MPL 153	Payable to persons disabled as a result of service in the armed forces and also to civilians disabled in World War II	

C. SUPPLEMENTARY BENEFITS

Benefit	Information leaflet	Who is eligible	Notes
1. Supplementary pension	SB 1	Payable to people over retirement age whose* income (including NI retirement pension) falls below assessed requirements	Non-contributory benefits. Intended to supplement other state benefits (e.g. where contribution requirements are not met) or private resources
2. Supplementary allowance	SB 9, SB 8 SB 2, SB 7	Payable to people aged over 16 years and not in full-time employment whose income falls below assessed requirements	The amount payable is worked out by taking the claimant's 'requirements'—made up of a basic scale plus allowances for dependents, and rent and mortgage interest and special needs— and deducting

Benefit	Information leaflet	Who is eligible	Notes
			from these his resources—what he is already receiving in the form of other benefits, interest on savings, value of property, etc.
			A lump sum 'exceptional needs' payment may be made in special circumstances
			Recipients of Supplementary Benefits are automatically entitled to certain other means-tested benefits and to exemption from certain charges e.g. free prescriptions
			Full details given in Supplementary Benefits Handbook obtainable from HMSO

D. OTHER BENEFITS

Benefit	Information leaflet	Who is eligible	Notes
1. Family Fund	Information from The Family Fund Beverley House, Shipton Rd, York Y03 6YB	Discretionary grants available to families caring for severely handicapped child under 15 years for special purposes, e.g. washing machine, car hire, holiday expenses, special footwear	Run by Joseph Rowntree Memorial Trust for the government. No means test, although circumstances are taken into account

2. Exemption from NHS charges	M 11	Persons over retirement age, children under 16 years, expectant and nursing mothers, recipients of Supplementary Benefits or FIS, other persons on low income
a) prescriptions		
b) spectacles		
c) dental treatment		
3. Educational benefits	Information and claim forms from Local Education Authority	
a) fares to school		a) depends on distance between home and school
b) school meals		b) families receiving FIS or SB and other low income families assessed by means test. Some or all children in the family
c) school milk		c) children under 11 years and all children in special schools
d) clothing grants		d) at the discretion of LEA subject to a means test
e) maintenance grants		e) children who stay on at school after compulsory school leaving age, subject to means test
		c) also available to children receiving day care with minders or in playgroups. Since d) and e) are at the discretion of the individual LEA, availability and amounts vary greatly
4. Welfare Foods (milk and vitamins)	FW 9	Free milk is available for: i) families with 3 or more children under school age
	FW 8	ii) expectant mothers with 2 children under school age
	M 11	iii) families receiving supplementary benefits or FIS and other low-income families
		Cheap baby milk and vitamins are available at child health clinics. Free milk is obtained from ordinary milkman using tokens instead of cash

Benefit	Information leaflet	Who is eligible	Notes
	FW 20	iv) children attending day nurseries playgroups or child minders v) handicapped children whether or not attending school	
5. Rent rebates and allowances	Information from rent rebate and allowances officer of local authority housing	People on supplementary benefit do not need to claim because allowance is made in their assessed level of benefit All other people living in local authority housing and privated rented accommodation are eligible subject to a means test. The amount paid is 60 per cent of the rent plus or minus an amount determined by how far income falls below or exceeds the prescribed amount	Administered by local authorities within nationally determined guidelines
6. Rate rebate	Information and application forms from local council or town hall	Recipients of supplementary benefit cannot claim separately because the amount is included in their assessed benefit level All other householders, whether tenants or owner occupiers, are eligible, subject to a means test	Operates on a similar basis to the rent rebate and allowances scheme. Payable for each half-yearly rate period (1 April to 30 Sept; 1 Oct. to 31 March); apply at the beginning of each half year

7. Tax allowances

FB 2
Fuller
information
from Inland
Revenue Tax
Office

A number of tax allowances are especially
relevant to district nurses' patients, who are
tax payers:

e.g.

i) dependent relative's allowance
ii) daughter's services allowance
iii) housekeeper allowance
iv) blind person's allowance

Appendix 4

A Synoptic History of District Nursing

1850–1900

Health Services and related legislation	Related Nursing events	District Nursing	Contemporary Events
Population: 18 million	1854 Miss Nightingale takes a party of nurses to Scutari	1854 Mrs Fry's Institute	1854 Cholera epidemic (Dr Snow and the Broad St. pump)
1855 John Simon at the Board of Health	1860 Foundation of the Nightingale Nursing School	1859 Mr Rathbone employs a 'district nurse'	1854-56 *The Crimean War*
1858 Registration of Doctors Board of Health dissolved	1862 Manchester & Salford Ladies Health Society	1864 District Nursing Ass. in Liverpool, Manchester and Salford	1864 The Geneva Convention
1866 Sanitary Act	1865 Ladies Medical College—gives instruction in midwifery	1868 Mrs Ranyard founds the Bible Women and Nurses Mission	1867 2nd Reform Act (male franchise extended)
1867 Metropolitan Poor Act (Poor Law able to build hospitals)			1870 Franco—Prussian War (Red Cross used)
1870 Education Act (Foster)	1887 British Nursing Ass. founded	1874 Metropolitan Nursing Ass. for District Nurse Training set up	1876 Royal Sanitary Inst. founded by Chadwick
1872 Public Health Acts	1890 First Preliminary Training School	1887 Queen Victoria Jubilee Institute for Nurses founded. (Rosalind Paget the first Superintendent)	1882 Koch discovers the tubercle bacillus
1875 (urban and rural sanitary authorities)	1894 Training course for Health Visitors in Buckinghamshire	1888 Rural Nursing Ass. set up	1890 Diphtheria anti toxin used
1886 Idiots Act	1892 The first School Nurse (Amy Hughes)	1889 The Jubilee Institute receives a Royal Charter	1892 Booth's report *Life and Labour* in London
1888 Local Government Act (creates County and County Borough authorities)	1899 The International Council of Nurses founded		1898 *The Boer War* (Queen Alexandra Military Nursing Service used)
1890 Lunacy Act (lays down regulations about 'certification')			

1900–1950

1901 *Population 33 million*
1902 Education Act (Balfour—schools under LEAs)
1907 School Medical Inspections
1907 Notification of Births Act (permissive)
1908 Old Age Pensions Act
1908 Children's Act (Child Life Protection)
1911 National Insurance Act (Lloyd George)
1918 Maternity & Child Welfare Act
1918 Education Act (Fisher) (school health service extended)
1919 Ministry of Health formed
1920 Dawson Report on the Health Services
1929 Local Government Act
1944 Education Act (Butler)
1945 Family Allnces. Act
1946 National Health Service Act
1948 National Assistance Act

1902 Midwives Act
1904 Committee on Nursing Registration
1916 College of Nursing Founded
1919 Nurses Registration Act (General Nursing Council)
1925 Regulations for Health Visitor training—first examinations with the RSI
1925 Student Nurses Ass.
1932 The Lancet Commission on Nursing
1937 Interdepartmental Com. on Nursing (Athlone)
1943 Rushcliffe Committee on pay
1943 Nurses Act (Assistant Nurse)
1942-45 Horder Committee
1947 Working Party on Recruitment & Training

1902 Village nurse midwifery training in East London
1912 Highlands & Islands medical service
1918 Maternity & Child Welfare Act requires home nurses for infectious cases
1925 Queen Victoria Jubilee Inst. becomes Queen's Inst. of District Nursing
1928 Supplementary Charter issued to the Queen's Inst.
1946 National Health Service Act—district nurses now part of the local authority health services
1947 Queen's Inst. offers training to male nurses

1901 *Edward VII*
1904 Report of the Interdepartmental Committee on Physical Deterioration
1904-9 Royal Commission on the Poor Law
1910 *George V*
1914-18 *First World War*
1918 Representation of the People Act (votes for women)
1926 The General Strike
1931 Gold Standard suspended
1933 Unemployment 22 per cent
1933 Nazi revolution in Germany
1935 Italy invades Ethiopia
1936 *George VI*
1938 Nazis seize Austria. Munich Agreement
1939 Florey prepares stable penicillin
1939-45 *Second World War*
1942 Beveridge Report
1945 Labour Government (Attlee)

1950–1980

Health Services and related legislation	Related Nursing events	District Nursing	Contemporary Events
1951 *Population 44 million*	1951 Midwives Act	1955 Working Party on the Training of District Nurses	1952 Conservative victory
1951 Min. of Health becomes Min. of Housing & Local Gov.	1956 Inquiry into Health Visiting (Jameson)	Panel of Assessors—National Cert. of District Nursing	1953 *Elizabeth II*
1956 Guillebaud Report on NHS costs	1962 Health Visitors & Social Workers Training Council	1959 Revision of GNC syllabus student nurses to have	1956 Suez crisis
1959 The Mental Health Act	1964 Reform of Nursing Education (Platt)	experience in the community	1957 The Treaty of Rome
1962 The Hospital Plan	1966 Committee on Senior Nursing Structure (Salmon)	1963 Future Scope of General Practice (Gillie Report	1957 Macmillan administration
1970 The Peel report on midwifery services	1969 Joint Board of Clinical Nursing Studies	recommends 'attachment')	1964 Labour administration (Wilson)
1970 Social Services Act	1972 Committee on Nursing	1969 Mayston Report Nursing Officer grade introduced	1970 Conservative administration (Heath)
1971 Industrial Relations Act	1974 Halsbury Report	1970 Arrangements for extending District Nurse	1973 Yom Kippur War—oil and sterling crisis
1972 White Paper on a Reorganised Health Service	1979 EEC Regulations on Nursing	training to enrolled nurses Circular 8/70	1973 Britain joins the EEC
1974 Reorganisation of the Health Services	1979 Nurses, Midwives and Health Visitors Act	1972 Revised syllabus	1974 'The Three Day Week'
1974 Reorganisation of Local Government Act	1980 New UK Central Council for Nurses, Midwives and	1974 Panel of Assessors Issue Handbook for Training and	1974 Labour administration (Wilson)
1974 Health and Safety at Work Act	Health Visitors set up with National Boards	Education Centres	1975 The Social Contract
1975 Employment Protection Act		1976 Working Party report of the Panel of Assessors.	1979 Conservative administration (Thatcher)
1979 Report of the Royal Commission on the NHS		Proposed that new curriculum replace the old	1980 Unemployment 2 million
1979 Consultative document on NHS reorganisation		syllabus	1980 The Gulf War
1980 The Health Services Act		1981 New Curriculum mandatory	1981 Cuts in public services

Appendix 5

Curriculum in District Nursing

For State Registered Nurses and Registered General Nurses

Issued by: The Panel of Assessors for District Nurse Training, Clifton House, Euston Road, London NW1 2RS.

Aim of the course in district nursing

The aim of the course is to prepare a district nurse who is competent to undertake nursing duties in the community and able to accept individual responsibility for the professional standards of her own performance. To satisfy this aim the curriculum has been designed to emphasise the use of a problem-solving approach to district nursing and reference is made throughout to the 'nursing process'.

Course objectives

Four main objectives are incorporated in the outline curriculum and elaborated in the detailed guide. It is intended that the principles are applied throughout the course of study and not limited to specific units of learning:

Objective 1 To assess and meet the nursing needs of patients in the community.

Objective 2 To apply skills and knowledge and to impart them effectively to patients, relatives, other carers and the general public.

Objective 3 To be skilled in communications, establishing and maintaining good relationships and able to co-ordinate appropriate services for the patient, his family and others involved with delivery of care.

Objective 4 To have an understanding of management and organisation principles within the multi-disciplinary team and a positive approach to future developments to meet health care needs.

Entry requirements

The curriculum will make considerable demands upon students and candidates should preferably be in possession of 5 'O' levels of the General Certificate of Education. To ensure, however, that people with the right qualities for district nursing are not excluded solely on the grounds of lack of academic qualifications, a form of assessment should be devised to select candidates who have the competence and ability to undertake the course. Candidates should be registered nurses whose names appear in the General Part of the Register of the General Nursing Council for Scotland, or the Northern Ireland Council for Nurses and Midwives. Further nursing experience since registration is desirable.

Length of course

Examinations will take place in March and July. Courses should be planned to coincide with these examinations and should be for a duration of six months of which one third should be allocated to the provision of practical teaching and experience.

Plan of course

Correlation of theory and practice

Theory and practice should be correlated throughout the course.

Theory

There should be flexibility in planning the time-table to include study blocks or days but some concentration of study at the beginning and end of the course would be expected.

Practical experience

One third of the course should be allocated to practical experience. The student should be placed with a practical work teacher who would assume responsibility for planning the student's practical work programme, allocating a controlled caseload, and teaching the skills of district nursing within a primary health care team.

Associated training

It is desirable that training should take place in association with

health visitors and social work students. There are also obvious advantages to district nurse students if practical work teachers can be based in practices which are used for general medical practice vocational training and such practices should be utilised wherever possible.

Examination procedure

Examination for the Certificate in District Nursing will be based upon:

a. *Principles and practice of district nursing*

A 3 hour written paper prepared by the Panel of Assessors will be taken at the end of 6 months. Questions will be set on the principles and practice of district nursing and related subjects.

b. *Assessment of course work*

During the course the student will be required to undertake 4 assignments; it will be for the Centre to determine the type of assignment, e.g. extended essays, case studies, project work. These should be marked internally but external assessors should be appointed to check the assessment procedure and to examine some of the work produced by the students.

c. *Assessment of practical work*

The practical work teacher will be required to make a continuous assessment of the student's progress throughout the 6 months of the course and report upon the student's competance to practise as a district nurse. Students who do not receive a satisfactory practical work report may be referred by the Panel for a period of additional practical experience under supervision.

Award of the Panel's Certificate in District Nursing (SRN/RGN) will be dependent upon the student achieving a pass in (a), (b) and (c).

Approval of centres and courses

A formal application must be made to the Panel by any Centre wishing to conduct a course in district nursing. Guidance on approval procedures is issued separately.

OUTLINE CURRICULUM COURSE CONTENT

Skills	Knowledge	Attitudes
	Principles and practice of district nursing techniques. Development of social policy	
1. Information gathering	Interviewing methods. Principles and problems of confidentiality	Awareness of the need to preserve confidentiality
2. Observation	Effect of the environment on the individual. Sociological concepts and their significance in health and disease	Respect for the values held by all persons with whom she comes into contact
3. Assessment of physical, social and emotional needs	Criteria for assessment of total needs of individual and groups of patients. Normal and disordered body functions. Psychological concepts and their significance in health and disease. Needs of crisis groups	Demonstration of an enquiring mind
4. Planning of care	Problem solving techniques. Programmes of care to meet assessed needs. Referral techniques	Respect for the patients and carers perception of their needs

Outline Curriculum (Continued)

5. Implementing care	Organisation of the nursing environment. Dietetics. Drugs and other therapeutic measures for conditions commonly met in the community. Rehabilitation	Respect for patient's property
6. Evaluation	Methods of evaluating care. Prevention of further ill health. Promotion of health	Awareness of the need for continual re-assessment of care provided and willingness to modify previously made plans
7. Supportive care	Determinants of stress in the family situation	Acceptance of professional responsibility for the welfare of people other than patients
8. Imparting skill and knowledge	Introduction to principles of learning and teaching. Skills analysis. Demonstration and teaching techniques. Self analysis. Assessment of performance of others. Programmes of nurse education and training	Understanding of the importance of teaching and willingness to accept this responsibility
		Appreciation of the value of health education in its widest sense and the need to develop an individual approach as necessary
		Willingness to learn and relearn
9. Communication	The basic principles of written and verbal communication. Record keeping. Report writing	Awareness of communication as an important part of total patient care

Outline Curriculum (Continued)

Skills	Knowledge	Attitudes
10. Establishment and maintenance of effective relationships	The dynamics of individual and group relationships. The psychological and social needs of families. The role and function of the primary care team. The management structure of the National Health Service. An outline of central and local government	Acceptance of her responsibility as clinical nursing expert within the primary care team
11. Co-ordination of services	The policies, structure and contribution of other health, social and voluntary services	Appreciation of, and respect for, the skilled contribution of others concerned with patient care
12. Organisation and supervision of the nursing team	The principles of management as adapted to the needs of community care. Basic understanding of the principles of motivation	Appreciation of the importance of teamwork. Willingness to accept managerial responsibility
13. Appreciation of methods of critical investigation	Development of new procedures and techniques. Information retrieval and use of resources. Ethical, legal, professional implications of research	Awareness of the value of research and its contribution to better patient care. Respect for human dignity

Appendix 6
Selected Relevant Official Reports and Related Legislation

1842 *Report on the Sanitary Conditions of the Labouring Population* (Edwin Chadwick). Edinburgh University Press.

1892 *Report of Life and Labour in London* (Charles Booth). London: Macmillan.

1904 *Report of the Interdepartmental Committee on Physical Deterioration.*
Gave rise to much of the social legislation 1905–1913, including the School Health Service.

1909 *Report of the Poor Law Commission,* including the Minority Report by Beatrice Webb.
Minority report recommended a 'comprehensive health service based on local government'—blueprint for subsequent reports.

1911 *The National Insurance Act*
Established the 'insurance principle' as a means of providing a limited health service.

1919 *The Nurses Registration Act*
General Nursing Councils set up

1920 *Report on the Future Provision of Medical and Allied Services* (Dawson).

1937 *Report of the Interdepartmental Committee on Nursing* (Athlone).
Recommended the Assistant Nurse.

1942 *Report on Social Insurance and Allied Services* (Beveridge).
The basis of most post-war social legislation.

1946 *The National Health Service Act* NHS came into being July 1st 1948.

1955 *Report of the Working Party on the Training of District Nurses.*
Recommended the National Certificate of District Nursing.

1956 *Report of the Inquiry into Health Visiting* (Jameson).

1962 Health Visitors and Social Workers Training Council set up.

1963 *Report on the Future Scope of General Practice* (Gillie).
　　Encouraged attachment of nursing staff to general practice.

1966 *Report of the Committee on Senior Nursing Staff Structure* (Salmon).
　　Recommended a new simplified structure of nurse managers to match the National Health Service structure.

1968 *Report of Local Authority and Allied Social Services* (Seebohm).
　　Recommended setting up Social Services Departments.

1969 *Report on the Management Structure in the Local Authority Nursing Service* (Mayston). London: DHSS.

1971 *Report of the Committee on the Organisation of Group Practice* (Havard Davis).

1972 *Report of the Committee on Nursing* (Briggs).
　　Recommended a new comprehensive and progressive system of nurse training and new arrangements for post basic studies.

1974 *The Reorganisation of the Health Services Act.*
　　Set up a new structure with Area Health Authorities and District Management Teams.

1974 *Report of the Committee of Inquiry into Pay and Related Conditions for Nurses* (Halsbury).
　　Recommended a new structure for salary scales.

1976 *Report of the Working Party of the Panel of Assessors on the Education and Training of the District Nurse* (Carr). DHSS.

1976 *Report on the Future of Child Health Services. 'Fit for the Future'* (Court).

1979 EEC Directives for Nurses comes into force.

1979 *The Nurses Midwives and Health Visitors Act*
　　Replaced the General Nursing Councils, the Central Midwives Board and the Council for the Training and Education of Health Visitors.

1979 *Report of the Staffing of Mental Handicap Residential Care* (Jay).

1980 The new curriculum for district nurse training issued; comes into force 1981. London: DHSS.

1981/82 Arrangements for restructuring the National Health Service into District Health Authorities under the provisions of *The Health Services Act.* (1980).

Note. Unless otherwise specified, these reports are published by Her Majesty's Stationery Office, London.

Index